Current Topics in Microbiology and Immunology

Volume 412

Series editors

Honorary editors

More information about this series at http://www.springer.com/series/82

Georg Häcker
Editor

Biology of *Chlamydia*

Responsible series editor: Klaus Aktories

Springer

Editor
Georg Häcker
Institute of Microbiology and Hygiene
Universitätsklinikum Freiburg
Freiburg
Germany

ISSN 0070-217X ISSN 2196-9965 (electronic)
Current Topics in Microbiology and Immunology
ISBN 978-3-030-10031-5 ISBN 978-3-319-71232-1 (eBook)
https://doi.org/10.1007/978-3-319-71232-1

Softcover re-print of the Hardcover 1st edition 2018

Printed on acid-free paper

This Springer imprint is published by the registered company Springer
International Publishing AG part of Springer Nature
The registered company address is: Gewerbestrasse 11, 6330 Cham, Switzerland

Preface

Chlamydiae are obligate intracellular bacteria. They live in an intracellular vacuole (the inclusion) that they customise to permit delivery of nutrients and to provide protection against host cell defences. *Chlamydiae* have two developmental forms: one is infectious (the elementary body) but has little metabolism and the other one divides very actively but is not infectious (the reticulate body). Once a cell is infected, EBs differentiate to RBs; after a cycle of about two days, re-differentiated EBs are released, either by lysis of the host cell or by the active release of intact inclusions.

What seems rather complicated is a very successful strategy. The phylum *Chlamydiae* has been around for about two billion years, with the extant *Chlamydiae* in their extremely wide spectrum of bacterial species and vastly differing hosts having split into separate lines around 700 million years ago. Many species of unicellular and multicellular hosts have their specialised *Chlamydia* but infection across these borders also occurs. The two species commonly found in humans are *Chlamydia pneumonia* (which is very common but causes only mild disease in most cases) and *C. trachomatis*, with a lower but still very substantial prevalence and great clinical importance, especially in causing infertility in female patients and scarring damage to the eyes.

We can categorise *chlamydia*l infection biology and research into *Chlamydia* into two areas, both under intensive research. The first considers the interaction of the bacteria with the individual host cell: how does *Chlamydia* manage to set up its inclusion, which is accepted by the host cell basically like another organelle? The inclusion is embedded by the cytoskeleton, it is supplied with all the necessary nutrients, and it is able to set up an equilibrium with the host cell's innate defences; how does that work?

The second issue is about the infection of multicellular hosts like humans: what are the mechanisms on either side that determine immune recognition, immunopathology and potentially anti-infective protection? The biggest clinical problem of *C. trachomatis* infection is damage to tissue, either in the female genital tract (worldwide) or to the eye (blinding trachoma, especially in Africa). Human chlamydial infection may be very prolonged affairs; it is much under investigation whether *Chlamydia* can be persistent in vivo, lying low within one host cell, or whether chronic infections reflect slowly propagating bacteria in vivo (or even re-infection).

Progress in all of these areas is rapid, and this book is the endeavour to present important developments and current thinking. The first four articles address questions of *chlamydial* microbiology and the bacterial interaction with the (human) host cell: the unusual cell wall of *Chlamydia*, where peptidoglycan was discovered only three years ago, is the focus of one article.

The next two chapters address questions of the early establishment of the bacteria in a host cell. The elementary body, the infectious form of *Chlamydia*, long considered an inactive particle, has in recent years been found to be a highly specialised form of *Chlamydia*, and its characteristics and abilities are discussed. The second of the two chapters will illustrate the ways how *Chlamydia* interacts with the host cytoskeleton; these interactions have been found to be crucial for uptake and establishment of the inclusion as well as for its maintenance and ultimately the release of the bacteria.

The enigma how *Chlamydia* manages to escape the host cell's defence mechanisms is the focus of the following article. Even epithelial cells—the regular host cell of *Chlamydia*—have numerous systems, such as apoptosis, autophagy, inflammasome and interferon signalling that can serve in the defence against microbial invaders. *Chlamydia* has to deal with these machineries, and that chapter discusses current views on this issue.

The genomic structure of *Chlamydia trachomatis* is at the centre of the next article. It focusses on the question how recent technological advances, in particular through whole-genome sequencing, have changed our perception of the genomic structure of the bacteria. Apart from the population structure, the appreciation of what is a successful strain and a new understanding of the relationship between strains causing distinct forms of disease has only become clear through these studies. One important underlying mechanism was found to be the unexpectedly large extent of recombination between chlamydial strains.

This surprising capacity for recombination has been one of the areas of discovery that have also informed the recent endeavours to manipulate the genome of *Chlamydia trachomatis*. For a long time, many papers on *Chlamydia* included the wistful statement that *Chlamydia* is not genetically tractable. This is no longer the case. Progress has been made, and some genetically modified bacteria have been characterised. The newly developed techniques will help us understand chlamydial virulence. However, we are still a long way off routine manipulation. The article on genetic dissection of *chlamydial* virulence provides an honest appraisal of exciting yet small advances and sketches out the way ahead.

Turning to the infection of the complex (especially human) host, three articles cover a number of questions that are highly relevant to human infection. One of the striking features of human genital infection with *Chlamydia trachomatis* is the chronic infection: unless the infection is cleared right away, as it is in some patients, the infection may be persistent with spontaneous rates of clearance of as low as

50% per year. One article in the book investigates the reasons and likely mechanisms of persistence and of the individually differential response to the infection.

As already mentioned, the clinically biggest problem of human infection with *Chlamydia trachomatis* is the damage to the infected tissue, which frequently is associated with female infertility but also with eye scarring. It is clear that this is at least in part immunopathology: both innate and adaptive immunity contribute to the damage. Current state of knowledge in this field, in particular from animal models, is summarised in the article on the immunopathogenesis of chlamydial infection.

The last chapter covers the prospect for a vaccine. With few exceptions, vaccines tend to be less than completely successful against bacteria, and past endeavours do not suggest that *Chlamydia* will be much different. Nevertheless, there has been progress: understanding correlates of protection and the development of subunit vaccines has been moving forward, and the opportunities and problems will be discussed in this chapter.

Like many other areas of science, research into *Chlamydia* has benefitted from new methods and has been fertilised by the interaction of specialists with different backgrounds. I do believe that this collection of articles, prepared by experts in the relevant fields, will be a great repository of up-to-date information in a fast developing area.

Freiburg, Germany
October 2017

Georg Häcker

Contents

Deconstructing the Chlamydial Cell Wall

Anna Klöckner, Henrike Bühl, Patrick Viollier and Beate Henrichfreise

Abstract The evolutionary separated Gram-negative *Chlamydiales* show a biphasic life cycle and replicate exclusively within eukaryotic host cells. Members of the genus *Chlamydia* are responsible for many acute and chronic diseases in humans, and *Chlamydia*-related bacteria are emerging pathogens. We revisit past efforts to detect cell wall material in *Chlamydia* and *Chlamydia*-related bacteria in the context of recent breakthroughs in elucidating the underlying cellular and molecular mechanisms of the chlamydial cell wall biosynthesis. In this review, we also discuss the role of cell wall biosynthesis in chlamydial FtsZ-independent cell division and immune modulation. In the past, penicillin susceptibility of an invisible wall was referred to as the "chlamydial anomaly." In light of new mechanistic insights, chlamydiae may now emerge as model systems to understand how a minimal and modified cell wall biosynthetic machine supports bacterial cell division and how cell wall-targeting beta-lactam antibiotics can also act bacteriostatically rather than bactericidal. On the heels of these discussions, we also delve into the effects of other cell wall antibiotics in individual chlamydial lineages.

Contents

A. Klöckner · H. Bühl · B. Henrichfreise (✉)
Institute for Pharmaceutical Microbiology, University of Bonn, Meckenheimer Allee 168, 53115 Bonn, Germany
e-mail: bhenrich@uni-bonn.de

P. Viollier
Department of Microbiology and Molecular Medicine, Institute of Genetics and Genomics in Geneva (IGE3), University of Geneva, Geneva, Switzerland

Current Topics in Microbiology and Immunology (2018) 412:1–34
DOI 10.1007/82_2016_34

Published Online: 21 September 2016

1 Introduction

1.1 The Bacterial Cell Wall

In free-living bacteria, the cell wall is the major stress-bearing element and protects the organism from osmotic lysis (Höltje 1998; Scheffers and Pinho 2005). The cell wall (also named murein sacculus) resembles an exoskeleton in that it wraps the cells and endows it with its characteristic shape. Synthesis of the bacterial cell wall takes place during cell growth and at the site of cell division organized by the MreB actin and the FtsZ tubulin, respectively. The cell wall is composed of peptidoglycan (PG), a tightly woven meshwork of linear glycan chains fortified by peptide bridges that contain D-amino acids (DAAs).

PG is unique to bacteria and serves as an important target for therapeutic intervention as most bacteria cannot proliferate without a cell wall. About 50 % of prescribed antibiotics inhibit PG biosynthesis (Walsh 2003; Kresse et al. 2007) including the clinically most relevant beta-lactams, but many other antibiotics also target this essential pathway. For instance, amino acid analogs such as fosfomycin and D-cycloserine block early cytoplasmic steps of PG biosynthesis, whereas bacitracin sequesters bactoprenol-PP, an universal and essential cytoplasmic membrane carrier for bacterial cell envelope precursors that are subsequently polymerized into lipoteichoic acids (LTA), lipopolysaccharide (LPS), and/or capsules in various monoderm (Gram-positive) or diderm (Gram-negative) bacteria. In Gram-negative bacteria, the PG is sandwiched in the periplasm between the cytoplasmic and the LPS containing outer membrane layers. The scaffold of the cell wall consists of PG, a polymer of linear glycan strands cross-linked via peptide bridges. The functional unit carried by the PG precursor lipid II is an β-1,4-linked aminosugar of *N*-acetylglucosamine (GlcNAc) and *N*-acetylmuramic acid (MurNAc) (Höltje 1998), harboring a pentapeptide side chain on the lactoyl group of the MurNAc moiety (Schleifer and Kandler 1972). The pentapeptide side chain contains L- and D-amino acids and one dibasic acid, which allows peptide cross-linking. In Gram-negative bacteria, this dibasic moiety is typically mesodiaminopimelic acid (mDAP), whereas Gram-positive bacteria mainly possess L-Lys, and thus, the most common pentapeptide side chain sequence is L-Ala-D-Glu-mDAP/L-Lys-D-Ala-D-Ala (Schleifer and Kandler 1972). As the PG sacculus protects bacteria from osmotic lysis, the selective pressure for PG would be reduced for bacteria that have found another way to assemble an osmoprotective envelope layer and/or that proliferate in isotonic environment where they are protected from lysis such as the cytoplasm of eukaryotic host cells.

1.2 Chlamydiae

Bacteria belonging to the order *Chlamydiales* are obligate intracellular organisms comprising *Chlamydia* and *Chlamydia*-related bacteria with a major economic and public health importance. *Chlamydia trachomatis* is the most common bacterial agent of sexually transmitted diseases (STD) and the world's leading cause of preventable blindness (Wright et al. 2008; Taylor and Haggerty 2011). *Chlamydia pneumoniae* is considered to cause infections in the upper and lower respiratory tracts and seems to be associated with various chronic diseases (Teh et al. 2012; Darveaux and Lemanske 2014; Grayston et al. 2015). The genus *Chlamydia* includes also important animal pathogens, such as *Chlamydia abortus* and *Chlamydia psittaci* involved in abortion in cattle and respiratory diseases in avian species, respectively (Vanrompay et al. 1995; Nunes and Gomes 2014). *Chlamydia*-related bacteria (also known as *Chlamydia*-like bacteria or environmental chlamydiae) are emerging pathogens. *Waddlia chondrophila* is associated with animal abortion and human miscarriage (Baud et al. 2007, 2014). Members of the genera *Simkania* and *Parachlamydia* are suspected to cause respiratory tract infections (Friedman et al. 2003; Greub 2009). A major concern with chlamydiae is the transmission of diseases from animal to human.

Members of the *Chlamydiales* are characterized by an extraordinary life cycle which alternates between two morphological forms, the elementary body (EB) and the reticulate body (RB) (Bedson and Bland 1932; Moulder 1991). The extracellular and metabolically less active EBs are responsible for the dissemination of the bacteria inside the infected tissue or to other hosts. Once internalized into a host cell, EBs ($\sim$0.3 μm in diameter) remain in special vacuoles named inclusions and differentiate to the intracellular, osmotically instable, metabolically more active RBs ($\sim$1 μm in diameter). These bodies undergo repeated cycles of binary fission before they redifferentiate to EBs, which are released and able to restart the cell cycle (Abdelrahman and Belland 2005). In the case of adverse conditions, such as nutrient starvation, the developmental cycle is interrupted, resulting in the appearance of aberrant bodies (ABs), a stress-activated and persistent state in which they survive treatment with certain antibiotics (Wyrick 2010). Treatment of *Chlamydia* with penicillin, a PG synthesis targeting beta-lactam antibiotic, leads to an inclusion containing non-dividing enlarged, less electron-dense ABs, which are capable to reenter the life cycle after removal of the antibiotic (Matsumoto and Manire 1970; Lambden et al. 2006; Skilton et al. 2009). Beta-lactams are bactericidal to many free-living bacteria blocking transpeptidase activity of penicillin-binding proteins (PBPs), which is crucial for cross-linking in the cell wall (Rogers et al. 1980; Russell and Chopra 1990) and leading to lysis from uncontrolled PG remodeling (Cho et al. 2014). The bacteriostatic effects of beta-lactam antibiotics on intracellular chlamydiae reflect an altered function of PG in the isotonic niche and a different composition/regulation of the PG-remodeling machine which apparently lacks orthologs of lytic transglycosylases and bifunctional PBPs. Only few growing bacteria such as mycoplasma and L-form bacteria which lack a cell wall (and do not inactivate or expel beta-lactams) are fully refractory to penicillin and other cell wall antibiotics (Taylor-Robinson and Bébéar 1997; Leaver et al. 2009; Errington 2013). Cell wall research in chlamydiae has been discussed from different perspectives in brilliant reviews (Moulder 1993; Ghuysen and Goffin 1999; McCoy and Maurelli 2006; Pavelka 2007; Mohammadi and Breukink 2014; Jacquier et al. 2015b). Here, we reassess genomic, biochemical, and cytological data on the discovery of cell wall material and effects of cell wall antibiotics in genomically reduced bacteria of the genus *Chlamydia* and in the deep branching *Chlamydia*-related bacteria in light of recent breakthroughs in understanding the role of a rudimentary cell wall biosynthesis/cell division machinery in chlamydial FtsZ-less cytokinesis and immune modulation.

2 On the Traces of PG in Chlamydiae

2.1 Early Experiments

Since the discovery of chlamydiae in 1907, innumerous taxonomic changes throughout decades took place. The obligate intracellular lifestyle and inability to multiply in cell-free media mistakenly led to the assumption that these organisms resemble viruses. In 1966, they were finally characterized as bacteria (Halberstaedter and von Prowazek 1907; Moulder 1966) not least because they were shown to be sensitive to antibiotics, such as chloramphenicol, tetracyclines, and penicillin (Hurst 1953). Early studies claimed the colorimetric detection of muramic acid, the hallmark of PG, in *C. psittaci* and *C. trachomatis* (Jenkin 1960; Perkins and Allison 1963) (Fig. 1); however, further attempts to confirm these result failed. Manire and Tamura (1967) could not detect muramic acid from purified EBs using a modified amino acid analysis system which allows the detection of amino sugars such as muramic acid (Manire and Tamura 1967). Later attempts to immunostain the cell wall using anti-PG antibodies were as unsuccessful as were all efforts to purify chlamydial PG sacculi or to detect periplasmic densities between the inner and the outer membranes using transmission electron microscopy (Tamura et al. 1971; Matsumoto 1979; Caldwell et al. 1981; Barbour et al. 1982; Moulder 1993; Hatch 1996). Almost all fruitless attempts to detect cell wall material in *Chlamydia* were performed in EBs and based on the fallacy that the more rigid and stable

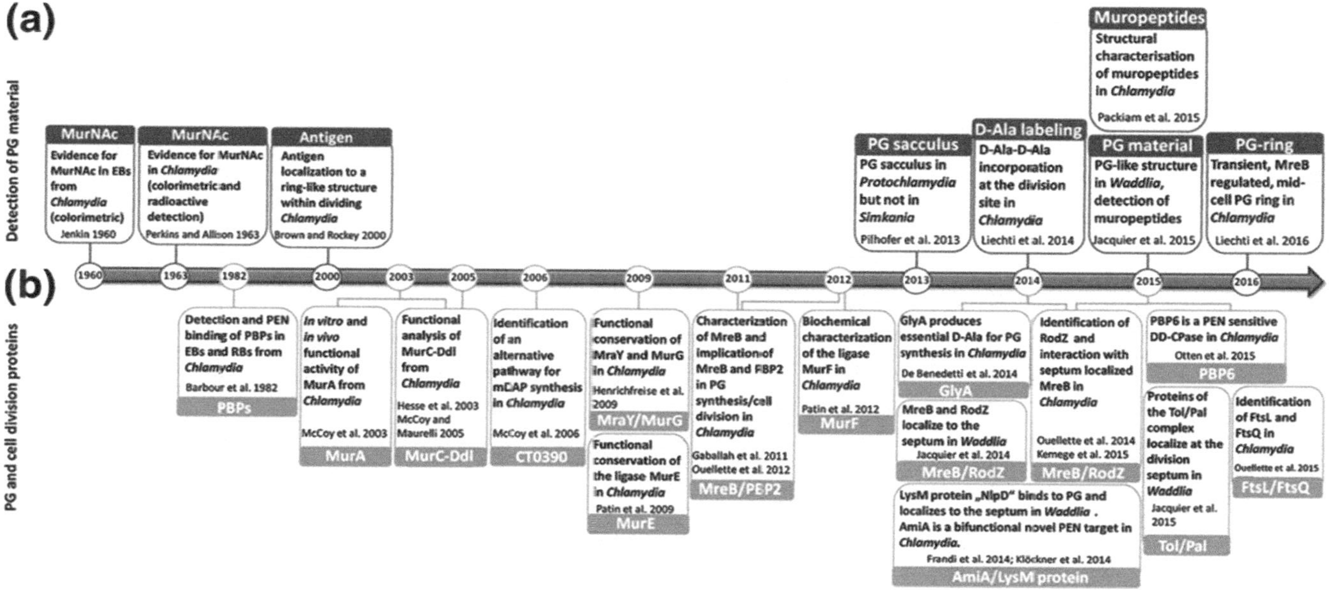

Fig. 1 Toward resolving the chlamydial anomaly. Selected steps in detecting chlamydial PG (**a**) and analyzing the involved protein machineries on a molecular level (**b**)

developmental form, the EBs, and not the fragile replicative RBs were expected to contain PG (Tamura and Manire 1967; Chopra et al. 1998). Only one study is reported trying to detect PG in particular in RBs of *C. trachomatis* albeit without any proof of the polymer in these morphological forms (Barbour et al. 1982). In those days, the failure to detect PG led to the assumption that even if EBs do contain PG, the quantities are insufficient to form a conventional sacculus providing structural stability (Fox et al. 1990; Moulder 1993; Chopra et al. 1998) and cysteine-rich disulfide-cross-linked proteins in the envelope were suggested to be the functional equivalent of a PG cell wall in *Chlamydia* (Hatch 1996).

2.2 Visualize the Invisible—The Discovery of PG Material in Chlamydiae

After more than 50 years of failure to detect chlamydial PG (Fig. 1), Pilhofer et al. proved for the first time existence of PG material in *Protochlamydia amoebophila*, a deeply rooting *Chlamydia*-related species (Pilhofer et al. 2013) making a major leap forward to resolve the mysterious "chlamydial anomaly." Natural contrast staining by electron cryotomography revealed densities between the two membrane layers that resembled the PG of Gram-negative bacteria. Additionally, they were able to isolate an intact sacculus, digest it with PG-cleaving enzymes, and conduct mass spectrometric analysis of the muropeptides, revealing two yet unknown modifications adding extra masses of 129 and 203 Da compared to canonical muropeptides. These findings showed that *P. amoebophila* is indeed surrounded by a novel type of PG sacculus (Pilhofer et al. 2013) (Fig. 2). Surprisingly, the researchers could not detect PG and were unable to isolate a PG sacculus in *Simkania negevensis*, another *Chlamydia*-related species (Pilhofer et al. 2013). Consistent with a less complete set of cell wall synthesis genes compared to other *Chlamydia*-related bacteria and in common with *Chlamydia*, *Simkania* lacks all the enzymes (UppP, YeiU, YbjG, and PgpB) known to catalyze bactoprenol-PP carrier dephosphorylation in *Escherichia coli* (Tatar et al. 2007), whereas *Protochlamydia*, *Parachlamydia*, and *Waddlia* retained UppP (Fig. 3). Moreover, *Simkania* and *Chlamydia* lack MurI glutamate racemase homologs as well as a regular Alr or DadX alanine racemase essential for PG synthesis (see below). A recent study on another *Chlamydia*-related bacterial genus revealed strong evidence for the presence of a cell wall. In *Waddlia*, PG-like material could be extracted from replicating cells, and after treatment with cell wall hydrolases, released muropeptides were detected by HPLC (Jacquier et al. 2015a). The nucleotide-binding oligomerization domain-containing proteins Nod1 and Nod2 are two cytosolic pattern recognition receptors of the human innate immune system and sense cell wall fragments (see below) (Girardin et al. 2003; McCoy and Maurelli 2006; Welter-Stahl et al. 2006). Further bolstering the presence of PG, the extracted material was recognized by

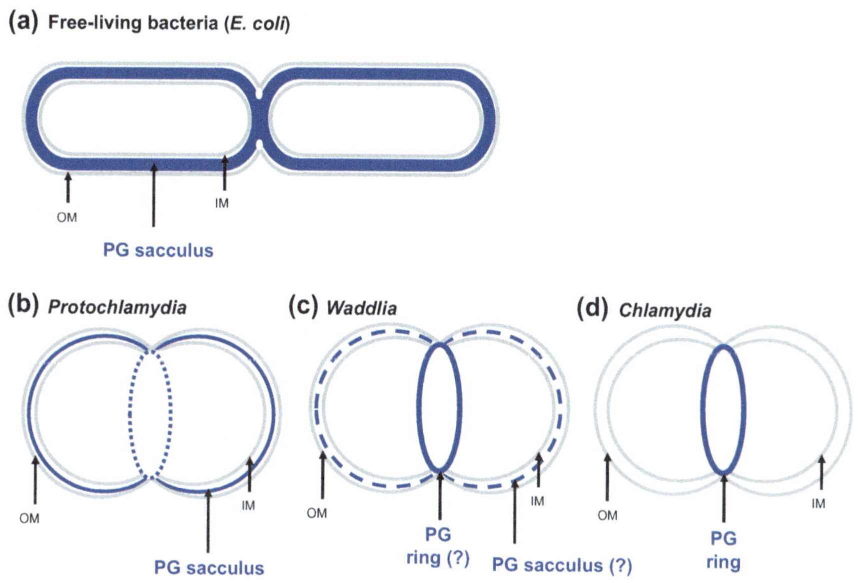

Fig. 2 Model on evolutionary reduction of PG structures in deeply rooting *Chlamydia*-related bacteria and in *Chlamydia*. Free-living bacteria such as *E. coli* (**a**) are wrapped by a shape-determining PG sacculus for osmotic stabilization, and synthesis of septal PG protects dividing cells against lysis. In chlamydiae, a stepwise rationalization of the energy cost-intensive pathway of PG biosynthesis during adaptation to a small host range leads to a minimal PG structure only needed at certain times and locations to facilitate cell division and to control immune modulation in the genus *Chlamydia*. In *Protochlamydia* (**b**) but not in *Simkania*, a modified PG sacculus was discovered (Pilhofer et al. 2013) and a recent study provided strong evidence for a cell wall in *Waddlia* (**c**) (Jacquier et al. 2015a). The structure of septal PG in *Protochlamydia* is unknown, whereas in *Waddlia*, localization of the PG-binding "NlpD" and Pal proteins suggests a *circular structure* (Frandi et al. 2014; Jacquier et al. 2015a) comparable to the narrow PG ring in *Chlamydia* transiently formed during cell division (**d**) (Liechti et al. 2014, 2016). *IM* inner membrane; *OM* outer membrane

human Nod1 and Nod2 receptors at rates comparable with those of *E. coli* PG (Jacquier et al. 2015a).

Shortly after the detection of a modified PG sacculus in *Protochlamydia*, a new method to make sites of PG biosynthetic activity in *Chlamydia* visible revolutionized the field. Liechti et al. succeeded in detecting PG biosynthesis in *C. trachomatis* by using special D-amino acid dipeptide probes that are incorporated during precursor assembly in the cytoplasm and can be subsequently labeled in the periplasm by a novel click chemistry method (Liechti et al. 2014). In contrast to *Protochlamydia* (Pilhofer et al. 2013), previous efforts to label *Chlamydia* with D-amino acid probes failed probably because the modified amino acids are not a substrate of the *Chlamydia* D-Ala-D-Ala ligase Ddl (Liechti et al. 2014). The elegant method described by Liechti et al. bypassed the Ddl enzyme via supply of D-Ala-D-Ala dipeptide analogs modified with alkyne or azide functional groups (Liechti et al. 2014). In replicating *C. trachomatis*, they demonstrated the uptake and incorporation of these dipeptide probes resulting in a fluorescently labeled ring-like structure at the division plane similar to previous observations in 2000 (Brown and Rockey 2000; Liechti et al. 2014). Brown and Rockey used antiserum raised against mycobacterial PG to immunostain an antigen of unknown identity and composition at the apparent septum in RBs of *C. trachomatis* and *C. psittaci* in a ring-like shape, whereas in EBs the distribution was diffuse and irregular (Brown and Rockey 2000). Lysozyme treatment abolished the labeling signal within chlamydial inclusions providing first evidence of glycan strands in the absence of common transglycosylases (Liechti et al. 2014).

In 2015, Packiam et al. defined the structure of *C. trachomatis* PG by making use of the aforementioned perception of *Chlamydia* through human Nod factors from the innate immune system and provided first direct structural confirmation of PG material in *Chlamydia* (Packiam et al. 2015). Nod2-depending activation of NF-κB in *Chlamydia*-infected cells was used as a biomarker to identify specific lysate fractions from *C. trachomatis*-infected cell cultures containing chlamydial PG fragments (Packiam et al. 2015). Next, a novel technique comprising a double-filtration step linked to a reverse-phase HPLC was used to isolate these muropeptides from the identified Nod2-activating fractions. Using the new technique, muramyl di- and tripeptides in *Chlamydia*-infected cell lysate fractions were detected. Additionally, mass spectrometric analysis of large muropeptide fragments containing up to three disaccharide units confirmed that transglycosylation reactions

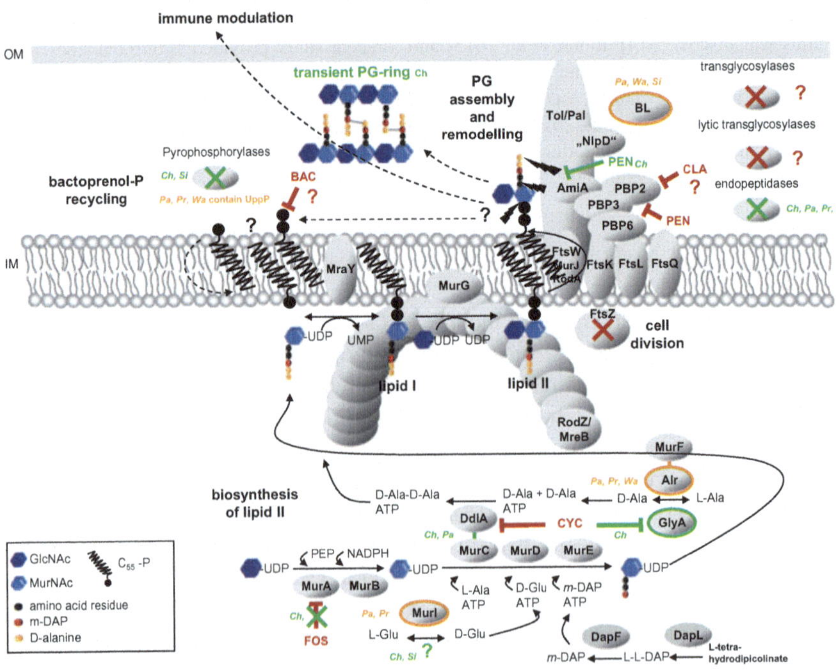

◀ **Fig. 3** Proposed model on PG biosynthesis and cell division machineries in chlamydiae. The rudimentary chlamydial cell wall biosynthesis and cell division machineries differ from *E. coli* and among chlamydial lineages. A complete cycle of lipid II biosynthesis, including translocation of the building block into the periplasm, incorporation into a PG structure, and recycling of the bactoprenol carrier, is indispensable for maintaining coordinated cell division. A characteristic of *Chlamydia* and *Simkania* is the absence of amino acid racemases Alr and MurI, and GlyA was found to function as alternative D-Ala racemase in *Chlamydia* (De Benedetti et al. 2014). The proteins MurC and DdlA are fused in *Chlamydia* and *Parachlamydia* but not in *Waddlia, Simkania,* and *Protochlamydia*. Export of lipid II to the periplasm could be facilitated by FtsW, MurJ, and/or RodA as surprisingly all putative flippases are retained in chlamydiae. Once in the periplasm, lipid II is incorporated into a transient septal PG ring in *Chlamydia* (Liechti et al. 2016) and most likely into a PG sacculus additionally to septal PG in *Waddlia* (Jacquier et al. 2015a). In *Protochlamydia* but not in *Simkania,* the presence of a PG sacculus was recently proven (Pilhofer et al. 2013). The only PBPs found in chlamydiae are homologs of monofunctional PBPs (PBP2 and PBP3) and of a carboxypeptidase (PBP6). Common transglycosylases, connecting the sugar backbone of the cell wall, are missing in all chlamydiae. Moreover, all chlamydiae apparently lack lytic transglycosylases and endopeptidases, which are major cell wall-remodeling enzymes, whereas evidence for endopeptidase activity of *Waddlia* "NlpD" was provided (Frandi et al. 2014). *Chlamydia* "NlpD" has carboxypeptidase activity (Klöckner et al. 2014). All pyrophosphorylases (UppP, YeiU, YbjG, PgpB) responsible for the recycling of the bactoprenol carrier in *E. coli* are missing in *Chlamydia* and *Simkania* albeit *Waddlia, Protochlamydia,* and *Parachlamydia* retained UppP. Chlamydiae possess only five cell division proteins, FtsI (PBP3), FtsK, FtsL, FtsQ, and FtsW, and AmiA, a protein required for cell separation in *E. coli.* In *Chlamydia,* AmiA is a bifunctional target protein of penicillin (Klöckner et al. 2014). The Tol-Pal transenvelope complex, involved in maintaining integrity of the outer membrane and facilitating concerted constriction of all envelope layers during cytokinesis, is conserved among chlamydiae (Jacquier et al. 2015a). Actin-like protein MreB, in combination with RodZ, functionally replaces FtsZ in orchestration of PG synthesis and cell division in chlamydiae (Gaballah et al. 2011; Ouellette et al. 2012; Jacquier et al. 2014; Ouellette et al. 2014; Kemege et al. 2015; Liechti et al. 2016) which do not encode this tubulin-like protein. Antibiotics that (may) block certain steps of the PG biosynthesis pathway are shown in red (see paragraph 5 for detailed information). Steps that remain to be clarified are highlighted by *question marks* and *dashed arrows*. (*BAC*) bacitracin, (*BL*) beta-lactamase, (*CA*) clavulanic acid, (*CYC*) D cycloserine, (*FOS*) fosfomycin, (*PEN*) penicillin, (*Ch*) *Chlamydia*, (*Pa*) *Parachlamydia*, (*Pr*) *Protochlamydia*, (*Si*) *Simkania*, (*Wa*) *Waddlia*

occur in *Chlamydia* despite the lack of commonly used transglycosylase homologs (Packiam et al. 2015) disproving the "glycanless peptidoglycan" hypothesis for *Chlamydia* (Ghuysen and Goffin 1999). Also, cross-linked muropeptides featuring two mDAP residues linked via alanine were detected, indicating the presence of PBP-catalyzed transpeptidation reactions in *C. trachomatis* (Packiam et al. 2015).

Only recently, super-resolution microscopy and use of the above-described clickable D-amino acid dipeptide probes revealed *a* ≤ 140-nm-wide PG ring in four *Chlamydia* species (*C. trachomatis, C. psittaci, Chlamydia muridarum,* and *Chlamydia caviae*) (Liechti et al. 2016). Formation of the PG ring occurred only in dividing RBs following cell constriction at the division septum and was perturbed in the presence of an inhibitor of MreB (Liechti et al. 2016), an actin-like protein that was previously proposed to functionally replace FtsZ in orchestration of PG synthesis and cell division in chlamydiae which do not encode this tubulin-like protein (Gaballah et al. 2011; Ouellette et al. 2012; Jacquier et al. 2014; Ouellette et al. 2014) (see below). Liechti et al. proposed that the transient presence of a narrow PG ring is an adaptation to the pathogenic lifestyle of *Chlamydia* within its vertebrate host and prevents PG recognition by the innate immune system in the infectious EB form (Liechti et al. 2016).

All in all, in the last three years, outstanding studies achieved multifaceted insight into the presence of PG (like) material in *Chlamydia*-related bacteria and *Chlamydia*. Detailed knowledge of the chlamydial rudimentary PG and cell division machineries is indispensable to understand cell wall antibiotic-induced persistence in *Chlamydia* and to reveal the mechanisms of the minimal cell wall machine executing de novo PG ring synthesis in RBs, remodeling during constriction, and degradation of PG in *Chlamydia*. For this purpose, *Chlamydia*-related bacteria provide invaluable evolutionary insight into how the energy cost-intensive pathway of PG biosynthesis was stepwise rationalized during adaptation to a small host range leading to a minimal PG structure only needed at certain times and locations to facilitate division and to control immune modulation appropriately.

3 Functional and Genomic Studies of the Chlamydial PG Biosynthesis Pathway

In the course of the evolutionary adaptation to an intracellular lifestyle, chlamydiae highly reduced their genome size (Collingro et al. 2011). Nevertheless, genome analyses revealed a nearly complete set of genes for the synthesis of cell wall precursor lipid II in chlamydiae (Stephens et al. 1998), and transcriptional activity of the genes peaks during RB division (16–18 h p.i.) (Nicholson et al. 2003; Belland et al. 2003), suggesting that the pathway is essential in chlamydial biology (Fig. 3). In line, proteomic comparison of RBs and EBs revealed that MurE, an enzyme involved in lipid II synthesis, is exclusively found in RBs. An evolutionary relationship between chlamydiae and plants including horizontal transfer from genes such as PG biosynthesis gene CT390 (see below) from chlamydiae to Archaeplastida has been controversially discussed (Born and Blanchard 1999; Ball et al. 2013; Facchinelli et al. 2013; Subtil et al. 2014). However, a recent study revealed no compelling evidence from gene trees that chlamydiae played a role in establishing the primary plastid endosymbiosis before the emergence of the Archaeplastida (Domman et al. 2015). In this regard, it is noteworthy that chloroplast organelles in various plants are thought to produce PG as well, as PG biosynthetic genes are encoded in plant genomes, and recently, PG was detected in moss chloroplasts (Hofmann 2016). Moreover, chloroplasts from glaucophyte algae for which evolutionary studies suggest that they branched of early from the Archaeplastida encode functional PG-remodeling enzymes and produce PG (Miyagishima et al. 2014).

3.1 Cytoplasmic and Membrane-Bound Steps of Chlamydial PG Biosynthesis

The PG biosynthesis in bacteria takes place in three different cellular compartments and requires numerous biosynthetic enzymes. It starts in the cytoplasm with the formation of the soluble precursor UDP-MurNAc-pentapeptide, catalyzed by the Mur enzymes A-F (Fig. 3). With the exception of MurB and MurD, all Mur enzymes from *Chlamydia* have been shown to be functional in the extensively reduced genomes of the intracellular pathogens (Hesse et al. 2003; McCoy et al. 2003; McCoy and Maurelli 2005; Patin et al. 2009, 2012). MurA is an UDP-*N*-acetylglucosamine enolpyruvyl transferase and adds enolpyruvate to *N*-acetylglucosamine (GlcNAc) which is reduced by MurB to MurNAc (van Heijenoort 2001; McCoy et al. 2003). Subsequently, five amino acids are added to the UDP-activated amino sugar to form the pentapeptide side chain. In *E. coli*, MurC adds L-Ala in position 1 (Vollmer and Bertsche 2008). Purified MurC from *C. trachomatis* that is fused to Ddl among *Chlamydia* and *Parachlamydia* lacks selectivity for alanine over glycine or serine (Hesse et al. 2003). Consistently, structure analyses on *C. trachomatis* muropeptides harvested from cell culture uncovered the presence of L-Ala or Gly in position 1 of peptide side chains (Packiam et al. 2015). *Chlamydia* rationalized pathways for alanine and serine but harbors an enzyme for reversible conversion of serine into glycine, the serine hydroxymethyltransferase GlyA which additionally shows alanine racemase activity (see below). Availability of L-Ala and analogs from the in vivo or in vitro cell culture environment might be reflected in a mixture of amino acids in the variable position 1 of the chlamydial peptide side chains. In the next step, D-Glu is attached by MurD. Mass spectrometric analyses proved the presence of Glu in *Chlamydia* (Packiam et al. 2015), but in the absence of a Glu racemase homolog in *Chlamydia,* the source of the non-proteinogenic D-Glu enantiomer is elusive. *Chlamydia* has an exceptional synthesis pathway for mDAP located in position 3 of the pentapeptide side chain, which is an important substrate for cross-linking activity of PBP transpeptidases. The amino acid is produced via the aminotransferase pathway which they share with plants and is not found in other bacteria (Pavelka 2007). L,L-diaminopimelate aminotransferase DapL (CT390) directly converts L-tetrahydrodipicolinate into L,L-diaminopimelate. Subsequently, DapF epimerizes the dibasic acid to mDAP which is linked to the UDP-MurNAc dipeptide by ligase MurE from *C. trachomatis* (McCoy et al. 2006).

In free-living bacteria, such as *E. coli*, the non-proteinogenic amino acid D-Ala is synthesized by the pyridoxal-5′-phosphate (PLP) cofactor-dependent racemases Alr and DadX and connected by ligase Ddl to produce D-Ala-D-Ala. MurF attaches the D-Ala-D-Ala dipeptide to the amino acid in position 3 (mDAP) to complete the pentapeptide side chain of the soluble UDP-MurNAc-pentapeptide precursor. The Ddl domain of the fusion protein MurC/Ddl from *C. trachomatis* specifically uses the D-Ala and not the L-Ala enantiomer to produce alanine dipeptides (McCoy and Maurelli 2005), and chlamydial MurF is capable of ligating D-Ala-D-Ala and the

UDP-MurNAc-tripeptide precursor in vitro (Fig. 3) (Patin et al. 2012). D-Ala is unique and essential in bacterial PG biosynthesis because PBP transpeptidases, the molecular targets of beta-lactams, depend on mDAP and D-Ala-D-Ala moieties to cross-link PG sugar strands (DD-transpeptidation, see below). In *Chlamydia*, the source of D-Ala and thus the presence of substrates for PBPs were unclear for years as the pathogen lacks common alanine racemases to produce the essential component in lipid II biosynthesis. Recently, PLP cofactor-dependent GlyA, the only protein of the methionine pathway (folate branch) that is retained in *Chlamydia* genomes, was shown to confer self-synthesis of D-Ala in *Chlamydia* (De Benedetti et al. 2014). Notably, the weak alanine racemase activity of *C. pneumoniae* GlyA did not completely compensate D-Ala requirements of an *E. coli* racemase mutant to build an entire PG sacculus but might be sufficient in cell wall-lacking *Chlamydia* to produce the recently detected narrow PG ring during cell division (Liechti et al. 2014, 2016) and to release immunogenic cell wall material.

Comparative analysis of *Chlamydia*-related genomes revealed that *Protochlamydia* (in which a PG sacculus was found), *Waddlia* (containing PG material in amounts that can be detected with conventional methods), and *Parachlamydia* (not investigated as to the presence of PG yet) harbor homologs of the highly active Ala racemases Alr and DadX. In contrast, in *Simkania* that contains neither Alr nor DadX but the weak racemase GlyA, the attempts to detect a PG sacculus failed. These findings implicate a PG sacculus in *Protochlamydia* and the presence of a reduced PG ring in *Simkania* as recently detected in *C. trachomatis* (Fig. 2) (Liechti et al. 2016).

Once the UDP-activated MurNAc pentapeptide is assembled, the soluble precursor is linked to a membrane carrier (bactoprenol) to form the first membrane-bound precursor lipid I. The reaction is catalyzed by the integral membrane protein MraY. Next, the membrane-associated MurG enzyme adds another sugar unit (GlucNAc) producing the completed cell wall building block lipid II. Proof of activity for chlamydial MraY and MurG, catalyzing the final steps in forming PG building blocks, corroborated functional conservation of the lipid II synthesis pathway in *Chlamydia* and opened the way to analyze functions of the rudimentary pathway in chlamydial cell division and immune response modulation (Henrichfreise et al. 2009).

In free-living bacteria, building block lipid II is flipped to the outside and incorporated in the existing cell wall by the activity of PBPs releasing bactoprenol-PP. Despite a reduced genome size, *Chlamydia* retained three seemingly redundant proteins, FtsW, MurJ, and RodA implicated in flipping lipid II in free-living bacteria (Young 2014).

3.2 *Periplasmic Steps of Chlamydial PG Biosynthesis*

A concerted action of cell wall assembling and degrading is needed to maintain an intact PG sacculus over the whole cell cycle and to prevent in particular cell lysis during growth and division of walled bacteria. Numerous synthases such as transpeptidases, transglycosylases, and degrading enzymes like endopeptidases, lytic transglycosylases, carboxypeptidases, and amidases are involved and tightly coordinated to avoid spatial or temporal imbalance of the incorporation and remodeling processes. In the *Chlamydia* life cycle, PG synthesis is temporally limited to the stage of replication and spatially reduced to a narrow ring structure at the division site (Fig. 2). Next, the transient ring is reduced in diameter synchronic to progressing constriction and afterward completely degraded by an unknown turnover machinery (Liechti et al. 2016). *Chlamydia* seems to harbor only a limited number of enzymes to synthesize and degrade PG. Transglycosylation during nascent ring synthesis and lytic transglycosylation during size reduction and degradation following completed constriction remain elusive in the absence of homologs known to catalyze these enzymatic steps in other bacteria. Moreover, only two putative monofunctional transpeptidases for cross-linking (PBP2 and PBP3) glycan strands and one carboxypeptidase PBP (PBP6) are found in *Chlamydia*. Genes to encode common endopeptidases, which are antagonists of the transpeptidases and cut cross-linked peptide side chains, could not be found in *Chlamydia* either, whereas evidence for endopeptidase action of "NlpD" was provided for *Waddlia* (Frandi et al. 2014). In *E. coli*, three cell division amidases are needed for proper cell separation and tightly controlled through regulatory proteins. *Chlamydia* conserved only one of these septal PG hydrolases and does not code for any known regulatory factor.

3.2.1 Penicillin-Binding Proteins

In line with the detection of three proteins in chlamydial cell lysates to bind radiolabeled penicillin in the early 1980s (Barbour et al. 1982), *Chlamydia* genomes encode two high molecular weight (HMW) PBPs and one low molecular weight PBP. The two HMW PBPs PBP2 and PBP3 (FtsI) are homologs of monofunctional transpeptidases that cross-link peptides of neighboring PG strands via mDAP and D-Ala-D-Ala moieties in free-living bacteria such as *E. coli*. The PG synthases are anchored to the cytoplasmic membrane and consist of two periplasmic domains, an *N*-terminal domain which has been involved in folding and dimerization (Goffin et al. 1996; Sauvage et al. 2014) of the proteins and the C-terminal penicillin-binding domain. Typical for acyl-serine transferases the latter domain contains the three motifs SxxK, S(Y)xN, and K(H,R)T(S)G that are essential for substrate recognition and catalysis (Sauvage et al. 2008). PBP2 incorporates cell wall material outside the septum, whereas PBP3 is part of the divisome and plays a vital role in incorporation of lipid II at the septum in *E. coli*. However, there is increasing evidence that PBP2 is temporally involved in mid-cell PG biosynthesis in *E. coli* (Den Blaauwen et al. 2003; Vats and Rothfield 2007; van der Ploeg et al. 2013) and the *C. trachomatis* homolog of PBP2 has recently been shown to interact with PBP3 and the cell division protein FtsK (Ouellette et al. 2012). Expression of PBP3 from *C. trachomatis* is controlled through non-coding RNA CTIG270 by inducing degradation of *ftsI* mRNA (Abdelrahman et al. 2011). Chlamydial PBP2 contains a unique insert of about 400 amino acid residues with yet unknown function (Ouellette et al. 2012).

The susceptibility of *Chlamydia* to beta-lactams, their ability to synthesize D-Ala with an alternative alanine racemase (De Benedetti et al. 2014), and their ability to incorporate exogenously added D-Ala-D-Ala into a distinct ring-like septal PG structure (Liechti et al. 2014) together indicate that the homologs of monofunctional transpeptidases play a critical role in the cell biology of these obligate intracellular pathogens. Noteworthy, incorporation of labeled precursors was also seen under beta-lactam treatment but rarely showed proper ring morphology in the non-dividing enlarged ABs (Liechti et al. 2014). These findings suggest that PG glycan strand formation is uncoupled from transpeptidation and carboxypeptidation in *Chlamydia,* but PBP-driven cross-linking is needed for shaping the ring and maintaining functional cell division (Liechti et al. 2016).

Low molecular weight PBPs from free-living bacteria are DD-carboxypeptidases or endopeptidases and lack the ability to incorporate lipid II into the PG meshwork and to cross-link adjacent glycan strands. Carboxypeptidases modulate the mature PG sacculus by removing terminal D-Ala from pentapeptide side chains which are not cross-linked (Ghosh et al. 2008). Thereby, the enzymes regulate the availability of D-Ala-D-Ala moieties for cross-linking through PBP transpeptidases and are thought to be involved in the maintenance of cell shape and septum formation (Nelson and Young 2000; Ghosh et al. 2008). Most walled bacteria harbor several apparently dispensable and enzymatically redundant low molecular weight PBPs. In contrast, cell wall-lacking *Chlamydia,* which produces only a transient PG ring during cell division, retained only a single low molecular weight PBP, a homolog to PBP6 from *E. coli*. PBP6 from *E. coli* was implicated in stabilizing PG in the stationary phase (Ghosh et al. 2008). Moreover, carboxypeptidases are thought to supply the monofunctional transpeptidase PBP3 with substrate during cell division in *E. coli* (Ghosh et al. 2008). The PBP6 homolog from *C. pneumoniae* was recently shown to function as carboxypeptidase cutting D-Ala from the cell wall building block lipid II (Otten et al. 2015). The penicillin-sensitive activity was dependent on a functional SxxK motif as typically found for PBPs in prokaryotes.

3.2.2 Amidase AmiA—A Bifunctional Target Protein of Penicillin

In *E. coli*, cell division amidases are essentially involved in septal PG hydrolysis and cell separation (Uehara and Bernhardt 2011). The enzymes remove the entire peptide side chain from the PG sugar backbone cutting between L-Ala in position 1 of the peptide and the MurNAc unit (Vollmer et al. 2008). The only chlamydial homolog of these amidases, AmiA, has been studied in *Waddlia* and *Chlamydia* (Frandi et al. 2014; Klöckner et al. 2014). Both homologs showed amidase activity and supported daughter cell separation in *E. coli* triple amidase knockout mutants. In contrast to AmiA from free-living bacteria, AmiA from *C. pneumoniae* used not only PG polymers but also cell wall precursor lipid II as a substrate and showed novel dual activity acting as amidase and carboxypeptidases. The latter function was blocked by penicillin and assigned to an SxxK motif that is typical for PBPs. Identification of AmiA as a so far unknown target of penicillin in *Chlamydia* paved the way to analyze AmiA homologs as potential determinants engaged in the effect of penicillin in other pathogens. In cell division amidases from Gram-negative bacteria, the active sites are occupied by a conserved α-helix (Yang et al. 2012). The amidases possess low basal in vitro activity and require the activation by EnvC and NlpD. These LytM-containing septal ring factors are thought to interact with the autoinhibitory domains to promote release of the regulatory domain and to activate their corresponding partner enzymes (EnvC activates AmiA and AmiB, while NlpD promotes AmiC activity) (Yang et al. 2012). Chlamydial AmiA homologs lack an autoinhibitory domain and are by default active enzymes (Frandi et al. 2014; Klöckner et al. 2014). Consistent with these findings, chlamydial genomes encode neither the amidase activators EnvC and NlpD nor FtsE and FtsX that are required to recruit AmiA to the division plane in *E. coli* (Yang et al. 2011). *E. coli* AmiA is distributed over the periplasm and kept in its off state, only hydrolyzing PG as part of the divisome following recruitment and activation via FtsE/X and EnvC (Yang et al. 2011). Immunolocalization in *Waddlia* revealed that AmiA is found throughout the periplasm with a possible enrichment at the division site in deeply constricted cells (Frandi et al. 2014). Nothing is known about the localization of AmiA in *Chlamydia* so far. How AmiA in chlamydiae is recruited to the divisome and how catalytic activities on lipid II and PG structures are regulated remain elusive.

3.2.3 "NlpD"—A Septal Lipid II/PG-Binding Hydrolase

Chlamydiae encode a protein that is misannotated as NlpD and that harbors two putative PG-binding LysM domains. As described above, *E. coli* NlpD belongs to the LytM factors and is an essential activator for the cell division amidase AmiC (Uehara et al. 2010). However, chlamydial "NlpD" (CPn0902 in *C. pneumoniae*) does not contain a LytM domain and a homologous protein cannot be found in other bacteria (Klöckner et al. 2014). *Waddlia* "NlpD" is recruited to the division plane at a later stage than MreB, and this localization is impaired in penicillin-treated cells. In support of the notion that "NlpD" from *Waddlia* interacts directly with a PG-like structure at the division plane, pelleting assays showed that the protein can bind *E. coli* PG in vitro and that this interaction is lost by mutations in the LysM PG-binding domains (Frandi et al. 2014). Interestingly, "NlpD" from *Waddlia* and *Chlamydia* confer hydrolytic activity on PG/precursors. Genetic experiments with *Waddlia* "NlpD" expressed in *E. coli* suggested that the LysM protein has or induces endopeptidase activity and the purified *C. pneumoniae* homolog had carboxypeptidase activity on cell wall building block lipid II (Frandi et al. 2014; Klöckner et al. 2014).

So far, besides PBP6, two additional uncommon carboxypeptidases have been found in *Chlamydia* increasing the number of carboxypeptidases to three and raising questions as to their functions in chlamydial cell biology. PBP6, AmiA, and "NlpD" might confer carboxypeptidase functions in chlamydial cell division in concerted action in that they control spatiotemporal dynamics of the formation of a robust PG structure at mid-cell by controlling the level of cross-linking. Moreover, the enzymes might contribute to the regulation of immunogenic muropeptide release in *Chlamydia*, as postulated for carboxypeptidases from free-living bacteria (Ghosh et al. 2008). Future work will address their roles in penicillin-induced persistence, immune modulation, and chlamydial cytokinesis.

4 Organization of the Chlamydial Division Septum

The presence of transpeptidase PBPs and PG degradation enzymes provided early indirect support for the existence of chlamydial PG. Additionally, immunolocalization of the PG-binding protein "NlpD" to the division septum in *Waddlia* (Frandi et al. 2014) further reinforced the notion that PG is present at the chlamydial division septum. As in other bacterial systems, septal PG is first synthesized and followed by its subsequent dissolution by PG hydrolases (Typas et al. 2012), events that must be tightly regulated in time and space for cytokinesis to proceed in the correct order and in a coordinated fashion on all envelope layers. The FtsZ tubulin that assembles beneath the cytoplasmic membrane at the future division site and that provides indirect linkages to the periplasmic PG layer (Erickson et al. 2010) is not encoded, neither in *Chlamydiae* nor in the related Planctomycetes (Jogler et al. 2012), indicating that the organization of cytokinesis is achieved by fundamentally different interactions in these two phyla. Moreover, FtsZ-interacting proteins that provide the docking sites for FtsZ on the inner membrane or that regulate its polymerization in time and space are also not encoded in these phyla. However, the MreB actin that also interacts indirectly with the periplasmic PG biosynthetic machinery and directly with cytoplasmic PG precursor biosynthesis proteins (White et al. 2010) is encoded in chlamydial and several Planctomycetes genomes (Jogler et al. 2012). Specific binding partners of MreB, such as the putative flippase RodA and RodZ transmembrane anchors for MreB in other systems (Vats et al. 2009; Matteï et al. 2010), are found in chlamydial genomes, while MreD is not present (Ouellette et al. 2014; Kemege et al. 2015). This genomic evidence already hinted that in chlamydiae, an actin-based system had functionally replaced the tubulin-based system that organizes the division septum in other bacteria (Gaballah et al. 2011; Ouellette et al. 2012). The fact that MreB had early on been shown to transiently localize to the division plane during the alpha-proteobacterial cell cycle (Figge et al. 2004; Slovak et al. 2006) provided further credence to this model. Chlamydial MreB was then indeed able to polymerize, to possess ATPase activity and to interact with cytoplasmic PG precursor biosynthetic enzyme MurF in vitro (Gaballah et al. 2011) and with the chlamydial RodZ (Ouellette et al. 2014; Kemege et al. 2015), FtsK (Ouellette et al. 2012), and possibly MraY and MurG homologs [found in *C. pneumoniae* but not in *C. trachomatis* (Gaballah et al. 2011; Ouellette et al. 2014)] in heterologous in vivo systems. Indirect interaction between MreB and RodA was shown to be facilitated via RodZ which interacts with the putative flippase in bacterial two-hybrid assays (Kemege et al. 2015). Moreover, known inhibitors of MreB polymerization also inhibited division and replication of *C. trachomatis*, *C. pneumoniae*, and *W. chondrophila* (Ouellette et al. 2012; Jacquier et al. 2014; Liechti et al. 2016).

Studies showing the immunolocalization of MreB and/or RodZ at the division plane in various *Chlamydiales* lineages provided cytological evidence for the MreB/RodZ-based system functioning in chlamydial cytokinesis (Jacquier et al. 2014; Kemege et al. 2015; Liechti et al. 2016). Remarkably, while MreB is robustly localized at the septum upon an early stage of *C. trachomatis* cytokinesis (Kemege et al. 2015; Liechti et al. 2016), septal signals were only visible at a late stage of constriction in *W. chondrophila* (Jacquier et al. 2014). These differences may underlie modifications in the assembly pathway of the division septum in distinct chlamydial lineages or simply the accessibility of epitopes recognized by the different antibodies to MreB that were used. RodZ is localized robustly during an early stage of *W. chondrophila* division (Jacquier et al. 2014), but no septal localization was observed in *C. trachomatis*, when probing for untagged RodZ using specific antiserum or even with an epitope-tagged derivative (Ouellette et al. 2014; Kemege et al. 2015). Septal MreB and/or RodZ are thus well positioned for the subsequent recruitment of other factors that recruits the PG biosynthetic machine. Recently, a possible structural homolog of *E. coli* FtsQ was localized to the *C. trachomatis* division septum (Ouellette et al. 2015) that is known to recruit the FtsI/PBP3 transpeptidase in other bacteria. The chlamydial homolog of FtsQ was found to interact with MreB, RodZ, and FtsK but not with FtsI, FtsW, or RodA in an *E. coli* bacterial two-hybrid assay (Ouellette et al. 2015). In *E. coli*, the FtsK DNA translocase recruits FtsQ (D'Ulisse et al. 2007) and MreB interacts with chlamydial FtsK (Ouellette et al. 2015). The order in which the components of the minimal PG and cell division machinery inclusive of Tol/Pal, PBP2, and PG-remodeling enzymes such as AmiA, "NlpD," and PBP6 assemble at the chlamydial division septum remains to be determined.

Interestingly, the interaction of MreB with the PG precursor biosynthesis protein MurF (Gaballah et al. 2011) and the indirect interaction with putative PG precursor flippase RodA (Kemege et al. 2015), along with the fact that inhibition of PG precursor biosynthesis not only blocks cell division but also diminishes septal RodZ signals in *W. chondrophila* (Jacquier et al. 2014; Liechti et al. 2016), suggest that the division machinery is stabilized at the division site during the act of PG synthesis. In support of this model, addition of an MreB inhibitor arrests PG biosynthesis in *Chlamydia* and RodZ localization in *W. chondrophila* (Jacquier et al. 2014; Liechti et al. 2016). Analogous models for self-reinforcing division protein recruitment have been proposed for *E. coli* (Gerding et al. 2009; Yahashiri et al. 2015). Septal PG is also required for the recruitment of PG-binding proteins "NlpD" and Pal in *W. chondrophila* (Frandi et al. 2014; Jacquier et al. 2015a). The latter is an outer membrane lipoprotein that is thought to ensure the integrity of the cell envelope during constriction by promoting the coordinated invagination of the outer membrane with the cytoplasmic membrane and PG (Gerding et al. 2007). Pal is also thought to interact with the inner membrane component TolA by proton-motive-force-driven structural transitions stemming from an energized TolAQR complex resembling the proton-conducting MotA/MotB, ExbB/ExbD, and AglR/AglS complexes of *E. coli* (Cascales et al. 2000). Whether TolA is also part of the MreB/RodZ complex or interacts with other chlamydial division proteins and is stabilized by the presence of active septal PG synthesis remain to be determined.

5 Antichlamydial Activity of Cell Wall Antibiotics—Cellular Effects and Molecular Targets

The minimum inhibitory concentration (MIC) is a measure for determining susceptibility of bacteria to antimicrobial compounds and is defined as the lowest concentration of the agent that inhibits visible growth (Andrews 2001). The obligate intracellular lifestyle makes analysis of chlamydial growth under antibiotic treatment more challenging than in free-living bacteria. Besides difficulties in propagating chlamydiae in cell culture, also the formation of aberrant chlamydial bodies in the presence of cell wall antibiotics leads to confusion.

5.1 Beta-Lactam Treatment of Chlamydiae

Already in the 1950s, two studies showed that penicillin inhibited cell division of *chlamydiae* grown in the yolk sac of chick embryos (Weiss 1950; Tajima et al. 1959). In cell culture, 100 units/ml of penicillin arrests cell division in *C. trachomatis* L2 RBs at the latest by the second binary fission resulting in up to four enlarged, non-infectious metabolically slowed ABs (Skilton et al. 2009).

These effects of beta-lactams on *C. trachomatis* led to slight modifications of the MIC definition for chlamydiae. The MIC was either the lowest concentration needed to prevent the development of normal inclusions filled with EBs (Walsh et al. 1987; Welsh et al. 1992), as seen for bactericidal antibiotics, or needed for the formation of abnormal inclusions filled with ABs (How et al. 1984; Storey and Chopra 2001), as observed with bacteriostatic cell wall antibiotics.

The characteristic beta-lactam ring structurally mimics D-Ala-D-Ala residues in the PG pentapeptide side chains. Beta-lactams do not target a single protein, but rather a group of DD-transpeptidases and DD-carboxypeptidases, known as PBPs with no mammalian homologs (Schneider and Sahl 2010). PBPs "mistakenly" use beta-lactams as a false substrate during cell wall biosynthesis, resulting in the acylation of the enzymes and blocking further transpeptidation reactions (Zapun et al. 2008).

In free-living bacteria that are PG wrapped, the bactericidal action of penicillin during growth is due to uncontrolled activity of PG hydrolases, while PBP-catalyzed biosynthesis steps of the bacterial cell wall are arrested (Tomasz 1979). Nevertheless, the precise effects of beta-lactams beyond blocking PBP-conferred transpeptidase activity are still not fully understood. Recently, triggering of a futile cycle of deregulated PG synthesis and hydrolysis, depletion of PG precursor pools and ultimately lysis by ectopic hydrolase activity were described for *E. coli* (Cho et al. 2014). *Chlamydia* genomes encode only one PG hydrolase, the cell division amidase AmiA, while *Waddlia* additionally harbors a putative endopeptidase ("NlpD"). Uncontrolled amidase activity of AmiA (and endopeptidase activity in *Waddlia*) does not lead to cell lysis in the isotonic niche making chlamydiac attractive non-model organisms to explore the mode of action of beta-lactams uncoupled from osmotic destabilization and cell lysis.

Neither uptake into the host cell nor establishment of an inclusion nor the EB to RB transition is prevented by penicillin treatment (Skilton et al. 2009). Penicillin or the aminopenicillin derivative amoxicillin induced non-dividing ABs that are metabolically slowed and refractory to the translation inhibitor azithromycin in cell culture (Wyrick and Knight 2004) and in murine infection models (Phillips-Campbell et al. 2014). At the same time, chromosomal and plasmid DNA replication is unaffected (Skilton et al. 2009) and the swollen ABs are filled with a minimum of 16 chromosomal copies at 60 h p.i. (Lambden et al. 2006) raising questions about the fate of the nucleic acid material during retransition of ABs back to the normal life cycle after removal of penicillin. Moreover, sphingomyelin transport into the inclusion and into the chlamydial cells, as measured by fluorescence accumulation upon addition of labeled ceramide, is not reduced during treatment with penicillin (Dille et al. 2014). Of interest, production of membrane vesicles is increased in penicillin- and IFN-gamma-induced ABs from *C. trachomatis* in cell culture and membrane vesicles can also be found in vivo in humans (Frohlich et al. 2014). Release of membrane vesicles is a universal mechanism in prokaryotes and implicated in the transportation of virulence factors, signaling molecules, and genetic material into target cells. A topical review from Frohlich et al. discusses the potential of chlamydial membrane vesicles to contribute to host–pathogen interactions in productive and persistent infections (Frohlich et al. 2014).

Kintner et al. tested commonly used beta-lactams revealing that these compounds induce chlamydial persistence in cell culture at clinically relevant concentration, as identified by the reversal formation of typical non-infectious ABs (Kintner et al. 2014). Experiments were performed without addition of eukaryotic translation inhibitor cycloheximide which might foster persistence or recovery after removal of the antibiotic (Ripa and Mårdh 1977). The study included penicillin derivatives, monobactams and cephalosporins, such as ceftriaxone which is recommended for the treatment of gonococcal infections that often occur in parallel with *C. trachomatis* genital tract infections. Beta-lactams are therapeutically used to treat a broad range of mild to life-threatening infections and may induce AB formation in patients with concurrent asymptomatic chlamydial infections, rendering the chlamydial cells resistant to the first-line antibiotic azithromycin as described above (Borel et al. 2014, 2016; Kintner et al. 2014).

Depending on the beta-lactam added to the cell culture, chlamydial inclusions were packed with different numbers and morphological types of enlarged ABs (Kintner et al. 2014), indicating that cell division is blocked after different numbers of binary fission probably due to differences in penetration, target affinity, or number of targets among the tested beta-lactams. In *E. coli*, the concentration of beta-lactams that causes bactericidal effects depends on the susceptibility of PBPs that are partially or fully saturated with the false substrate. The more PBPs are targeted due to a broader spectrum of the antibiotic, the lower the concentration required to induce cell death (Satta et al. 1995). Characterization of all putative target proteins on a molecular level including the novel penicillin target AmiA (Klöckner et al. 2014) is needed to understand underlying mechanisms of differences in the bacteriostatic effect of beta-lactams in *Chlamydia*.

A recent study showed that also the animal pathogenic *Chlamydia* species *Chlamydia pecorum* forms ABs upon treatment with penicillin in culture, regardless of inclusion/exclusion of cycloheximide, though recovery is more robust in the presence of the eukaryotic translation inhibitor (Leonard et al. 2016). Little is known about effects of beta-lactam antibiotics on *Chlamydia*-related bacteria. These genomically less reduced chlamydiae as compared to *Chlamydia* show an inconsistent pattern of penicillin sensitivity. *Simkania* resides in a vacuole featuring extensive contact sites with the ER which partially covers the inclusion (Mehlitz et al. 2014), and this emerging pathogen is refractory to penicillin and ampicillin (Kahane et al. 1993; Pilhofer et al. 2013), whereas *Waddlia* and *Protochlamydia* are susceptible and form ABs in the presence of penicillin (Pilhofer et al. 2013; Jacquier et al. 2014). Penicillin, amoxicillin, ceftriaxone, and imipenem do not kill *Parachlamydia* in amoebae culture up to concentrations of 32 mg/l (Maurin et al. 2002). Whether these beta-lactams instead induce formation of ABs is not reported. Of interest, *Parachlamydia*, *Waddlia*, and *Simkania* but not *Protochlamydia* (nor *Chlamydia*) encode homologs of AmpC beta-lactamases in their genomes.

Accessibility inside the host cell, affinity, and number of target proteins as well as production and substrate specificity of beta-lactamases that hydrolyze the beta-lactam ring may contribute to differences in the beta-lactam sensitivity among *Chlamydia*-related bacteria.

5.2 Beta-Lactamase Inhibitor Clavulanic Acid

As a result of prolonged and frequently inappropriate use of beta-lactams, an increased resistance to these drugs is reported (Zahar et al. 2009). A successful strategy to bypass beta-lactamase-mediated resistance is the combined use of beta-lactams with beta-lactamase inhibitors. A common clinically used beta-lactamase inhibitor is clavulanic acid with minimal, clinically irrelevant antibiotic activity. It has a weak antimicrobial activity in *E. coli* (MIC 25 μg/ml) due to its affinity for PBP2 from *E. coli* (Spratt et al. 1977). Surprisingly, *Chlamydia* exposed to low, clinically relevant concentrations of clavulanic acid (0.35 μg/ml) show the AB phenotype typically found in penicillin-induced persistence (Bowie 1986; Kintner et al. 2014). The PBP2 homolog in *Chlamydia* is involved in cell division (Ouellette et al. 2012), and clavulanic acid likely induces the persistent stage through inhibition of PBP2 function in chlamydial cytokinesis. Identification of the underlying target(s) on a molecular level could help to elucidate the riddle of bacteriostatic activity of a beta-lactamase inhibitor in *Chlamydia*. Nothing is known about the activity of clavulanic acid in *Chlamydia*-related species. Inhibition of the beta-lactamase activity in *Parachlamydia*, *Waddlia*, and *Simkania* should be precluded as AmpC enzymes are resistant to clavulanic acid (Livermore 1995).

5.3 *Fosfomycin, D-Cycloserine, and Bacitracin*

Besides inhibition of penicillin target proteins, chlamydial PG biosynthesis can be blocked at different stages of lipid II precursor biosynthesis in the cytoplasm and at the cell membrane. Fosfomycin, a phosphonic antibiotic, inactivates the cytosolic UDP-*N*-acetylglucosamine enolpyruvyl transferase MurA, catalyzing one of the initial steps of the lipid II biosynthesis pathway, and prevents formation of MurNAc from GlcNAc and phosphoenolpyruvate (Kahan et al. 1974). Blocking the important PG synthesis step has a bactericidal effect and leads to cell death in free-living bacteria such as *E. coli* (Michalopoulos et al. 2011). In *Waddlia* and *Protochlamydia*, fosfomycin has a bacteriostatic activity preventing cell division and inducing AB formation (Jacquier et al. 2014). Fosfomycin prevents septum localization of the MreB regulator RodZ and the PG-binding protein Pal in *Waddlia* (Jacquier et al. 2014, 2015a). Surprisingly, fosfomycin has no effect on *Chlamydia* and *Simkania* growth and morphology (McCoy et al. 2003; Pilhofer et al. 2013). Resistance to fosfomycin is also reported in other bacteria, like *E. coli*, and caused by a Cys115 to Asp substitution in MurA, a mutation that is intrinsically present in MurA homologs from *Chlamydia* but not in *Chlamydia*-related bacteria (Kim et al. 1996; McCoy et al. 2003). In support of this, purified MurA from *C. trachomatis* is not inhibited by fosfomycin (McCoy et al. 2003), whereas reasons for fosfomycin resistance in *Simkania* remain elusive.

D-cycloserine is an amino acid derivative and a structural analog of D-Ala, an essential amino acid in the lipid II pentapeptide side chain. The antibiotic is well known as competitive inhibitor of D-Ala ligase Ddl and alanine racemases in bacteria (Strominger et al. 1960; Lambert and Neuhaus 1972). In 1963, Moulder et al. reported antichlamydial activity of D-cycloserine in chick embryo yolk sacs infected with *Chlamydia* and proved that this effect is reversible by the addition of D-Ala (Moulder et al. 1963). Moreover, purified MurC-Ddl fusion protein from *C. trachomatis* had D-cycloserine-sensitive D-Ala ligase activity (McCoy and Maurelli 2005). Additionally, a recent study showed that D-cycloserine blocks the activity of the alternative alanine racemase GlyA identifying besides MurC-Ddl, a second target of D-cycloserine in *Chlamydia* (De Benedetti et al. 2014).

The antibiotic bacitracin was isolated from a *Bacillus licheniformis* strain in 1945 (Johnson et al. 1945). The cyclic polypeptide specifically inhibits dephosphorylation of the membrane carrier bactoprenol-PP resulting in the accumulation of cell wall precursor UDP-MurNAc-pentapeptide in the cytoplasm (Siewert and Strominger 1967), prevention of lipid II export, and arrest of cell wall biosynthesis (Newton and Abraham 1950; Maxted 1953). Moreover, bactoprenol is a universal carrier for sugar components of polymers in the bacterial envelope such as teichoic acids in Gram-positive bacteria or LPS in the outer membrane of Gram-negative bacteria (Guo et al. 2008). Bacitracin is active against Gram-positive bacteria but does not reach its target in the periplasm of Gram-negative bacteria because of poor penetration through the outer membrane. Treatment of *Chlamydia* with bacitracin clears chlamydial infection in cell culture models. The underlying mechanisms of the effect are not clear. Attachment and entry of *Chlamydia* require interaction with protein disulfide isomerase (PDI) of the host cell. Bacitracin is capable of inhibiting the early stages of the chlamydial infectivity cycle and might have an effect on entry through inhibition of PDI but not on chlamydial lipid II carrier recycling as shown for free-living bacteria (Abromaitis and Stephens 2009). However, in vitro evidence for the specificity of bacitracin for PDI is rare, and the mechanism how bacitracin blocks the protein is unknown (Karala and Ruddock 2010). Whether bacitracin can penetrate through the structurally modified outer membrane in chlamydiae (Kosma 1999) (see below) as seen for O-antigen-defective mutants in other species (Nikaido 2003) and has an additional effect on bactoprenol-PP recycling possibly interfering with synthesis of the PG ring in *Chlamydia* or the cell wall in *Protochlamydia* and *Waddlia* remain to be clarified. A collateral blockage in LPS synthesis can be excluded as LPS in *Chlamydia* differs from other Gram-negative bacteria. Among others, the structure lacks O-antigen sugars (Kosma 1999), the only LPS components to be flipped over the cytoplasmic membrane using the bactoprenol carrier system—initiated by attaching sugar units to bactoprenol catalyzed by the MraY homolog WecA (Price and Momany 2005), a protein which is also rationalized from *Chlamydia* genomes.

6 Role of PG Components in Chlamydial Immune Modulation

As a major component of the bacterial cell envelope, PG is well known to serve as stimulus of the human first-line defense against invading pathogens. Not only PG in the bacterial envelope but also released PG material (muropeptides) contribute to the recognition of bacteria through binding to different components of the human innate immune system (Sukhithasri et al. 2013). Chlamydiae get into contact with PG-sensing proteins of the host defense during two stages of the life cycle: first, as extracellular EBs which could be recognized on the surface of epithelial or endothelial tissues via Toll-like receptors (TLR), or by Mannose-binding lectin (MBL) and the more recently described PG recognition proteins (PGRPs or PGLYRPs) in blood or mucosa secretions before internalization takes place (Tydell et al. 2006; Dziarski et al. 2012; Sukhithasri et al. 2013). Moreover, defensins and lysozyme could contribute to extracellular first-line defense against chlamydiae via sensing or targeting chlamydial PG or precursors. Next, intracellular detection could proceed via both Nod factors in the cytoplasm and TLRs which localize to the inclusion membrane (O'Connell et al. 2006).

The surface pathogen recognition receptor TLR2 is involved in acute inflammatory response to chlamydial infections, and its activation is inhibited by chloramphenicol but not by ampicillin (O'Connell et al. 2006). The chlamydial effector molecules for TLR2 sensing are unknown. TLR2 may possess affinity to PG and LPS (Erridge et al. 2004; Nagarajan 2012). Thus, contribution of both bacterial envelope structures is conceivable. As TLR2 also colocalizes with the inclusion membrane with the receptor domain oriented into the inclusion lumen, the innate immune PRR seems to be involved not only in surface recognition but also into intracellular recognition of chlamydiae (O'Connell et al. 2006). Serum protein MBL recognizes PG via the GlcNAc moiety (Nadesalingam et al. 2005) and activates the complement system (Rantala et al. 2011). The innate immune system protein impedes infection with *C. trachomatis* in cell culture (Swanson et al. 1998) but recognizes glycoproteins in the outer membrane rather than PG. Human PGLYRPs are sensors for PG, LPS, and effectors of antimicrobial defense (Dziarski et al. 2012). PGLYRP-1, PGLYRP-3, and PGLYRP-4 exploit a bacterial stress response to kill bacteria, whereas PGLYRP-2 is an amidase that hydrolyzes PG (see below) (Kashyap et al. 2011). Recently, antichlamydial activity was reported for recombinant PGLYRP and associated with chlamydial two-component stress response system CtcB CtcC (Bobrovsky et al. 2016). The alpha-defensin HNP-1 possesses intermediate affinity to lipid II and beta-defensin hBD3 has LPS-binding capacity and intermediate affinity to lipid II (Wilmes and Sahl 2014). Both cationic and amphiphilic peptides contribute to first-line host defense against invading pathogens and combine antibiotic activities with modulation of immune responses. So far, involvement of HNP-1 in response to *C. trachomatis* infections has been reported. The concentration of HNP-1 in urethral secretions of infected men is elevated, and the defensin shows antichlamydial activity in cell culture (Porter et al. 2005). Detection of *Chlamydia* in the EB stage via PG recognition can be most likely ruled out as the temporary PG ring is completely degraded before RB to EB transition (Liechti et al. 2016). Whether EBs from cell wall-wrapped *Chlamydia*-related emerging pathogens contain host defense-stimulating PG material remains to be investigated.

Infections with *Chlamydia* are also sensed by the human cytosolic innate immunity PRRs Nod1 and Nod2, which recognize cell wall fragments to signal through a MyD88-independent pathway and mediate activation of the transcription factor NF-κB (McCoy and Maurelli 2006). Moreover, extracted *Waddlia* muropeptides have been shown to stimulate activation of Nod1 and Nod2 (Jacquier et al. 2015a). Nod1 specifically recognizes mDAP-containing muropeptides, whereas Nod2 depends on the presence of MurNAc for activation (Girardin et al. 2003; McCoy and Maurelli 2006; Welter-Stahl et al. 2006). *C. trachomatis* muropeptides not only contain alanine but also glycine residues in position 1 of the pentapeptide side chain (Packiam et al. 2015), an alteration which has been shown to affect Nod2 recognition (Inohara et al. 2003).

Besides functioning in cell division, AmiA may also play a role in modulating host response and thus contribute to chlamydial pathogenicity. Comparable to mammalian PGLYRP2 (PG recognition protein-L), which has amidase activity and may function as scavenger to reduce host proinflammatory response to PG (Humann and Lenz 2009), the amidase activity of chlamydial AmiA may block Nod2 sensing as the cytoplasmic PRR is not capable of binding released peptide side chains disconnected from MurNAc. Treatment with the cell wall antibiotics D-cycloserine and penicillin leads to increased activation of the Nod2 factor implicating that also other beta-lactams including ceftriaxone, the recommended treatment of gonococci that often cause coinfections with *C. trachomatis,* leads to exacerbated inflammation through Nod2 signaling (Packiam et al. 2015). Of interest, the amidase function of AmiA, which should counteract Nod2 activation, is not inhibited by penicillin (Klöckner et al. 2014), suggesting that the accumulating PG components under penicillin treatment are not a substrate of the hydrolase.

Activation of Nod factors in the host cytoplasm implies transport of immunogenic muropeptides. Such an export over the inclusion membrane requires maintenance of a specific and so far unknown mechanism unique to the otherwise highly economizing chlamydiae. Hence, stimulation of the host cell response through export of muropeptides into the host cytoplasm should be beneficial for the intracellular stage of chlamydiae. However, modulation of the muropeptide cocktail might be conferred by amidase and carboxypeptidase activities to contribute to long-term residence inside the host cell.

7 Missing Bricks in the Ring—Future Research and Perspectives

Toward deeper mechanistic understanding of the minimal and modified cell wall biosynthetic machinery in chlamydiae, several steps in PG biosynthesis and remodeling need to be elucidated. A major mystery in the field represents how transglycosylation of the recently reported sugar strands in chlamydial PG (Packiam et al. 2015) is executed since no proteins that could act as transglycosylases are found in chlamydial genomes. Moreover, lytic transglycosylases and endopeptidases, the antagonists of transglycosylases and transpeptidases, which are essential to degrade the transient PG ring in *Chlamydia* and/or the PG sacculus in *Chlamydia*-related species remain to be uncovered. Another open question is how the complete cycle of lipid II synthesis, translocation and incorporation, including recycling of the membrane carrier can be maintained in *Chlamydia* as the genus does not possess proteins that function as bactoprenol-PP pyrophosphorylases in other bacteria. The elusive racemase, transglycosylase, lytic transglycosylase, and endopeptidase and pyrophosphorylase activities could be conferred by proteins with different primary structures or by related but very promiscuous enzymes.

The pathway for PG synthesis has been highly rationalized in the course of evolutionary adaptation to a small range of vertebrate hosts in *Chlamydia*, and a narrow PG ring is only synthesized during cell division at the septum and apparently directly degraded afterward. These findings suggest fine-tuned mechanisms of regulation for PG biosynthetic and remodeling processes which need to be in turn tightly synchronized with the cell division machinery. Surprisingly, AmiA, the only cell division amidase found in chlamydiae, is not constrained by an autoinhibitory loop as shown for the *E. coli* enzymes AmiA/B/C (Yang et al. 2012; Rocaboy et al. 2013) implicating non-canonical regulatory mechanisms in the intracellular pathogens.

In *E. coli*, the transmembrane protein MreD is needed to connect the cytoplasmic actin-like MreB to PBP2-driven cross-linking of cell wall material on the outside. Functional analysis of the unique insert in chlamydial PBP2 may help to clarify how the MreD-lacking MreB-based system facilitates controlled polymerization reactions of precursor lipid II into the PG ring during cell division in *Chlamydia*. Moreover, the exact order of assembly of the divisome components remains to be determined in chlamydiae, a process for which involvement of PG precursor lipid II and the PG ring is conceivable by binding and recruiting cell division proteins throughout all envelope layers. The PG ring might additionally have a mechanic role during constriction. Feeding experiments with labeled dipeptide probes in *Chlamydia*-related bacteria as done before in *Chlamydia* could reveal how widespread the septal PG ring is and help to explore the evolutionary reduction of PG structures in chlamydial lineages.

Future research is needed to elucidate which PG synthesis and remodeling steps operate in chlamydiae and possibly other obligate intracellular pathogens, while also unearthing important deviations from the canonical FtsZ-dependent cell division and septal PG control mechanisms of free-living model bacteria. This work will also provide a basis for the design of novel anti-infective strategies against productive and persistent infections with *Chlamydia* and yield better understanding of cell wall antibiotics-induced persistence and controlled host response modulation through release of immunogenic PG material.

Acknowledgments Support was received by the intramural funding scheme of the Medical Faculty of Bonn, BONFOR. H.B. received a PhD fellowship from the Jürgen Manchot foundation. B.H. is associated member of the DFG Cluster of Excellence ImmunoSensation.

References

Abdelrahman YM, Belland RJ (2005) The chlamydial developmental cycle. FEMS Microbiol Rev 29:949–959

Abdelrahman YM, Rose LA, Belland RJ (2011) Developmental expression of non-coding RNAs in Chlamydia trachomatis during normal and persistent growth. Nucleic Acids Res 39:1843–1854

Abromaitis S, Stephens RS (2009) Attachment and entry of Chlamydia have distinct requirements for host protein disulfide isomerase. PLoS Pathog 5:e1000357

Andrews JM (2001) Determination of minimum inhibitory concentrations. J Antimicrob Chemother 48:5–16

Ball SG, Subtil A, Bhattacharya D et al (2013) Metabolic effectors secreted by bacterial pathogens: essential facilitators of plastid endosymbiosis? Plant Cell 25:7–21

Barbour AG, Amano K, Hackstadt T et al (1982) Chlamydia trachomatis has penicillin-binding proteins but not detectable muramic acid. J Bacteriol 151:420–428

Baud D, Goy G, Osterheld MC et al (2014) Role of Waddlia chondrophila placental infection in miscarriage. Emerg Infect Dis 20:460–464

Baud D, Thomas V, Arafa A et al (2007) Waddlia chondrophila, a potential agent of human fetal death. Emerg Infect Dis 13:1239–1243

Bedson SP, Bland JOW (1932) A morphological study of psittacosis virus, with the description of a developmental cycle. Br J Exp Pathol 13:461–466

Belland RJ, Zhong G, Crane DD et al (2003) Genomic transcriptional profiling of the developmental cycle of Chlamydia trachomatis. Proc Natl Acad Sci USA 100:8478–8483

Bobrovsky P, Manuvera V, Polina N et al (2016) Recombinant human peptidoglycan recognition proteins reveal antichlamydial activity. Infect Immun IAI.01495–15

Borel N, Leonard C, Slade J et al (2016) Chlamydial antibiotic resistance and treatment failure in veterinary and human medicine. Curr Clin Microbiol Reports 3:10–18

Borel N, Pospischil A, Hudson AP et al (2014) The role of viable but non-infectious developmental forms in chlamydial biology. Front Cell Infect Microbiol 4:97

Born TL, Blanchard JS (1999) Structure/function studies on enzymes in the diaminopimelate pathway of bacterial cell wall biosynthesis. Curr Opin Chem Biol 3:607–613

Bowie WR (1986) In vitro activity of clavulanic acid, amoxicillin, and ticarcillin against Chlamydia trachomatis. Antimicrob Agents Chemother 29:713–715

Brown WJ, Rockey DD (2000) Identification of an antigen localized to an apparent septum within dividing Chlamydiae. Infect Immun 68:708–715

Caldwell HD, Kromhout J, Schachter J (1981) Purification and partial characterization of the major outer membrane protein of Chlamydia trachomatis. Infect Immun 31:1161–1176

Cascales E, Gavioli M, Sturgis JN et al (2000) Proton motive force drives the interaction of the inner membrane TolA and outer membrane pal proteins in Escherichia coli. Mol Microbiol 38:904–915

Cho H, Uehara T, Bernhardt TG (2014) Beta-lactam antibiotics induce a lethal malfunctioning of the bacterial cell wall synthesis machinery. Cell 159:1300–1311

Chopra I, Storey C, Falla TJ et al (1998) Antibiotics, peptidoglycan synthesis and genomics: the chlamydial anomaly revisited. Microbiology 144:2673–2678

Collingro A, Tischler P, Weinmaier T et al (2011) Unity in variety—the pan-genome of the Chlamydiae. Mol Biol Evol 28:3253–3270

D'Ulisse V, Fagioli M, Ghelardini P et al (2007) Three functional subdomains of the Escherichia coli FtsQ protein are involved in its interaction with the other division proteins. Microbiology 153:124–138

Darveaux JI, Lemanske RF (2014) Infection-related asthma. J Allergy Clin Immunol Pract 2:658–663

De Benedetti S, Bühl H, Gaballah A et al (2014) Characterization of serine hydroxymethyltransferase GlyA as a potential source of D-alanine in Chlamydia pneumoniae. Front Cell Infect Microbiol 4:19

Den Blaauwen T, Aarsman MEG, Vischer NOE et al (2003) Penicillin-binding protein PBP2 of Escherichia coli localizes preferentially in the lateral wall and at mid-cell in comparison with the old cell pole. Mol Microbiol 47:539–547

Dille S, Herbst K, Volceanov L et al (2014) Golgi fragmentation and sphingomyelin transport to Chlamydia trachomatis during penicillin-induced persistence do not depend on the cytosolic presence of the Chlamydial protease CPAF. PLoS ONE 9:e103220

Domman D, Horn M, Embley TM et al (2015) Plastid establishment did not require a chlamydial partner. Nat Commun 6:6421

Dziarski R, Kashyap DR, Gupta D (2012) Mammalian peptidoglycan recognition proteins kill bacteria by activating two-component systems and modulate microbiome and inflammation. Microb Drug Resist 18:280–285

Erickson HP, Anderson DE, Osawa M (2010) FtsZ in bacterial cytokinesis: cytoskeleton and force generator all in one. Microbiol Mol Biol Rev 74:504–528

Erridge C, Pridmore A, Eley A et al (2004) Lipopolysaccharides of bacteroides fragilis, Chlamydia trachomatis and Pseudomonas aeruginosa signal via toll-like receptor 2. J Med Microbiol 53:735–740

Errington J (2013) L-form bacteria, cell walls and the origins of life. Open Biol 3:120143

Facchinelli F, Colleoni C, Ball SG et al (2013) Chlamydia, cyanobiont, or host: who was on top in the ménage à trois? Trends Plant Sci 18:673–679

Figge RM, Divakaruni AV, Gober JW (2004) MreB, the cell shape-determining bacterial actin homologue, co-ordinates cell wall morphogenesis in Caulobacter crescentus. Mol Microbiol 51:1321–1332

Fox A, Rogers JC, Gilbart J et al (1990) Muramic acid is not detectable in Chlamydia psittaci or Chlamydia trachomatis by gas chromatography-mass spectrometry. Infect Immun 58:835–837

Frandi A, Jacquier N, Théraulaz L et al (2014) FtsZ-independent septal recruitment and function of cell wall remodelling enzymes in chlamydial pathogens. Nat Commun 5:4200

Friedman MG, Dvoskin B, Kahane S (2003) Infections with the chlamydia-like microorganism *Simkania negevensis*, a possible emerging pathogen. Microbes Infect 5:1013–1021

Frohlich KM, Hua Z, Quayle AJ et al (2014) Membrane vesicle production by Chlamydia trachomatis as an adaptive response. Front Cell Infect Microbiol 4:73

Gaballah A, Kloeckner A, Otten C et al (2011) Functional analysis of the cytoskeleton protein MreB from Chlamydophila pneumoniae. PLoS ONE 6:e25129

Gerding MA, Liu B, Bendezú FO et al (2009) Self-enhanced accumulation of FtsN at division dites and roles for other proteins with a SPOR domain (DamX, DedD, and RlpA) in Escherichia coli cell constriction. J Bacteriol 191:7383–7401

Gerding MA, Ogata Y, Pecora ND et al (2007) The trans-envelope Tol-Pal complex is part of the cell division machinery and required for proper outer-membrane invagination during cell constriction in *E. coli*. Mol Microbiol 63:1008–1025

Ghosh AS, Chowdhury C, Nelson DE (2008) Physiological functions of D-alanine carboxypeptidases in *Escherichia coli*. Trends Microbiol 16:309–317

Ghuysen JM, Goffin C (1999) Lack of cell wall peptidoglycan versus penicillin sensitivity: new insights into the chlamydial anomaly. Antimicrob Agents Chemother 43:2339–2344

Girardin SE, Boneca IG, Viala J et al (2003) Nod2 is a general sensor of peptidoglycan through muramyl dipeptide (MDP) detection. J Biol Chem 278:8869–8872

Goffin C, Fraipont C, Ayala JA et al (1996) The non-penicillin-binding module of the tripartite penicillin- binding protein 3 of *Escherichia coli* is required for folding and/or stability of the penicillin-binding module and the membrane-anchoring module confers cell septation activity on the folded. J Bacteriol 178:5402–5409

Grayston JT, Belland RJ, Byrne GI et al (2015) Infection with Chlamydia pneumoniae as a cause of coronary heart disease: the hypothesis is still untested. Pathog Dis 73:1–9

Greub G (2009) Parachlamydia acanthamoebae, an emerging agent of pneumonia. Clin Microbiol Infect 15:18–28

Guo H, Yi W, Song JK et al (2008) Current understanding on biosynthesis of microbial polysaccharides. Curr Top Med Chem 8:141–151

Halberstaedter L, von Prowazek S (1907) Ueber Zelleinschlüsse parasitärer Natur beim Trachom. Arb aus dem Kais Gesundheitsamt 26:44–47

Hatch TP (1996) Disulfide cross-linked envelope proteins: the functional equivalent of peptidoglycan in chlamydiae? J Bacteriol 178:1–5

Henrichfreise B, Schiefer A, Schneider T et al (2009) Functional conservation of the lipid II biosynthesis pathway in the cell wall-less bacteria Chlamydia and Wolbachia: why is lipid II needed? Mol Microbiol 73:913–923

Hesse L, Bostock J, Dementin S et al (2003) Functional and biochemical analysis of Chlamydia trachomatis MurC, an enzyme displaying UDP-N-acetylmuramate: amino acid ligase activity. J Bacteriol 185:6507–6512

Hofmann N (2016) Invisible no longer: peptidoglycan in moss chloroplasts. Plant Cell tpc.00521.2016

Höltje JV (1998) Growth of the stress-bearing and shape-maintaining murein sacculus of *Escherichia coli*. Microbiol Mol Biol Rev 62:181–203

How S, Hobson D, Hart C (1984) Studies in vitro of the nature and synthesis of the cell wall of Chlamydia trachomatis. Curr Microbiol 10:269–274

Humann J, Lenz LL (2009) Bacterial peptidoglycan degrading enzymes and their impact on host muropeptide detection. J Innate Immun 1:88–97

Hurst EW (1953) Chemotherapy of virus diseases. Br Med Bull 9:180–185

Inohara N, Ogura Y, Fontalba A et al (2003) Host recognition of bacterial muramyl dipeptide mediated through NOD2: implications for Crohn's disease. J Biol Chem 278:5509–5512

Jacquier N, Frandi A, Pillonel T et al (2014) Cell wall precursors are required to organize the chlamydial division septum. Nat Commun 5:3578

Jacquier N, Frandi A, Viollier PH et al (2015a) Disassembly of a medial transenvelope structure by antibiotics during intracellular division. Chem Biol 22:1217–1227

Jacquier N, Viollier PH, Greub G (2015b) The role of peptidoglycan in chlamydial cell division: towards resolving the chlamydial anomaly. FEMS Microbiol Rev 39:262–275

Jenkin HM (1960) Preparation and properties of cell walls of the agent of meningopneumonitis. J Bacteriol 80:639–647

Jogler C, Waldmann J, Huang X et al (2012) Identification of proteins likely to be involved in morphogenesis, cell division, and signal transduction in Planctomycetes by comparative genomics. J Bacteriol 194:6419–6430

Johnson BA, Anker H, Meleney FL (1945) Bacitracin: a new antibiotic produced by a member of the B. subtilis Group. Science 102:376–377

Kahan FM, Kahan JS, Cassidy PJ et al (1974) The mechanism of action of fosfomycin (phosphonomycin). Ann NY Acad Sci 235:364–386

Kahane S, Gonen R, Sayada C et al (1993) Description and partial characterization of a new Chlamydia-like microorganism. FEMS Microbiol Lett 109:329–333

Karala A-R, Ruddock LW (2010) Bacitracin is not a specific inhibitor of protein disulfide isomerase. FEBS J 277:2454–2462

Kashyap DR, Wang M, Liu LH et al (2011) Peptidoglycan recognition proteins kill bacteria by activating protein-sensing two-component systems. Nat Med 17:676–683

Kemege KE, Hickey JM, Barta ML et al (2015) *Chlamydia trachomatis* protein CT009 is a structural and functional homolog to the key morphogenesis component RodZ and interacts with division septal plane localized MreB. Mol Microbiol 95:365–382

Kim DH, Lees WJ, Kempsell KE et al (1996) Characterization of a Cys115 to Asp substitution in the *Escherichia coli* cell wall biosynthetic enzyme UDP-GlcNAc enolpyruvyl transferase (MurA) that confers resistance to inactivation by the antibiotic fosfomycin. Biochemistry 35:4923–4928

Kintner J, Lajoie D, Hall J et al (2014) Commonly prescribed β-lactam antibiotics induce C. trachomatis persistence/stress in culture at physiologically relevant concentrations. Front Cell Infect Microbiol 4:44

Klöckner A, Otten C, Derouaux A et al (2014) AmiA is a penicillin target enzyme with dual activity in the intracellular pathogen Chlamydia pneumoniae. Nat Commun 5:4201

Kosma P (1999) Chlamydial lipopolysaccharide. Biochim Biophys Acta 1455:387–402

Kresse H, Belsey MJ, Rovini H (2007) The antibacterial drugs market. Nat Rev Drug Discov 6:19–20

Lambden P, Pickett M, Clarke I (2006) The effect of penicillin on Chlamydia trachomatis DNA replication. Microbiology 152:2573–2578

Lambert MP, Neuhaus FC (1972) Mechanism of D-cycloserine action: alanine racemase from *Escherichia coli* W. J Bacteriol 110:978–987

Leaver M, Domínguez-Cuevas P, Coxhead JM et al (2009) Life without a wall or division machine in *Bacillus subtilis*. Nature 457:849–853

Leonard CA, Dewez F, Borel N (2016) Penicillin G-induced chlamydial stress response in a porcine strain of *Chlamydia pecorum*. Int J Microbiol 2016:1–10

Liechti G, Kuru E, Packiam M et al (2016) Pathogenic Chlamydia lack a classical sacculus but synthesize a narrow, mid-cell peptidoglycan ring, regulated by MreB, for cell division. PLoS Pathog 12:e1005590

Liechti GW, Kuru E, Hall E et al (2014) A new metabolic cell-wall labelling method reveals peptidoglycan in Chlamydia trachomatis. Nature 506:507–510

Livermore DM (1995) Beta-Lactamases in laboratory and clinical resistance. Clin Microbiol Rev 8:557–584

Manire GP, Tamura A (1967) Preparation and chemical composition of the cell walls of mature infectious dense forms of meningopneumonitis organisms. J Bacteriol 94:1178–1183

Matsumoto A (1979) Recent progress of electron microscopy in microbiology and its development in future: from a study of the obligate intracellular parasites, Chlamydia organisms. J Electron Microsc 28(Suppl):S57–S64

Matsumoto A, Manire GP (1970) Electron microscopic observations on the effects of penicillin on the morphology of Chlamydia psittaci. J Bacteriol 101:278–285

Matteï PJ, Neves D, Dessen A (2010) Bridging cell wall biosynthesis and bacterial morphogenesis. Curr Opin Struct Biol 20:749–755

Maurin M, Bryskier A, Raoult D (2002) Antibiotic susceptibilities of Parachlamydia acanthamoeba in amoebae. Antimicrob Agents Chemother 46:3065–3067

Maxted WR (1953) The use of bacitracin for identifying group A haemolytic streptococci. J Clin Pathol 6:224–226

McCoy AJ, Adams NE, Hudson AO et al (2006) L,L-diaminopimelate aminotransferase, a trans-kingdom enzyme shared by Chlamydia and plants for synthesis of diaminopimelate/lysine. Proc Natl Acad Sci 103:17909–17914

McCoy AJ, Maurelli AT (2006) Building the invisible wall: updating the chlamydial peptidoglycan anomaly. Trends Microbiol 14:70–77

McCoy AJ, Maurelli AT (2005) Characterization of Chlamydia MurC-Ddl, a fusion protein exhibiting D-alanyl-D-alanine ligase activity involved in peptidoglycan synthesis and D-cycloserine sensitivity. Mol Microbiol 57:41–52

McCoy AJ, Sandlin RC, Maurelli AT (2003) In vitro and in vivo functional activity of Chlamydia MurA, a UDP-N-Acetylglucosamine enolpyruvyl transferase involved in peptidoglycan synthesis and fosfomycin resistance. J Bacteriol 185:1218–1228

Mehlitz A, Karunakaran K, Herweg JA et al (2014) The chlamydial organism *Simkania negevensis* forms ER vacuole contact sites and inhibits ER-stress. Cell Microbiol 16:1224–1243

Michalopoulos AS, Livaditis IG, Gougoutas V (2011) The revival of fosfomycin. Int J Infect Dis 15:e732–e739

Miyagishima SY, Nakamura M, Uzuka A et al (2014) FtsZ-less prokaryotic cell division as well as FtsZ- and dynamin-less chloroplast and non-photosynthetic plastid division. Front Plant Sci 5:459

Mohammadi T, Breukink E (2014) The chlamydial anomaly clarified? ChemBioChem 15:1391–1392
Moulder JW (1991) Interaction of chlamydiae and host cells in vitro. Microbiol Rev 55:143–190
Moulder JW (1993) Why is Chlamydia sensitive to penicillin in the absence of peptidoglycan? Infect Agents Dis 2:87–99
Moulder JW (1966) The relation of the psittacosis group (Chlamydiae) to bacteria and viruses. Annu Rev Microbiol 20:107–130
Moulder JW, Novosel DL, Officer JE (1963) Inhibition of the growth of agents of the psittacosis group by D-cycloserine and its specific reversal by D-alanine. J Bacteriol 85:707–711
Nadesalingam J, Dodds AW, Reid KBM et al (2005) Mannose-binding lectin recognizes peptidoglycan via the N-acetyl glucosamine moiety, and inhibits ligand-induced proinflammatory effect and promotes chemokine production by macrophages. J Immunol 175:1785–1794
Nagarajan UM (2012) Immune recognition and host cell response during Chlamydia infection. In: Tan M, Bavoil PM (eds) Intracellular pathogens I: chlamydiales. ASM Press, Washington, DC, pp 217–239
Nelson DE, Young KD (2000) Penicillin binding protein 5 affects cell diameter, contour, and morphology of *Escherichia coli*. J Bacteriol 182:1714–1721
Newton GGF, Abraham EP (1950) Ayfivin and bacitracin: resolution of crude products into similar series of peptides. Biochem J 47:257–267
Nicholson TL, Olinger L, Chong K et al (2003) Global stage-specific gene regulation during the developmental cycle of Chlamydia trachomatis. J Bacteriol 185:3179–3189
Nikaido H (2003) Molecular basis of bacterial outer membrane permeability revisited. Microbiol Mol Biol Rev 67:593–656
Nunes A, Gomes JP (2014) Evolution, phylogeny, and molecular epidemiology of Chlamydia. Infect Genet Evol 23:49–64
O'Connell CM, Ionova IA, Quayle AJ et al (2006) Localization of TLR2 and MyD88 to Chlamydia trachomatis inclusions: evidence for signaling by intracellular TLR2 during infection with an obligate intracellular pathogen. J Biol Chem 281:1652–1659
Otten C, De Benedetti S, Gaballah A et al (2015) Co-solvents as stabilizing agents during heterologous overexpression in *Escherichia coli*—application to chlamydial penicillin-binding protein 6. PLoS ONE 10:e0122110
Ouellette SP, Karimova G, Subtil A et al (2012) Chlamydia co-opts the rod shape-determining proteins MreB and Pbp2 for cell division. Mol Microbiol 85:164–178
Ouellette SP, Rueden KJ, Abdelrahman YM et al (2015) Identification and partial characterization of potential FtsL and FtsQ homologs of Chlamydia. Front Microbiol 6:1264
Ouellette SP, Rueden KJ, Gauliard E et al (2014) Analysis of MreB interactors in Chlamydia reveals a RodZ homolog but fails to detect an interaction with MraY. Front Microbiol 5:279
Packiam M, Weinrick B, Jacobs WR et al (2015) Structural characterization of muropeptides from Chlamydia trachomatis peptidoglycan by mass spectrometry resolves "chlamydial anomaly". Proc Natl Acad Sci USA 112:11660–11665
Patin D, Bostock J, Blanot D et al (2009) Functional and biochemical analysis of the Chlamydia trachomatis ligase MurE. J Bacteriol 191:7430–7435
Patin D, Bostock J, Chopra I (2012) Biochemical characterisation of the chlamydial MurF ligase, and possible sequence of the chlamydial peptidoglycan pentapeptide stem. Arch Microbiol 194:505–512
Pavelka MS (2007) Another brick in the wall. Trends Microbiol 15:147–149
Perkins HR, Allison AC (1963) Cell-wall constituents of rickettsiae and psittacosis-lymphogranuloma organisms. J Gen Microbiol 30:469–480
Phillips-Campbell R, Kintner J, Schoborg RV (2014) Induction of the Chlamydia muridarum stress/persistence response increases azithromycin treatment failure in a murine model of infection. Antimicrob Agents Chemother 58:1782–1784
Pilhofer M, Aistleitner K, Biboy J et al (2013) Discovery of chlamydial peptidoglycan reveals bacteria with murein sacculi but without FtsZ. Nat Commun 4:2856

Porter E, Yang H, Yavagal S et al (2005) Distinct defensin profiles in Neisseria gonorrhoeae and Chlamydia trachomatis urethritis reveal novel epithelial cell-neutrophil interactions. Infect Immun 73:4823–4833
Price NP, Momany FA (2005) Modeling bacterial UDP-HexNAc: Polyprenol-P HexNAc-1-P transferases. Glycobiology 15:29–42
Rantala A, Lajunen T, Juvonen R et al (2011) Low mannose-binding lectin levels and MBL2 gene polymorphisms associate with Chlamydia pneumoniae antibodies. Innate Immun 17:35–40
Ripa KT, Mårdh PA (1977) Cultivation of *Chlamydia trachomatis* in cycloheximide-treated mccoy cells. J Clin Microbiol 6:328–331
Rocaboy M, Herman R, Sauvage E et al (2013) The crystal structure of the cell division amidase AmiC reveals the fold of the AMIN domain, a new peptidoglycan binding domain. Mol Microbiol 90:267–277
Rogers HJ, Perkins HR, Ward JB (1980) Structure of peptidoglycan. In: Rogers H, Perkins H, Ward J (eds) Microbial cell walls and membranes. Springer, Netherlands, pp 190–214
Russell AD, Chopra I (1990) Understanding antibacterial action and resistance, 2nd edn. Ellis Horwood, Chichester
Satta G, Cornaglia G, Mazzariol A et al (1995) Target for bacteriostatic and bactericidal activities of beta-lactam antibiotics against Escherichia coli resides in different penicillin-binding proteins. Antimicrob Agents Chemother 39:812–818
Sauvage E, Derouaux A, Fraipont C et al (2014) Crystal structure of penicillin-binding protein 3 (PBP3) from *Escherichia coli*. PLoS ONE 9:e98042
Sauvage E, Kerff F, Terrak M et al (2008) The penicillin-binding proteins: structure and role in peptidoglycan biosynthesis. FEMS Microbiol Rev 32:234–258
Scheffers DJ, Pinho MG (2005) Bacterial cell wall synthesis: new insights from localization studies. Microbiol Mol Biol Rev 69:585–607
Schleifer KH, Kandler O (1972) Peptidoglycan types of bacterial cell walls and their taxonomic implications. Bacteriol Rev 36:407–477
Schneider T, Sahl HG (2010) An oldie but a goodie—cell wall biosynthesis as antibiotic target pathway. Int J Med Microbiol 300:161–169
Siewert G, Strominger JL (1967) Bacitracin: an inhibitor of the dephosphorylation of lipid pyrophosphate, an intermediate in the biosynthesis of the peptidoglycan of bacterial cell walls. Proc Natl Acad Sci USA 57:767–773
Skilton RJ, Cutcliffen LT, Barlow D et al (2009) Penicillin induced persistence in Chlamydia trachomatis: high quality time lapse video analysis of the developmental cycle. PLoS ONE 4: e7723
Slovak PM, Porter SL, Armitage JP (2006) Differential localization of Mre proteins with PBP2 in Rhodobacter sphaeroides. J Bacteriol 188:1691–1700
Spratt BG, Jobanputra V, Zimmermann W (1977) Binding of thienamycin and clavulanic acid to the penicillin-binding proteins of *Escherichia coli* K-12. Antimicrob Agents Chemother 12:406–409
Stephens RS, Kalman S, Lammel C et al (1998) Genome sequence of an obligate intracellular pathogen of humans: *Chlamydia trachomatis*. Science 282:754–759
Storey C, Chopra I (2001) Affinities of β-lactams for penicillin binding proteins of Chlamydia trachomatis and their antichlamydial activities. Antimicrob Agents Chemother 45:303–305
Strominger JL, Ito E, Threnn RH (1960) Competitive inhibition of enzymatic reactions by oxamycin. J Am Chem Soc 82:998–999
Subtil A, Collingro A, Horn M (2014) Tracing the primordial Chlamydiae: extinct parasites of plants? Trends Plant Sci 19:36–43
Sukhithasri V, Nisha N, Biswas L et al (2013) Innate immune recognition of microbial cell wall components and microbial strategies to evade such recognitions. Microbiol Res 168:396–406
Swanson AF, Ezekowitz RAB, Lee A et al (1998) Human mannose-binding protein inhibits infection of HeLa cells by *Chlamydia trachomatis*. Infect Immun 66:1607–1612
Tajima M, Samejima T, Yoshitoshi N (1959) Morphology of meningopneumonitis virus exposed to penicillin as observed with the electron microscope. J Bacteriol 77:23–34

Tamura A, Manire GP (1967) Preparation and chemical composition of the cell membranes of developmental reticulate forms of meningopneumonitis organisms. J Bacteriol 94:1184–1188

Tamura A, Matsumoto A, Manire GP et al (1971) Electron microscopic observations on the structure of the envelopes of mature elementary bodies and developmental reticulate forms of *Chlamydia psittaci*. J Bacteriol 105:355–360

Tatar LD, Marolda CL, Polischuk AN et al (2007) An *Escherichia coli* undecaprenyl-pyrophosphate phosphatase implicated in undecaprenyl phosphate recycling. Microbiology 153:2518–2529

Taylor BD, Haggerty CL (2011) Management of *Chlamydia trachomatis* genital tract infection: screening and treatment challenges. Infect Drug Resist 4:19–29

Taylor-Robinson D, Bébéar C (1997) Antibiotic susceptibilities of mycoplasmas and treatment of mycoplasmal infections. J Antimicrob Chemother 40:622–630

Teh B, Grayson ML, Johnson PDR et al (2012) Doxycycline versus macrolides in combination therapy for treatment of community-acquired pneumonia. Clin Microbiol Infect 18:e71–e73

Tomasz A (1979) The mechanism of the irreversible antimicrobial effects of penicillins: how the beta-lactam antibiotics kill and lyse bacteria. Annu Rev Microbiol 33:113–137

Tydell CC, Yuan J, Tran P et al (2006) Bovine peptidoglycan recognition protein-S: antimicrobial activity, localization, secretion, and binding properties. J Immunol 176:1154–1162

Typas A, Banzhaf M, Gross CA et al (2012) From the regulation of peptidoglycan synthesis to bacterial growth and morphology. Nat Rev Microbiol 10:123–136

Uehara T, Bernhardt TG (2011) More than just lysins: peptidoglycan hydrolases tailor the cell wall. Curr Opin Microbiol 14:698–703

Uehara T, Parzych KR, Dinh T et al (2010) Daughter cell separation is controlled by cytokinetic ring-activated cell wall hydrolysis. EMBO J 29:1412–1422

van der Ploeg R, Verheul J, Vischer NOE et al (2013) Colocalization and interaction between elongasome and divisome during a preparative cell division phase in *Escherichia coli*. Mol Microbiol 87:1074–1087

van Heijenoort J (2001) Recent advances in the formation of the bacterial peptidoglycan monomer unit. Nat Prod Rep 18:503–519

Vanrompay D, Ducatelle R, Haesebrouck F (1995) *Chlamydia psittaci* infections: a review with emphasis on avian chlamydiosis. Vet Microbiol 45:93–119

Vats P, Rothfield L (2007) Duplication and segregation of the actin (MreB) cytoskeleton during the prokaryotic cell cycle. Proc Natl Acad Sci USA 104:17795–17800

Vats P, Shih YL, Rothfield L (2009) Assembly of the MreB-associated cytoskeletal ring of *Escherichia coli*. Mol Microbiol 72:170–182

Vollmer W, Bertsche U (2008) Murein (peptidoglycan) structure, architecture and biosynthesis in *Escherichia coli*. Biochim Biophys Acta 1778:1714–1734

Vollmer W, Joris B, Charlier P et al (2008) Bacterial peptidoglycan (murein) hydrolases. FEMS Microbiol Rev 32:259–286

Walsh C (2003) Where will new antibiotics come from? Nat Rev Microbiol 1:65–70

Walsh M, Kappus EW, Quinn TC (1987) In vitro evaluation of CP-62,993, erythromycin, clindamycin, and tetracycline against Chlamydia trachomatis. Antimicrob Agents Chemother 31:811–812

Weiss E (1950) The effect of antibiotics on agents of the psittacosis-lymphogranuloma group: I. The effect of penicillin. J Infect Dis 87:249–263

Welsh LE, Gaydos CA, Quinn TC (1992) In vitro evaluation of activities of azithromycin, erythromycin, and tetracycline against *Chlamydia trachomatis* and *Chlamydia pneumoniae*. Antimicrob Agents Chemother 36:291–294

Welter-Stahl L, Ojcius DM, Viala J et al (2006) Stimulation of the cytosolic receptor for peptidoglycan, Nod1, by infection with *Chlamydia trachomatis* or *Chlamydia muridarum*. Cell Microbiol 8:1047–1057

White CL, Kitich A, Gober JW (2010) Positioning cell wall synthetic complexes by the bacterial morphogenetic proteins MreB and MreD. Mol Microbiol 76:616–633

Wilmes M, Sahl HG (2014) Defensin-based anti-infective strategies. Int J Med Microbiol 304:93–99

Wright HR, Turner A, Taylor HR (2008) Trachoma. Lancet 371:1945–1954

Wyrick PB (2010) Chlamydia trachomatis persistence in vitro: an overview. J Infect Dis 201 (Suppl 2):S88–S95

Wyrick PB, Knight ST (2004) Pre-exposure of infected human endometrial epithelial cells to penicillin in vitro renders *Chlamydia trachomatis* refractory to azithromycin. J Antimicrob Chemother 54:79–85

Yahashiri A, Jorgenson MA, Weiss DS (2015) Bacterial SPOR domains are recruited to septal peptidoglycan by binding to glycan strands that lack stem peptides. Proc Natl Acad Sci USA 112:11347–11352

Yang DC, Peters NT, Parzych KR et al (2011) An ATP-binding cassette transporter-like complex governs cell-wall hydrolysis at the bacterial cytokinetic ring. Proc Natl Acad Sci USA 108: e1052–e1060

Yang DC, Tan K, Joachimiak A et al (2012) A conformational switch controls cell wall-remodelling enzymes required for bacterial cell division. Mol Microbiol 85:768–781

Young KD (2014) Microbiology. A flipping cell wall ferry. Science 345:139–140

Zahar JR, Lortholary O, Martin C et al (2009) Addressing the challenge of extended-spectrum beta-lactamases. Curr Opin Investig Drugs 10:172–180

Zapun A, Contreras-Martel C, Vernet T (2008) Penicillin-binding proteins and beta-lactam resistance. FEMS Microbiol Rev 32:361–385

One Face of *Chlamydia trachomatis*: The Infectious Elementary Body

Mathilde M. Cossé, Richard D. Hayward and Agathe Subtil

Abstract The lifestyle of *Chlamydiae* is unique: the bacteria alternate between two morphologically distinct forms, an infectious non-replicative elementary body (EB), and a replicative, non-infectious reticulate body (RB). This review focuses on recent advances in understanding the structure and function of the infectious form of the best-studied member of the phylum, the human pathogen *Chlamydia trachomatis*. Once considered as an inert particle of little functional capacity, the EB is now perceived as a sophisticated entity that encounters at least three different environments during each infectious cycle. We review current knowledge on its composition and morphology, and emerging metabolic activities. These features confer resistance to the extracellular environment, the ability to penetrate a host cell and ultimately enable the EB to establish a niche enabling bacterial survival and growth. The bacterial and host molecules involved in these processes are beginning to emerge.

Contents

M.M. Cossé · A. Subtil (✉)
Unité de Biologie cellulaire de l'infection microbienne, Institut Pasteur,
25 rue du Dr Roux, 75015 Paris, France
e-mail: agathe.subtil@pasteur.fr

M.M. Cossé · A. Subtil
CNRS UMR3691, Paris, France

R.D. Hayward
Institute of Structural and Molecular Biology, Birkbeck and University
College London, Malet Street, London, WC1E 7HX, UK

Current Topics in Microbiology and Immunology (2018) 412:35–58
DOI 10.1007/82_2016_12

Published Online: 20 May 2016

In the first half of the twentieth century, Sir Samuel Phillips Bedson (1886–1969) made several seminal contributions to the thriving field of microbiology (Downie 1971). As a prominent pioneer in the description of *Chlamydia* biology, he proposed, based only on rudimentary light microscopy observations, that the agent of psittacosis (now known as *Chlamydia psittaci*) exhibited a "morphological change from the small infecting elementary body (EB) to the large form or initial body" (Bedson and Gostling 1954). At the time, Bedson believed what he observed through the lenses of his microscope to be a virus, and it was more than a decade later until the chlamydiae were definitively classified as bacteria (Moulder 1966). Nevertheless, his description of two morphologically distinct forms was confirmed with the advent of the electron microscope and the ultramicrotome. Today, the small form remains designated as the EB, while the second larger one is termed the reticulate body (RB). Most importantly, Bedson introduced the concept that the infectious agent underwent a "developmental cycle," which is now recognized as a hallmark of the chlamydiae (AbdelRahman and Belland 2005; Omsland et al. 2014). All the members of this phylum are obligate intracellular pathogens and symbionts of eukaryotic cells. The developmental cycle begins with the adhesion of the EB to a eukaryotic host cell. Subsequently, EB force their own actin-dependent internalization. The remainder of the cycle occurs within the host cell, within a specialized membrane-bound compartment termed "the inclusion." Once inside this compartment, the EB differentiates into the RB. This is the only replicative form of the bacteria, which divides by binary fission and within a few days yields several hundred bacteria per infected cell. The cycle is completed by the redifferentiation of RBs into EBs, and their release in the extracellular space, from where they initiate a novel cycle.

For half a century, the EB has been considered as a largely "passive" element of the developmental cycle, unable to divide, with its range of activity limited to adhesion to the host cell, followed by internalization. In contrast, the ability of replicative RBs to manipulate host metabolism, and some of the mechanisms involved, were rapidly recognized (Hackstadt et al. 1997; Schachter 1988). Over the last 15 years, we have gained new insights into the morphology and composition of EBs. Most importantly, our perception of their properties has radically changed with the realization that these "particles" have active roles in the infectious process. This chapter will review the current knowledge of EBs and describes the initial steps of *Chlamydia* infection, until EB differentiation into RBs. We will focus predominantly on *C. trachomatis*, the agent of trachoma and genital tract infection (Batteiger 2012). However, data suggest that the principal properties of EBs are conserved across the *Chlamydiae* (Omsland et al. 2014). Where relevant, data obtained from species other than *C. trachomatis* will also be introduced.

1 The Infectious Particle: Not so Elementary, My Dear Bedson!

1.1 A Morphology Tailored for Specific Needs

Early investigators focused their attention on EBs rather than RBs for two reasons. For one thing, EBs were easier to purify, because they were much less fragile. Secondly, with the ultimate aim to define protective antigens to design a vaccine against *Chlamydia* infection, it made sense to study primarily the extracellular form of the bacteria. Blocking the adhesion or entry step performed by EBs would prevent *Chlamydia* infection, since RBs do not have the capacity to invade host cells.

Transmission electron microscopy revealed that EBs are small (0.3 μm in diameter), and this contributed largely to their initial erroneous classification as viruses. Images also showed a highly condensed nucleoid, not observed in RBs. Two histone-like proteins Hc1 and Hc2 (encoded by *hctA* and *hctB*, respectively) were identified, that were expressed specifically in EBs, concomitant with nucleoid compaction (Brickman et al. 1993; Hackstadt et al. 1991). By analogy with the role of histones in eukaryotic cells, these proteins are responsible for nucleoid compaction in EBs and are sufficient to induce genome compaction following their expression in *Escherichia coli* (Barry et al. 1992; Brickman et al. 1993; Christiansen et al. 1993). These two chlamydial histone-like proteins have distinct properties (Brickman et al. 1993; Pedersen et al. 1996), the regulation of their expression differ to some extent (Grieshaber et al. 2006) and Hc2 is specific to the *Chlamydiaceae* (Collingro et al. 2011). Whether other proteins participate to the unique organization of the nucleoid in EBs remains unknown.

A second characteristic feature of EB morphology is the composition and structure of the outer membrane. EBs are enveloped by the chlamydial outer membrane complex (COMC), which is defined as the insoluble fraction during extraction with the weak anionic detergent sodium lauryl sarcosinate (Sarkosyl). The COMC comprises a shell of proteins cross-linked through intra- and inter-molecular disulphide bonds. This dense network confers rigidity and limits permeability, resulting in the resistance of EBs to physical or osmotic stress (Hackstadt et al. 1985). In contrast, while several COMC components remain in RBs, the cysteine residues within component proteins become reduced, and consequently a tight network does not assemble. This simple change in COMC properties is central to the biology of the bacterium, as COMC rigidity confers resistance to the fluctuating environmental conditions encountered outside the host cell. EBs can exploit this simple strategy because they do not divide. Conversely, RBs need to divide, and reduction of the COMC disulphide bonding is central to the conversion of EBs to the replicative state. In the intracellular space within the inclusion lumen, RBs are exposed to a quite constant environment. The relative fragility of RBs, which becomes obvious during purification protocols, is not challenged in the inclusion lumen. The COMC is comprised of many proteins, but is dominated by only a few, which are more abundant. These include the major outer membrane protein (MOMP, representing 60 % of the weight of the outer membrane) and the cysteine-rich proteins OmcA and OmcB [reviewed in (Hatch 1999)]. Several studies, including more recent approaches taking advantage of proteomics (Birkelund et al. 2009; Liu et al. 2010), have aimed at defining the composition of the COMC. Although these studies all agree on the major components, discrepancies still exist regarding less abundant proteins, most likely due to variations in experimental procedures, since the COMC is defined by biochemical properties. Presumably, the incorporation of proteins into the COMC largely depends on the number of accessible free cysteine residues. In addition to providing rigidity, disulphide bonding may also regulate the activity of some outer membrane proteins. This is certainly the case for the major porin MOMP (Bavoil et al. 1984), but remains for the most part unexplored for other components.

Besides proteins, the principal component of the outer leaflet of the outer membrane of Gram-negative bacteria is the lipopolysaccharide. This is also the case in *Chlamydia*, although lipooligosaccharide (LOS) is predominant (Rund et al. 1999). Another more striking difference is the absence of peptidoglycan in EBs (Liechti et al. 2014), a polymer that plays a crucial structural role in other bacteria. It is likely that the rigidity provided by the chlamydial COMC is sufficient to eliminate the metabolic cost of synthesizing additional cell envelope components.

The differences in the structure of the EB and RB envelope were not readily apparent when conventional ultrathin section methods were used (Tamura et al. 1971), but became evident when observed using cryo-electron microscopy, where the thickness of the outer membrane in EBs appeared nearly twice that of RBs (Huang et al. 2010). Cryo-electron tomography has recently allowed striking refinements in the description of EB morphology (Nans et al. 2014; Pilhofer et al. 2014). Although seminal early imaging had revealed the presence of asymmetrically distributed electron dense structures on the surface of EBs, the nature of these "projections" remained unknown (Gregory et al. 1979; Matsumoto 1981; Nichols et al. 1985). The polymorphic membrane protein D (PmpD) exists as an oligomer, with a distinct 23-nm flower-like structure and an asymmetric distribution, reminiscent of the surface projections or rosettes described by Matsumoto and others (Swanson et al. 2009). PmpD belongs to a family of membrane proteins, which functions in adhesion (see Sect. 2.3), and it remains possible that other Pmp family members might also form protruding complexes on the EB surface. Besides outer membrane protein complexes and COMC components, the prominent appendages of the infectious bacteria are macromolecular type 3 secretion (T3S) complexes. T3S are conserved amongst many medically important bacterial pathogens, and T3S structure has been investigated extensively. T3S directs the translocation of bacterial effector protein substrates across both bacterial membranes and a third eukaryotic membrane (Galan et al. 2014). Immunogold electron microscopy using an antibody raised against the protein comprising the needle that protrudes from the outer membrane proximal face of the T3S apparatus, was consistent with a non-homogenous distribution of these complexes on the bacterial surface (Betts et al. 2008). Furthermore, recent observations by cryo-electron tomography demonstrated that EBs indeed exhibit two distinct poles. One hemisphere is characterized by a pronounced expansion of the periplasmic space, which accommodates an array of T3S complexes. The opposing pole often more proximal to the nucleoid is characterized by a complex membranous structure, arising from an invagination of the inner membrane (Nans et al. 2014; Nichols et al. 1985) (Fig. 1).

1.2 Non-dividing, But Not Inactive

Originally coined to describe a virus-like particle, the name EB persisted: after all, the term "elementary" seemed appropriate for an inert particle lacking many characteristics shared by other bacteria. It fitted the notion that this form behaved like a dormant spore, well adapted to resist damage in the extracellular environment, but with little if any discernible metabolic activity. In short, the EB was believed to have only a passive role in the chlamydial developmental cycle. Half a century later, the EB has won more consideration. The first move in this direction came from the discovery by the Hackstadt group of a protein translocated from EBs into the host cell during invasion, revealing an active role for the infectious form in this initial step for the first time (Clifton et al. 2004) (see Sect. 2.4). Transcriptomics and proteomics have since demonstrated that EBs are endowed with strong metabolic abilities and a specific cohort of proteins likely engaged in triggering invasion (Albrecht et al. 2011; Saka et al. 2011; Skipp et al. 2016). The development of an axenic medium supporting RNA and protein synthesis in EBs confirmed their metabolic abilities and definitively altered perceptions of this "elementary" particle (Omsland et al. 2012).

Before further considering recent advances in understanding the structure and function of EBs, it is important to emphasize that the generic name "EB" likely encompasses several bacterial states. Historically, EB analysis has started with the purification of particles of a certain density from infected cultures using a gradient. This procedure isolates particles of homogenous size and morphology. However, because RB-to-EB conversion is asynchronous, a mixture of "young" and "old" EBs are acquired, which might differ in their metabolic activities. Secondly, the environmental conditions encountered by EBs within the inclusion, or following release into the extracellular environment, are very different. Additionally, upon internalization in the host cells, EBs rapidly sense the change in the environment and respond to it by initiating differentiation into RBs. Some of the metabolic abilities of EBs are probably only required in this third, highly specialized context. Thus, EBs encounter at least three distinct environments: the inclusion lumen, which is shared with RBs that can supply some metabolic products required by

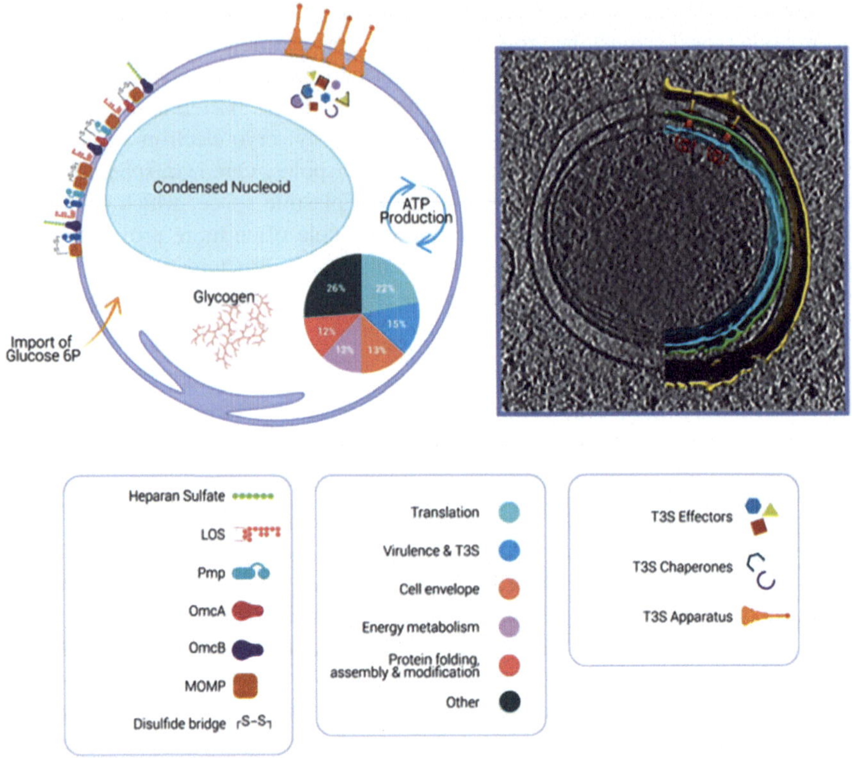

Fig. 1 Morphology and main properties of the *C. trachomatis* elementary body. *Left* Schematic view. The cellular envelope shows several remarkable features. The chlamydial outer membrane complex (COMC) is made of a dense network of heavily cross-linked proteins. Several of the outer membrane proteins, mainly OmcB and the Pmps, participate to the adhesion step. The periplasm is free of peptidoglycan. It enlarges at one pole to accommodate an array of T3S apparatuses. The inner membrane invaginates at the opposite pole and contains a number of proteins, including transporters. The nucleoid is condensed around histone-like proteins, but still allows for some transcriptional activity. In contrast to RBs, EBs contain glycogen. They produce ATP, and this activity is sustained mainly through the import of glucose-6-phosphate. Effector proteins, associated or not to chaperones, are ready for translocation through the T3S apparatuses upon contact with the host cell. The pie chart depicts the relative abundance of proteins associated with the indicated functions, adapted from Saka et al. (2011). *Top right* 10-nm slice from denoised cryo-electron tomogram of a plunge frozen *C. trachomatis* LGV2 elementary body in contact with the membrane of an early bacterial containing vacuole via the T3S. Right hand side shows overlay of 3-D surface rendering, highlighting features observed in the micrograph. Bacterial outer (*green*), inner (*cyan*) and host (*yellow*) membranes are shown. T3S (*top*) are shown in the rendering with secretin (*orange*), inner membrane ring (*blue*), sorting platform, export apparatus and ATPase (*red*) highlighted. Bacterial ribosomes are discernible in the upper cytoplasmic hemisphere, and the inner membrane invagination observed at the lower pole

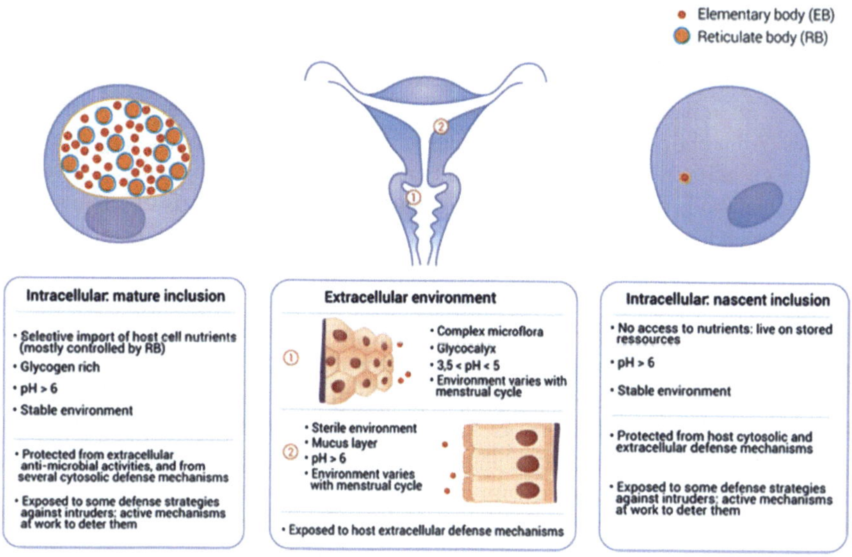

Fig. 2 EBs face different environments. EB genesis occurs in the mature inclusion (*left*, EBs are depicted as orange circles), separated from the host cytoplasm. RBs control the import of ions and small molecules through the inclusion membrane, providing a stable environment. In particular, RB activities lead to the accumulation of glycogen in the *C. trachomatis* inclusion lumen, before it is stored in the EBs themselves. It is very different from the extracellular conditions to which EBs are exposed before entering a new host cell (*centre*). In the lower genital tract, EBs are exposed to the genital flora, which generates a low pH. The squamous stratified epithelium is protected by an abundant glycocalyx. Upon ascending the genital tract, EBs face a sterile environment with close to neutral pH. The epithelium of the endometrium and the fallopian tubes are made of single columnar cells. The presence of ciliated cells, which provide mechanical clearance, and the secretion of a thick layer of mucus restrain EB adhesion and internalization. Both in the lower and the upper genital tracts, the extracellular environment changes during the menstruous cycle. Once internalized (*right*), EBs are transiently shielded from external resources and become exposed to some innate defence mechanisms. Within a couple of hours, novel genes are expressed to start establishing exchanges with the host cytoplasm

EBs; the extracellular space, where other microorganisms may be present and where EBs face a variety of extracellular antimicrobial activities; and the nascent tight bacterial containing vacuoles, against which the host cell have developed innate defence strategies (Fig. 2). Each of these environments have different pH, osmotic and nutritional compositions, and it is possible that EBs sense and adapt to them, although this has only been illustrated so far during the transition from the extracellular space to the early tight bacterial containing vacuole (see Sect. 2.6).

Early comparisons of the metabolic properties of EBs and RBs revealed striking differences between the two forms [reviewed recently by Omsland et al. (2014)]. For instance, the RNA-to-DNA ratio is three times lower in EBs than RBs (Tamura et al. 1967). Since EBs do not actively divide, the protein pool is not replenished to the same extent as in RBs, thus this lower RNA-to-DNA ratio is expected. DNA condensation in the EB nucleoid reduces access of components of the transcription machinery to the nucleic acid, which contributes to reduced transcriptional activity. However, transcription takes place in EBs (Sarov and Becker 1971), and beyond the mere quantitative aspect, RBs and EBs exhibit very different transcriptional profiles (Albrecht et al. 2011). Consistently, proteomics data also showed that EBs contain a specific set of proteins, with a high representation of proteins involved in energy metabolism, transcription and translation. This supports the view that energy-dependent activities play a central role in the biology of the infectious particle (Saka et al. 2011; Skipp et al. 2016; Vandahl et al. 2001) (Fig. 1).

The second category of proteins enriched in EBs was the components of the T3S machinery, and associated chaperones and effector substrates. This protein group represented ~14 % of the EB proteome compared to ~5 % of the RB (Saka et al. 2011). Consistent with these observations, many of the genes encoding elements of the T3S apparatus and effectors are strongly expressed at the end of the infectious cycle, when EBs predominate in the bacterial population (Albrecht et al. 2011). Thus, EBs are released primed with a battery of T3S complexes clustered on one pole of the outer membrane (Mueller et al. 2014). The large pool of ATP measured in EBs (Tipples and McClarty 1993) likely provides the energy for rapid effector translocation upon contact with the host cell plasma membrane.

1.3 A Metabolism Centred on Glucose Catabolism

Although sequencing of the *C. trachomatis* genome revealed an intrinsic ability to produce ATP, it was unclear whether this capacity was actually utilized by the EBs. Proteomic analysis of *C. pneumoniae* EBs revealed a large number of proteins involved in ATP-generating metabolic pathways such as glycolysis and the tricarboxylic acid cycle (Vandahl et al. 2001), a finding later confirmed by quantitative proteomics on *C. trachomatis* EBs (Saka et al. 2011; Skipp et al. 2016).

An axenic medium, that sustained transcriptional and translational activities, was used to distinguish the nutritional requirements of the two forms of the bacteria. Most notably, EBs were dependent upon glucose-6-phosphate (G6P) for ATP synthesis, as well as for transcription and translation, while RBs were entirely dependent upon exogenous ATP as an energy source (Omsland et al. 2012). These data definitively established the fact that EBs do indeed produce ATP. Whether this occurs when the bacteria are still within the large inclusion (an environment largely mimicked by the axenic media), in the early bacterial containing vacuoles after invasion, or whether they equally use this capacity during the extracellular stage of the developmental cycle, now requires further investigation (Omsland et al. 2014).

How do the EBs obtain glucose? The ability for the protein Uhpc of *C. pneumoniae* to transport G6P was demonstrated in *E. coli* (Schwoppe et al. 2002). Very recently, it was shown that *C. trachomatis* EBs import only G6P, but not glucose-1-phosphate or glucose (Gehre et al. 2016), consistent with the fact that *Chlamydiaceae* have dispensed with the gene encoding hexokinase, in contrast to the environmental chlamydiae (Collingro et al. 2011). Uhpc is more abundant in RBs, but is also detectable in EBs (Saka et al. 2011; Skipp et al. 2016) and likely mediates G6P import from the inclusion lumen. In *C. trachomatis* inclusions, glucose is stored in the lumen as glycogen. Glycogen accumulation proceeds via two pathways, the bulk uptake of host glycogen and de novo synthesis by secreted bacterial enzymes (Gehre et al. 2016). The polymer is also detectable in EBs, but not in RBs. Glycogen stores in EBs are likely to provide the energy required to sustain extracellular metabolism, as well as the rapid activities required during invasion, when transcription and translation must be initiated prior to the RBs possessing the means to hijack ATP pools from the host. However, ATP-driven metabolism rapidly takes over, with rapid transcription of the ADP/ATP translocase occurring within one hour of infection (Belland et al. 2003).

2 From the Generation to the Conversion of EBs: A Chronological Perspective

2.1 EB Biogenesis

Traditionally, the description of *Chlamydia* biology starts with the step of adhesion to the host cell, which defines the beginning of a new infectious cycle (AbdelRahman and Belland 2005). However, determinants of invasion were prepared at the end of the previous cycle, during the generation of the infectious progeny. Indeed, internalization occurs relatively fast with 75 % entry within 15 min for serovar L2 (Vromman et al. 2014), leaving the early bacterial containing vacuole immediately exposed to innate cellular defences. The bacterium must secure its niche faster than de novo protein synthesis allows, thus proteins required early during infection are synthesized at the end of the previous cycle and stored. Consequently, this section begins with a brief recapitulation of the current stage of knowledge on EB biogenesis.

The differentiation of RBs into EBs is asynchronous. The first EBs are observed about 18 hpi, while most of the bacteria are still in the replicative form and continue to divide for several hours. Mature inclusions contain a mixture of EBs and RBs, and other diverse forms, together referred to as intermediate bodies. EBs thus initially reside in a very controlled environment and likely benefit nutritionally from proximity to the surrounding RBs (Fig. 2). The signal(s) that trigger RB-to-EB differentiation are still unknown and are not reproduced in an axenic medium. Since the bacteria residing within one inclusion do not initiate the differentiation programme simultaneously, this might involve stochastic variations in the expression of a given sensor. In any event, alterations in the gene expression pattern are observed in the second half of the infectious cycle, with the expression of late genes (Belland et al. 2003), presumably driving the physiological and morphological changes during EB biogenesis. In particular, the expression of histone-like proteins leads to the compaction of the nucleoid, a phenotype observed by electron microscopy. Interestingly, inhibition of LOS synthesis does not impact upon RB replication but inhibited the expression of selected late-stage proteins and the generation of EBs, suggesting the existence of an outer membrane check point to proceed to EB transition (Nguyen et al. 2011). Also, muramidase is enriched in EBs, suggesting that peptidoglycan structures synthesized in the RB are degraded during the conversion (Skipp et al. 2016).

2.2 The Extracellular Episode

This is the least well documented episode of the EB journey. Different species of *Chlamydia* are exposed to very diverse extracellular environments, depending on the specific niche. Raman microspectroscopy revealed that extracellular *Protochlamydia amoebophila* showed metabolic activity and remained infectious for as long as three weeks after release (Haider et al. 2010). A second study showed that the availability of D-glucose is essential to sustain metabolic activity. Likewise, the infectivity of *C. trachomatis* declined more rapidly in the absence of nutrients (Sixt et al. 2013). While Haider et al. (2010) demonstrated amino acid uptake and protein synthesis after extracellular incubation of *C. trachomatis*, it is unknown how long *C. trachomatis* EBs can persist viably in the natural extracellular environment and to what extent an active metabolism sustains this. Ascension through the genital tract exposes the bacteria to different stimuli including the absence or presence of other microorganisms, and changes in pH, oxygen and nutrient concentration, or exposure to antimicrobial defence systems. A recent study showed that LL-37, a member of the cathelicidin family of antimicrobial peptides produced by mucosal epithelial cells and neutrophils, exhibited anti-chlamydial activity (Tang et al. 2015). This was blocked when the antimicrobial peptides were pre-incubated with a chlamydial protease named CPAF, known to be translocated into the host cytoplasm during infection. The authors proposed that CPAF may be released to counteract antimicrobial peptide activities during the extracellular stage of infection.

2.3 The Adhesion Step

In contrast, adhesion of EBs to host cells has been investigated extensively, with the hope that the identification of the factors involved in this crucial early step would enable the design of new inhibitory molecules that could act as potential therapeutics. *C. trachomatis* EBs normally target polarized epithelial cells of mucosal surfaces. In vitro, almost all the cell types that have been tested, whether polarized or not, can be infected with only very little variation in the attachment or entry efficiency (Guseva et al. 2007). While the molecular mechanisms underlying attachment are still not well understood, all the data to date suggest that chlamydial adhesion relies on multiple redundant adhesion molecules, both on the bacteria and on the host surface. This distinguishes the entry mechanism from those of *Listeria monocytogenes* and *Yersinia enterocolitica* where defined bacterial surface invasins engage specific host cell receptors to promote pathogen internalization. Considering the fact that a failure in bacterial adhesion would definitively interrupt the developmental cycle, it seems only logical that the bacteria have evolved several redundant mechanisms to attach to eukaryotic cells. Over the years, a number of molecules on the bacterial surface have demonstrated to possess adhesin-like properties in vitro. These have been recently reviewed in detail (Hegemann and Moelleken 2012).

One prominent mediator of bacterial attachment is actually derived from host molecules. Glycosaminoglycans (GAGs) are linear glycoside chains composed of negatively charged disaccharide repeat units, such as heparan sulphate. Proteoglycans, proteins with covalently attached GAGs, are abundant in the extracellular matrix and on the plasma surface of eukaryotic cells, and are used for adhesion of a number of viruses and bacteria. Compelling evidence indicated that chlamydiae bound exogenous heparan sulphate and exploited it in a tripartite configuration, to mediate invasion by engaging a host receptor (Chen and Stephens 1994). Later, it was shown that the N-terminal domain of the bacterial protein OmcB contained a heparin-binding domain, and that OmcB behaved as an adhesin (Moelleken and Hegemann 2008). Several studies had reported that different *C. trachomatis* biovars showed different requirements for GAGs (Hegemann and Moelleken 2012). The N-terminal domain of OmcB is variable, and the data obtained in vitro regarding OmcB adhesive properties from different species corresponded to the differences in the requirement for GAGs observed during infection studies. Thus, OmcB is likely the bacterial component of the tripartite interaction between the bacteria, GAGs and the host cell, although it cannot be ruled out that as yet unidentified bacterial molecules are also involved.

In addition to OmcB/GAGs, a number of molecules present on the surface of EBs have been implicated in their ability to bind eukaryotic cells, including MOMP, the major constituent of the COMC (Hegemann and Moelleken 2012). More recently, attention has turned to a family of polymorphic membrane proteins (Pmps), whose existence was revealed by genome sequencing (Stephens et al. 1998). *C. trachomatis* have a repertoire of 9 Pmps, while *C. pneumonia* have 21. They are autotransporters, present on the outer membrane of EBs, where they associate to varying degrees with the COMC (Liu et al. 2010) and undergo proteolytic cleavage (Hegemann and Moelleken 2012). Patients with *C. trachomatis* genital infection display different antibody profiles against individual or multiple Pmps (Tan et al. 2009), suggesting that these proteins are variably expressed. In vitro heterogeneity in the expression of the different Pmps was indeed observed, but the underlying mechanism is not known (Tan et al. 2010). Members of the family show little overall similarity, except for the presence of multiple tetrapeptide repeats of GGA(I,L,V) and FxxN. The Hegemann laboratory demonstrated that these motifs mediate adhesion to cell surface receptor(s), and incubation with recombinant Pmps led to a decrease in bacterial infectivity as would be predicted (Molleken et al. 2010). The adhesin-like properties of Pmps appear to be species specific as incubation with recombinant Pmps from *C. trachomatis* inhibited subsequent infection with *C. trachomatis* but not with *C. pneumoniae*, and vice versa (Becker and Hegemann 2014). In agreement with the view that Pmps exhibit species specificity, the epidermal growth factor (EGF) receptor was identified as the binding partner *C. pneumonia*e Pmp21, but did not mediate adhesion of *C. trachomatis* (Becker and Hegemann 2014; Molleken et al. 2013). Many questions about how Pmps operate at a molecular level remain open. Pre-incubation of cells with individual Pmps blocked infection to a similar degree, whether they were mixed together or employed alone. This indicates that Pmps of one species recognize the same host cell receptor or group of receptors. Also, Pmps may form hetero-oligomeric complexes on the bacterial surface (Swanson et al. 2009). This could reconcile why despite apparent redundancy between adhesive Pmps, interfering with adhesive properties of one specific Pmp, for instance by incubating with recombinant PmpX or using anti-PmpX serum, significantly impairs bacterial adhesion (Becker and Hegemann 2014). Intriguingly, a subset of Pmps is exclusively expressed by RBs (Albrecht et al. 2011; Saka et al. 2011; Skipp et al. 2005), indicating that their role in infection might not be restricted to EB adhesion alone.

Antibodies against LOS or the inhibition of LOS synthesis significantly reduce chlamydial infectivity (Fadel and Eley 2008), indicating that LOS is involved in adhesion, and/or in a subsequent step during bacterial internalization. A recent study showed that a small molecule that binds lipid A with high affinity inhibits both adhesion and entry, resulting in a strong inhibition of cellular infection (Osaka and Hefty 2014). It is not known whether the inhibitory effect observed on entry reflects a direct role of LOS in this step or is a indirect consequence of functional disruption to other outer membrane surface molecules important for entry, such as T3S systems.

Snapshots of surface attached EBs reveal that an array of T3S complexes is exposed on the EB pole facing the plasma membrane (Nans et al. 2014). This is consistent with the idea that this secretion system is activated upon attachment, and that the translocation of effectors triggers bacterial uptake. It is not yet known, however, whether the bacterial proteins that promote attachment show the same polarization as the secretion machineries. Finally, comparison of the T3S complexes from free or cell-attached *C. trachomatis* revealed a marked compaction of the basal body of the secretion apparatus when the needle tip contacted the host cell, indicating that the periplasmic domains of the basal body components compress during effector translocation (Nans et al. 2015).

Adhesion involves two partners, the bacterium and the host. It appears that several host proteins bind EBs, mirroring the diversity of bacterial adhesins [reviewed by (Hegemann and Moelleken 2012)]. The platelet-derived growth factor receptor (Elwell et al. 2008), the fibroblast growth factor 2 (Kim et al. 2011) and, more recently, the ephrinA2 receptor (Subbarayal et al. 2015) have been implicated in *C. trachomatis* adhesion to cells. These transmembrane receptors are signalling molecules, and some data indicate that their activity is also exploited to enhance bacterial invasion. Two chaperone proteins of the endoplasmic reticulum present at the plasma membrane have also been implicated in *C. trachomatis* adhesion, the protein disulphide isomerase (PDI) (Conant and Stephens 2007; Davis et al. 2002) and the glucose regulated protein 96 (Gp96) (Karunakaran et al. 2015), and in their absence bacterial adhesion is reduced. Part of this effect is likely indirect, as the absence of each of these chaperones negatively impacts the levels of several other proteins at the plasma membrane, including some of the other putative EB targets mentioned above. Interestingly, PDI has a second role in EB entry as its thiol-mediated oxidoreductase activity is necessary for invasion (Abromaitis and Stephens 2009). One attractive hypothesis is that this host isomerase reduces the abundant disulphide bonds present on the surface of EBs, in particular in components of the secretion apparatus, thereby contributing to the translocation of bacterial proteins required for invasion (see below) (Abromaitis and Stephens 2009; Betts-Hampikian and Fields 2011; Ferrell and Fields 2016).

2.4 The Entry Step

Entry of all chlamydiae relies on the plasticity of the actin cytoskeleton, as inhibitors of actin polymerization attenuate bacterial entry (Carabeo et al. 2002). *C. trachomatis* invasion is sustained by discreet and transient actin polymerization, which drives the engulfment of the particle into a tight membrane bounded vesicle, disconnected from the extracellular medium (Carabeo et al. 2007; Nans et al. 2014). Bacterial uptake is orchestrated by factors from both the bacteria and the host. On the host side, regulators of the actin network are activated upon infection, such as the small GTPase Rac1 (Carabeo et al. 2004), and regulators of plasma membrane trafficking such as the small GTPase Arf6 (Balañá et al. 2005). Rac1 interacts with the WAVE actin nucleation promoting factor complex, which in turn stimulates the Arp2/3 complex. Bacterial adhesion to signalling receptors may initiate part of these signalling cascades that trigger the activation of host actin regulators (Elwell et al. 2008). Concomitantly, the bacteria secrete effector proteins that also directly modify the host cytoskeleton and fully participate in the entry process. A significant contributor is the bacterial protein translocated actin-recruiting phosphoprotein (TarP) (Clifton et al. 2004). TarP is a multi-domain scaffold protein that interacts with the actin cytoskeleton at several levels, either directly via its intrinsic actin nucleation activity (Jewett et al. 2006, 2010), or indirectly by engaging actin (Jiwani et al. 2013), or actin-binding proteins such as focal adhesion kinase (Thwaites et al. 2014) and vinculin (Thwaites et al. 2015). Additionally, the N-terminal of *C. trachomatis* TarP is phosphorylated by host cell kinases (Jewett et al. 2008; Mehlitz et al. 2008), leading to the engagement of Rac1 guanine nucleotide exchange factors, and in turn to Rac1 activation (Lane et al. 2008). Less is known about the other immediate effectors (discussed below), but it is likely that, in addition to TarP, they contribute to the fine tuning of actin polymerization and depolymerization, as well as the membrane encapsulation of internalized bacteria.

TarP translocation is likely activated upon intimate attachment to the host cell, an event that probably serves as a trigger for T3S, although the molecular details of the mechanisms controlling this process remain unknown. Many questions remain regarding the control of T3S in chlamydiae [recently reviewed by (Ferrell and Fields 2016)], and it is likely that only a few of the pre-packed effectors, translocated into the host cell within the first minutes of infection, have been identified. In addition to TarP, the actions of two additional effectors are partially understood: CT694, which interacts with the cytoskeletal organizing protein AHNAK (Hower et al. 2009), and the translocated early phosphoprotein or TepP (CT875). Like TarP, TepP is phosphorylated in the host cytoplasm, allowing its interaction with the scaffolding protein CrkI/II. Cells infected with a *tepP* mutant showed altered expression of a subset of genes associated with the innate immune response, suggesting that this effector may serve to interfere with signalling cascades important for the regulation of the innate immune response to *Chlamydia* (Chen et al. 2014). Interestingly, TarP, CT694, CT695 [another immediate effector of unknown function (Mueller and Fields 2015)] and TepP share the same T3S chaperone, Slc1 (Brinkworth et al. 2011; Chen et al. 2014; Pais et al. 2013). In EBs, the majority of TarP, but only a minor proportion of TepP, is found pre-complexed with Slc1. Pre-engagement with its cognate chaperone could prime TarP for rapid translocation and explain why its translocation is detected earlier than that of TepP (Chen et al. 2014).

Finally, the urogenital serovars of *C. trachomatis* possess a supplementary gene in the plasticity zone, *ct166*. The encoded protein presents homology with the N-terminal glucosyltransferase domain of clostridial glucosylating toxins (CGTs). The glucosylation activity of these enzymes specifically blocks GTP-binding proteins of the Rho and Ras families. CT166 is detected within EBs, although the proof of its translocation into the host cytosol upon infection is still missing. However, ectopic production of the protein induces actin reorganization comparable to that induced by CGTs. Moreover, expression of CT166 *in trans* severely impaired chlamydial uptake (Thalmann et al. 2010). Thus, CT166 could locally mediate the glucosylation of Rac1 leading to its inactivation, and an associated reduction in actin polymerization once invasion is complete. In addition, it is also possible that CT166 glucosylates Ras, although the potential consequence of this awaits experimental validation in an infection system (Bothe et al. 2015).

A major challenge in the field is to define what determines the specificity of each chlamydial species for a host or for a particular tissue. Factors on the EB surface are likely part of the answer, since they show differences in their adhesion properties, especially through OmcB and the Pmp family. TarP also exhibits sequence polymorphism between species and has been proposed to be one potential determinant of host specificity (Lutter et al. 2010). Finally, the *ct166* gene, which is located in the plasticity zone and is not expressed in all species, might also modulate infectivity (Belland et al. 2001).

2.5 Still Space for Early Effectors

As mentioned above, once encapsulated within the tight early bacterial containing vacuole, the EB must secure this niche faster than de novo protein synthesis would allow (Fig. 3). This is probably the role of yet uncharacterized effectors, which might be translocated soon after the invasion step. In the absence of tools to specifically manipulate *Chlamydia* genome, several laboratories have searched for putative effector proteins based on the presence an N-terminal amino acid sequence recognized by the T3S machineries of other bacteria such as *Yersinia* or *Shigella*. Large-scale screens have identified a number of potential effectors (da Cunha et al. 2014; Subtil et al. 2005). An alternative strategy has been used to identify putative T3S chaperones, based on similarities with known chaperones of T3S in other bacteria and to identify interacting partner proteins that also constitute effector candidates (Pais et al. 2013). Validation of the candidates has long been a bottleneck, due to the need to obtain good antibodies to detect the putative effector. Even then, the arising data were not always conclusive, since effectors that are translocated at such a small dose become diluted in the host cytoplasm and consequently escape antibody-based detection. Recently, a strategy based on the detection of fluorescently labelled β-lactamase reporters has been successfully adopted to detect the translocation of chlamydial T3S effectors (Mueller and Fields 2015). It is likely that this method will accelerate the identification of novel effectors and enable new functional studies.

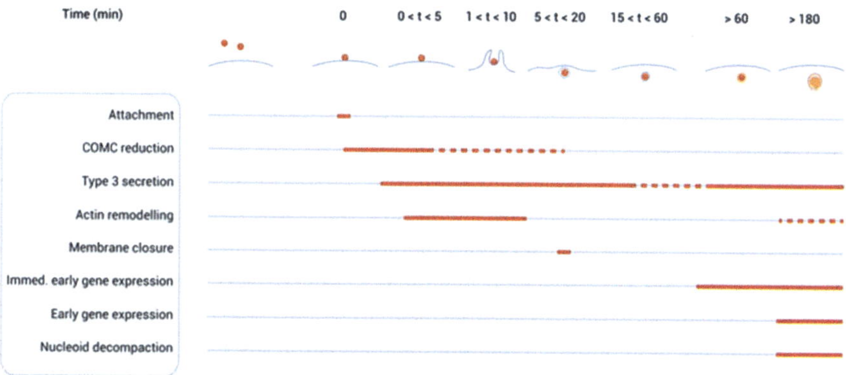

Fig. 3 Synopsis of *C. trachomatis* invasion in epithelial cells. Attachment of the infectious particle triggers the activation of T3S. Reduction of the disulphide bonds at the EB surface might be initiated at this stage, to allow for effector translocation. The time needed for completion of this step is not known. Early effector actions include manipulation of the host cytoskeleton and of membrane traffic. Signalling through host membrane receptors also contribute to membrane rearrangement and closure, resulting in the engulfment of the infectious particle in the nascent inclusion. T3S apparatuses may transiently disassemble, until a second wave of secretion begins, this time of neo-synthesized effectors (immediate early genes turned on). Nucleoid decompaction is only observed later. Mature inclusions show remodelling of peripheral actin (and of other cytoskeleton elements), when this is initiated is not known

What do we know about host cell defence against intruders, and the strategies used by *Chlamydia* to circumvent them? It has long been recognized that the *Chlamydia* inclusion engages in few interactions with endocytic compartments, thereby escaping the default pathway of fusion with late endocytic compartments. When bacterial protein synthesis is inhibited, the inclusion eventually fuses with late compartments, suggesting that bacterial effectors contribute to the escape from the default pathway (Scidmore et al. 1996). However, even under inhibited conditions, the fusion with acidic endosomal compartments occurred only later. Thus, it is possible that pre-synthesized effectors define the nascent inclusion as a non-endocytic compartment, acting prior to further effectors that are synthesized later in the infection cycle. Another very ancestral cellular defence strategy against microbial invasion is the autophagic machinery. Intracellular bacteria are recognized, and eliminated by this process, unless they have acquired escape strategies (Randow and Youle 2014). *C. trachomatis* appears to cope well with evading the host autophagic response, at least in cell culture models, since good EB preparations can result in close to one inclusion per EB (Omsland et al. 2012). The autophagosome marker LC3 associates with the inclusion membrane; however, it appears that it does so as a microtubule-associated protein rather than an autophagosome component (Al-Younes et al. 2011). In mouse embryonic fibroblasts deficient for conventional autophagy, the generation of infectious chlamydial progeny increases (Yasir et al. 2011). This effect occurs predominantly through acceleration of the bacterial growth rate, rather than by the formation or retention of more inclusions, suggesting that autophagy per se is unable to eliminate inclusions, at least in fibroblasts. By contrast, in macrophages and in the presence of interferon γ, autophagy appears to be mobilized for the elimination of inclusions (Al-Zeer et al. 2013). Thus, it appears that while the autophagy machinery can limit chlamydial development under some circumstances, *C. trachomatis* has developed strategies to significantly counteract this arm of the host defence. How this is achieved is not known. One classical signal to recruit the autophagy machinery is ubiquitination (Rogov et al. 2014). During invasion, a transient enrichment in ubiquitin was observed at the site of entry of *C. caviae*. This species encodes for a protein with deubiquitinase activity, *Chla*OTU, and it was proposed that *Chla*OTU is involved in the rapid dissipation of ubiquitin at the site of entry, presumably to avoid the formation of autophagic membranes around early bacterial containing vacuoles (Furtado et al. 2013). *C. trachomatis* has no *chlaOTU* gene; however, it encodes two deubiquitinases, which are translocated in the host cytoplasm during infection (Misaghi et al. 2006). ChlaDub1 is enriched in RBs, but it is also present in EBs (Saka et al. 2011). Whether this effector also functions at a very early stage of infection remains to be investigated.

Finally, host molecules recruited to early bacterial containing vacuoles directly or indirectly might promote inclusion biogenesis. For instance, the EphA2 receptor remains active after bacterial internalization and supports the activation of the PI3K/Akt signalling pathway that is required for normal chlamydial development (Subbarayal et al. 2015).

2.6 Setting Up the Decor Before Leaving the Stage to the RB

Following invasion, the bacteria undergo dramatic morphological changes, which only become apparent 2 hpi (Shaw et al. 2000). Nucleoid relaxation certainly contributes to the enhancement of gene transcription during the EB-to-RB transition, but this is only fully completed 6–8 hpi, although transcription is initiated less than 1 hpi (Belland et al. 2003). In fact, bacterial protein synthesis is needed for DNA decondensation itself. Early bacterial protein synthesis results in the production of a small metabolite that disrupts the association of the two histone-like proteins with DNA (Grieshaber et al. 2004, 2006). Thus, the selective early gene transcription, restricted to a subset of less than 30 genes called immediate early genes (Belland et al. 2003), is not regulated by nucleoid decondensation. These genes are transcribed by the σ^{66} RNA polymerase. Whether they are specifically activated, and how, is still an open question. Another possibility is that transcription of these genes may be constitutively active, while others remain repressed. Experimental data using in vitro transcription assays led the Tan laboratory to propose that early in the developmental cycle, DNA supercoiling levels are low (Niehus et al. 2008), allowing only the transcription of genes with supercoiling independent promoters (Cheng and Tan 2012). One of these immediate early gene is *euo*, which codes for a transcriptional repressor that silences the expression of σ^{66} and σ^{28} dependent late genes (Rosario et al. 2014). Scc4, a small protein that interacts with two subunits of the RNA polymerase, potentially links T3S and transcriptional regulation (Rao et al. 2009), as it also serves as a chaperone for the T3S substrate CopN (Silva-Herzog et al. 2011). Two recent papers confirmed that the dual functions of Scc4 may link T3S to the regulation of gene expression in *Chlamydia* (Hanson et al. 2015; Shen et al. 2015). However, when Scc4 regulates RNA polymerase during the bacterial developmental cycle is not yet clear. One study suggested that Scc4 regulates early transcription once released from CopN (Shen et al. 2015). This contradicts the initial characterization of Scc4 as a negative regulator of transcription, which suggested that transcriptional regulation by Scc4 is limited to late in the developmental cycle (Hanson et al. 2015).

One intriguing finding arising from recent cryo-EM studies was the seemingly early disappearance of T3S complexes once invasion was completed (Nans et al. 2014). This would mean that effector translocation is potentially paused early after entry and only resumes when novel T3S complexes are assembled. However, the immediate early genes include ten bacterial proteins that are translocated by a T3S mechanism into the inclusion membrane, called Inc proteins (Belland et al. 2003; Dehoux et al. 2011; Weber et al. 2015). Inc proteins do not accumulate in bacteria and are probably immediately translocated upon synthesis. Thus if indeed, T3S complexes are disassembled after invasion, they must be rapidly reassembled, possibly reusing former constituents or with subtly altered composition, as the genes coding for the components of the apparatus are not amongst the early transcribed genes. These "immediate" Inc proteins constitute a second generation of effectors, which, in continuity with the action of pre-packed effectors secreted during the invasion step, define the characteristics of the early inclusion membrane. Consequently, they dictate the interactions between the inclusion and the host, even before the EB-to-RB conversion is completed. Amongst the ten immediate Inc proteins, three have been functionally studied. IncD links the host lipid transfer protein CERT to the inclusion membrane, allowing for ceramide uptake directly from the endoplasmic reticulum (Agaisse and Derre 2014; Derre et al. 2011). CT229 interacts with Rab4, which is one of the several small Rab GTPases recruited to the inclusion membrane (Rzomp et al. 2006). Finally, CT850 interacts with dynein light chain DYNLT1, indicating that it might promote appropriate positioning of the inclusion at the microtubule-organizing centre (Mital et al. 2015).

3 Conclusion

Most bacteria exhibit morphological changes in response to environmental cues. What makes chlamydiae unusual is the pronounced dichotomy between its two forms, and the fact that cycling between them has become absolutely required. In the last decade, several unsuspected capacities have been discovered in EBs. One big challenge in the field remains to understand when these capacities are used, and to what extent EBs adapt to the different environments they face between two growth phases.

Acknowledgments We thank Dr. Andrea Nans for providing the EM image shown in Fig. 1. This work was supported by the European Research Council (NUChLEAR grant number 282046), the Agence Nationale pour la Recherche (Expendo ANR-14-CE11-0024-02), the Institut Pasteur and the Centre National de la Recherche Scientifique. Research on EB structure and inclusion biogenesis is supported by projects grants MR/N000846/1 and MR/I008696/1 from the Medical Research Council to R.D.H.

References

AbdelRahman YM, Belland RJ (2005) The chlamydial developmental cycle. FEMS Microbiol Rev 29:949–959

Abromaitis S, Stephens RS (2009) Attachment and entry of *Chlamydia* have distinct requirements for host protein disulfide isomerase. PLoS Pathog 5:e1000357

Agaisse H, Derre I (2014) Expression of the effector protein IncD in *Chlamydia trachomatis* mediates recruitment of the lipid transfer protein CERT and the endoplasmic reticulum-resident protein VAPB to the inclusion membrane. Infect Immun 82:2037–2047

Albrecht M, Sharma CM, Dittrich MT, Muller T, Reinhardt R, Vogel J, Rudel T (2011) The transcriptional landscape of *Chlamydia pneumoniae*. Genome Biol 12:R98

Al-Younes HM, Al-Zeer MA, Khalil H, Gussmann J, Karlas A, Machuy N, Brinkmann V, Braun PR, Meyer TF (2011) Autophagy-independent function of MAP-LC3 during intracellular propagation of *Chlamydia trachomatis*. Autophagy 7:814–828

Al-Zeer MA, Al-Younes HM, Lauster D, Abu Lubad M, Meyer TF (2013) Autophagy restricts *Chlamydia trachomatis* growth in human macrophages via IFNG-inducible guanylate binding proteins. Autophagy 9:46–58

Balañá ME, Niedergang F, Subtil A, Alcover A, Chavrier P, Dautry-Varsat A (2005) ARF6 GTPase controls bacterial invasion by actin remodelling. J Cell Sci 118:2201–2210

Barry CE 3rd, Hayes SF, Hackstadt T (1992) Nucleoid condensation in *Escherichia coli* that express a chlamydial histone homolog. Science 256:377–379

Batteiger BE (2012) *Chlamydia* infection and epidemiology. In: Tan M, Bavoil PM (eds) Intracellular pathogens I; Chlamydiales. ASM press, Washington, DC

Bavoil P, Ohlin A, Schachter J (1984) Role of disulfide bonding in outer membrane structure and permeability in *Chlamydia trachomatis*. Infect Immun 44:479–485

Becker E, Hegemann JH (2014) All subtypes of the Pmp adhesin family are implicated in chlamydial virulence and show species-specific function. Microbiol Open 3:544–556

Bedson SP, Gostling JV (1954) A study of the mode of multiplication of psittacosis virus. Br J Exp Pathol 35:299–308

Belland RJ, Scidmore MA, Crane DD, Hogan DM, Whitmire W, McClarty G, Caldwell HD (2001) *Chlamydia trachomatis* cytotoxicity associated with complete and partial cytotoxin genes. Proc Natl Acad Sci USA 98:13984–13989

Belland RJ, Zhong GM, Crane DD, Hogan D, Sturdevant D, Sharma J, Beatty WL, Caldwell HD (2003) Genomic transcriptional profiling of the developmental cycle of *Chlamydia trachomatis*. Proc Natl Acad Sci USA 100:8478–8483

Betts HJ, Twiggs LE, Sal MS, Wyrick PB, Fields KA (2008) Bioinformatic and biochemical evidence for the identification of the type III secretion system needle protein of *Chlamydia trachomatis*. J Bacteriol 190:1680–1690

Betts-Hampikian HJ, Fields KA (2011) Disulfide bonding within components of the Chlamydia type III secretion apparatus correlates with development. J Bacteriol 193:6950–6959

Birkelund S, Morgan-Fisher M, Timmerman E, Gevaert K, Shaw AC, Christiansen G (2009) Analysis of proteins in *Chlamydia trachomatis* L2 outer membrane complex, COMC. FEMS Immunol Med Microbiol 55:187–195

Bothe M, Dutow P, Pich A, Genth H, Klos A (2015) DXD motif-dependent and -independent effects of the *Chlamydia trachomatis* cytotoxin CT166. Toxins 7:621–637

Brickman TJ, Barry CE 3rd, Hackstadt T (1993) Molecular cloning and expression of hctB encoding a strain-variant chlamydial histone-like protein with DNA-binding activity. J Bacteriol 175:4274–4281

Brinkworth AJ, Malcolm DS, Pedrosa AT, Roguska K, Shahbazian S, Graham JE, Hayward RD, Carabeo RA (2011) *Chlamydia trachomatis* Slc1 is a type III secretion chaperone that enhances the translocation of its invasion effector substrate TARP. Mol Microbiol 82:131–144

Carabeo RA, Grieshaber SS, Fischer E, Hackstadt T (2002) *Chlamydia trachomatis* induces remodeling of the actin cytoskeleton during attachment and entry into HeLa cells. Infect Immun 70:3793–3803

Carabeo RA, Grieshaber SS, Hasenkrug A, Dooley C, Hackstadt T (2004) Requirement for the Rac GTPase in *Chlamydia trachomatis* invasion of non-phagocytic cells. Traffic 5:418–425

Carabeo RA, Dooley CA, Grieshaber SS, Hackstadt T (2007) Rac interacts with Abi-1 and WAVE2 to promote an Arp2/3-dependent actin recruitment during chlamydial invasion. Cell Microbiol 9:2278–2288

Chen JC-R, Stephens RS (1994) Trachoma and LGV biovars of *Chlamydia trachomatis* share the same glycosaminoglycan-dependent mechanism for infection of eukaryotic cells. Mol Microbiol 11:501–507

Chen Y-S, Bastidas RJ, Saka HA, Carpenter VK, Richards KL, Plano GV, Valdivia RH (2014) The *Chlamydia trachomatis* type III secretion chaperone Slc1 engages multiple early effectors, including TepP, a tyrosine-phosphorylated protein required for the recruitment of CrkI-II to nascent inclusions and innate immune signaling. PLoS Pathog 10:e1003954

Cheng E, Tan M (2012) Differential effects of DNA supercoiling on *Chlamydia* early promoters correlate with expression patterns in midcycle. J Bacteriol 194:3109–3115

Christiansen G, Pedersen LB, Koehler JE, Lundemose AG, Birkelund S (1993) Interaction between the *Chlamydia trachomatis* histone H1-like protein (Hc1) and DNA. J Bacteriol 175:1785–1795

Clifton DR, Fields KA, Grieshaber NA, Dooley CA, Fischer ER, Mead DJ, Carabeo RA, Hackstadt T (2004) A chlamydial type III translocated protein is tyrosine-phosphorylated at the site of entry and associated with recruitment of actin. Proc Natl Acad Sci USA 101: 10166–10171

Collingro A, Tischler P, Weinmaier T, Penz T, Heinz E, Brunham RC, Read TC, Bavoil PM, Sachse K, Kahane S, Friedman MG, Rattei T, Myers GS, Horn M (2011) Unity in variety—the pan-genome of the *Chlamydiae*. Mol Biol Evol 28:3253–3270

Conant CG, Stephens RS (2007) *Chlamydia* attachment to mammalian cells requires protein disulfide isomerase. Cell Microbiol 9:222–232

da Cunha M, Milho C, Almeida F, Pais SV, Borges V, Mauricio R, Borrego MJ, Gomes JP, Mota LJ (2014) Identification of type III secretion substrates of *Chlamydia trachomatis* using *Yersinia enterocolitica* as a heterologous system. BMC Microbiol 14:40

Davis CH, Raulston JE, Wyrick PB (2002) Protein disulfide isomerase, a component of the estrogen receptor complex, is associated with *Chlamydia trachomatis* serovar E attached to human endometrial epithelial cells. Infect Immun 70:3413–3418

Dehoux P, Flores R, Dauga C, Zhong G, Subtil A (2011) Multi-genome identification and characterization of chlamydiae-specific type III secretion substrates: the Inc proteins. BMC Genom 12:109

Derre I, Swiss R, Agaisse H (2011) The lipid transfer protein CERT interacts with the *Chlamydia* inclusion protein IncD and participates to ER-Chlamydia inclusion membrane contact sites. PLoS Pathog 7:e1002092

Downie AW (1971) Obituary. S. P. Bedson, 1886–1969. J Gen Microbiol 65:1–3

Elwell CA, Ceesay A, Kim JH, Kalman D, Engel JN (2008) RNA interference screen identifies Abl kinase and PDGFR signaling in *Chlamydia trachomatis* entry. PLoS Pathog 4:e1000021

Fadel S, Eley A (2008) Is lipopolysaccharide a factor in infectivity of *Chlamydia trachomatis*? J Med Microbiol 57:261–266

Ferrell JC, Fields KA (2016) A working model for the type III secretion mechanism in *Chlamydia*. Microbes Infect 18:84–92

Furtado AR, Essid M, Perrinet S, Balañá ME, Dautry-Varsat A, Yoder N, Dehoux P, Subtil A (2013) The chlamydial OTU-domain like protein *Chla*OTU is an early type III secretion effector targeting ubiquitin and NDP52. Cellular Microbiol 15:2064–2079

Galan JE, Lara-Tejero M, Marlovits TC, Wagner S (2014) Bacterial type III secretion systems: specialized nanomachines for protein delivery into target cells. Annu Rev Microbiol 68:415–438

Gehre L, Gorgette O, Prévost MC, Ducatez M, Giebel AM, Nelson DE, Ball SG, Subtil A (2016) Sequestration of host metabolism by an intracellular pathogen. eLife. doi:10.7554/eLife.12552

Gregory WW, Gardner M, Byrne GI, Moulder JW (1979) Arrays of hemispheric surface projections on *Chlamydia psittaci* and *Chlamydia trachomatis* observed by scanning electron microscopy. J Bacteriol 138:241–244

Grieshaber NA, Fischer ER, Mead DJ, Dooley CA, Hackstadt T (2004) Chlamydial histone-DNA interactions are disrupted by a metabolite in the methylerythritol phosphate pathway of isoprenoid biosynthesis. Proc Natl Acad Sci USA 101:7451–7456

Grieshaber NA, Sager JB, Dooley CA, Hayes SF, Hackstadt T (2006) Regulation of the *Chlamydia trachomatis* histone H1-like protein Hc2 is IspE dependent and IhtA independent. J Bacteriol 188:5289–5292

Guseva NV, Dessus-Babus S, Moore CG, Whittimore JD, Wyrick PB (2007) Differences in *Chlamydia trachomatis* serovar E growth rate in polarized endometrial and endocervical epithelial cells grown in three-dimensional culture. Infect Immun 75:553–564

Hackstadt T, Todd WJ, Caldwell HD (1985) Disulfide-mediated interactions of the chlamydial major outer membrane protein: role in the differentiation of chlamydiae? J Bacteriol 161:25–31

Hackstadt T, Baehr W, Ying Y (1991) *Chlamydia trachomatis* developmentally regulated protein is homologous to eukaryotic histone H1. Proc Natl Acad Sci USA 88:3937–3941

Hackstadt T, Fischer ER, Scidmore MA, Rockey DD, Heinzen RA (1997) Origins and functions of the chlamydial inclusion. Trends Microbiol 5:288–293

Haider S, Wagner M, Schmid MC, Sixt BS, Christian JG, Hacker G, Pichler P, Mechtler K, Muller A, Baranyi C, Toenshoff ER, Montanaro J, Horn M (2010) Raman microspectroscopy reveals long-term extracellular activity of Chlamydiae. Mol Microbiol 77:687–700

Hanson BR, Slepenkin A, Peterson EM, Tan M (2015) *Chlamydia trachomatis* type III secretion proteins regulate transcription. J Bacteriol 197:3238–3244

Hatch TP (1999) Developmental biology. In: Stephens RS (ed) *Chlamydia*: intracellular biology, pathogenesis, and immunity. American Society for Microbiology, Washington, DC, pp 29–67

Hegemann JH, Moelleken K (2012) Chlamydial adhesion and adhesins. In: Tan M, Bavoil PM (eds) Intracellular pathogens I: *Chlamydiales*. American Society for Microbiology, Washington, DC, pp 97–125

Hower S, Wolf K, Fields KA (2009) Evidence that CT694 is a novel *Chlamydia trachomatis* T3S substrate capable of functioning during invasion or early cycle development. Mol Microbiol 72:1423–1437

Huang Z, Chen M, Li K, Dong X, Han J, Zhang Q (2010) Cryo-electron tomography of *Chlamydia trachomatis* gives a clue to the mechanism of outer membrane changes. J Electron Microsc (Tokyo) 59:237–241

Jewett TJ, Fischer ER, Mead DJ, Hackstadt T (2006) Chlamydial TARP is a bacterial nucleator of actin. Proc Natl Acad Sci USA 103:15599–15604

Jewett TJ, Dooley CA, Mead DJ, Hackstadt T (2008) *Chlamydia trachomatis* tarp is phosphorylated by src family tyrosine kinases. Biochem Biophys Res Commun 371:339–344

Jewett TJ, Miller NJ, Dooley CA, Hackstadt T (2010) The conserved tarp actin binding domain is important for chlamydial invasion. PLoS Pathog 6:e1000997

Jiwani S, Alvarado S, Ohr RJ, Romero A, Nguyen B, Jewett TJ (2013) *Chlamydia trachomatis* Tarp harbors distinct G and F actin binding domains that bundle actin filaments. J Bacteriol 195:708–716

Karunakaran K, Subbarayal P, Vollmuth N, Rudel T (2015) Chlamydia-infected cells shed Gp96 to prevent chlamydial re-infection. Mol Microbiol 98:694–711

Kim JH, Jiang S, Elwell CA, Engel JN (2011) *Chlamydia trachomatis* co-opts the FGF2 signaling pathway to enhance infection. PLoS Pathog 7:e1002285

Lane BJ, Mutchler C, Al Khodor S, Grieshaber SS, Carabeo RA (2008) Chlamydial entry involves TARP binding of guanine nucleotide exchange factors. PLoS Pathog 4:e1000014

Liechti GW, Kuru E, Hall E, Kalinda A, Brun YV, VanNieuwenhze M, Maurelli AT (2014) A new metabolic cell-wall labelling method reveals peptidoglycan in *Chlamydia trachomatis*. Nature 506:507–510

Liu X, Afrane M, Clemmer DE, Zhong G, Nelson DE (2010) Identification of *Chlamydia trachomatis* outer membrane complex proteins by differential proteomics. J Bacteriol 192:2852–2860

Lutter EI, Bonner C, Holland MJ, Suchland RJ, Stamm WE, Jewett TJ, McClarty G, Hackstadt T (2010) Phylogenetic analysis of *Chlamydia trachomatis* Tarp and correlation with clinical phenotype. Infect Immun 78:3678–3688

Matsumoto A (1981) Isolation and electron microscopic observations of intracytoplasmic inclusions containing *Chlamydia psittaci*. J Bacteriol 145:605–612

Mehlitz A, Banhart S, Hess S, Selbach M, Meyer TF (2008) Complex kinase requirements for *Chlamydia trachomatis* Tarp phosphorylation. FEMS Microbiol Lett 289:233–240

Misaghi S, Balsara ZR, Catic A, Spooner E, Ploegh HL, Starnbach MN (2006) *Chlamydia trachomatis*-derived deubiquitinating enzymes in mammalian cells during infection. Mol Microbiol 61:142–150

Mital J, Lutter EI, Barger AC, Dooley CA, Hackstadt T (2015) *Chlamydia trachomatis* inclusion membrane protein CT850 interacts with the dynein light chain DYNLT1 (Tctex1). Biochem Biophys Res Commun 462:165–170

Moelleken K, Hegemann JH (2008) The Chlamydia outer membrane protein OmcB is required for adhesion and exhibits biovar-specific differences in glycosaminoglycan binding. Mol Microbiol 67:403–419

Molleken K, Schmidt E, Hegemann JH (2010) Members of the Pmp protein family of *Chlamydia pneumoniae* mediate adhesion to human cells via short repetitive peptide motifs. Mol Microbiol 78:1004–1017

Molleken K, Becker E, Hegemann JH (2013) The *Chlamydia pneumoniae* invasin protein Pmp21 recruits the EGF receptor for host cell entry. PLoS Pathog 9:e1003325

Moulder JW (1966) The relation of the psittacosis group (Chlamydiae) to bacteria and viruses. Annu Rev Microbiol 20:107–130

Mueller KE, Fields KA (2015) Application of β-lactamase reporter fusions as an indicator of effector protein secretion during infections with the obligate intracellular pathogen *Chlamydia trachomatis*. PLoS ONE 10:e0135295

Mueller KE, Plano GV, Fields KA (2014) New frontiers in type III secretion biology: the Chlamydia perspective. Infect Immun 82:2–9

Nans A, Saibil HR, Hayward RD (2014) Pathogen-host reorganization during *Chlamydia* invasion revealed by cryo-electron tomography. Cell Microbiol 16:1457–1472

Nans A, Kudryashev M, Saibil HR, Hayward RD (2015) Structure of a bacterial type III secretion system in contact with a host membrane *in situ*. Nat Comm 6:10114

Nguyen BD, Cunningham D, Liang X, Chen X, Toone EJ, Raetz CR, Zhou P, Valdivia RH (2011) Lipooligosaccharide is required for the generation of infectious elementary bodies in *Chlamydia trachomatis*. Proc Natl Acad Sci USA 108:10284–10289

Nichols BA, Setzer PY, Pang F, Dawson CR (1985) New view of the surface projections of *Chlamydia trachomatis*. J Bacteriol 164:344–349

Niehus E, Cheng E, Tan M (2008) DNA supercoiling-dependent gene regulation in Chlamydia. J Bacteriol 190:6419–6427

Omsland A, Sager J, Nair V, Sturdevant DE, Hackstadt T (2012) Developmental stage-specific metabolic and transcriptional activity of *Chlamydia trachomatis* in an axenic medium. Proc Natl Acad Sci USA 109:19781–19785

Omsland A, Sixt BS, Horn M, Hackstadt T (2014) Chlamydial metabolism revisited: interspecies metabolic variability and developmental stage-specific physiologic activities. FEMS Microbiol Rev 38:779–801

Osaka I, Hefty PS (2014) Lipopolysaccharide-binding alkylpolyamine DS-96 inhibits *Chlamydia trachomatis* infection by blocking attachment and entry. Antimicrob Agents Chemother 58:3245–3254

Pais SV, Milho C, Almeida F, Mota LJ (2013) Identification of novel type III secretion chaperone-substrate complexes of *Chlamydia trachomatis*. PLoS ONE 8:e56292

Pedersen LB, Birkelund S, Christiansen G (1996) Purification of recombinant *Chlamydia trachomatis* histone H1-like protein Hc2, and comparative functional analysis of Hc2 and Hc1. Mol Microbiol 20:295–311

Pilhofer M, Aistleitner K, Ladinsky MS, Konig L, Horn M, Jensen GJ (2014) Architecture and host interface of environmental chlamydiae revealed by electron cryotomography. Environ Microbiol 16:417–429

Randow F, Youle RJ (2014) Self and nonself: how autophagy targets mitochondria and bacteria. Cell Host Microbe 15:403–411

Rao X, Deighan P, Hua Z, Hu X, Wang J, Luo M, Wang J, Liang Y, Zhong G, Hochschild A, Shen L (2009) A regulator from *Chlamydia trachomatis* modulates the activity of RNA polymerase through direct interaction with the beta subunit and the primary sigma subunit. Genes Dev 23:1818–1829

Rogov V, Dötsch V, Johansen T, Kirkin V (2014) Interactions between autophagy receptors and ubiquitin-like proteins form the molecular basis for selective autophagy. Mol Cell 53:167–178

Rosario CJ, Hanson BR, Tan M (2014) The transcriptional repressor EUO regulates both subsets of Chlamydia late genes. Mol Microbiol 94:888–897

Rund S, Lindner B, Brade H, Holst O (1999) Structural analysis of the lipopolysaccharide from *Chlamydia trachomatis* serotype L2. J Biol Chem 274:16819–16824

Rzomp KA, Moorhead AR, Scidmore MA (2006) The GTPase Rab4 interacts with *Chlamydia trachomatis* inclusion membrane protein CT229. Infect Immun 74:5362–5373

Saka HA, Thompson JW, Chen YS, Kumar Y, Dubois LG, Moseley MA, Valdivia RH (2011) Quantitative proteomics reveals metabolic and pathogenic properties of *Chlamydia trachomatis* developmental forms. Mol Microbiol 82:1185–1203

Sarov I, Becker Y (1971) Deoxyribonucleic acid-dependent ribonucleic acid polymerase activity in purified trachoma elementary bodies: effect of sodium chloride on ribonucleic acid transcription. J Bacteriol 107:593–598

Schachter J (1988) The intracellular life of *Chlamydia*. Curr Top Microbiol Immunol 138:109–139

Schwoppe C, Winkler HH, Neuhaus HE (2002) Properties of the glucose-6-phosphate transporter from *Chlamydia pneumoniae* (HPTcp) and the glucose-6-phosphate sensor from *Escherichia coli* (UhpC). J Bacteriol 184:2108–2115

Scidmore MA, Rockey DD, Fischer ER, Heinzen RA, Hackstadt T (1996) Vesicular interactions of the *Chlamydia trachomatis* inclusion are determined by chlamydial early protein synthesis rather than route of entry. Infect Immun 64:5366–5372

Shaw EI, Dooley CA, Fischer ER, Scidmore MA, Fields KA, Hackstadt T (2000) Three temporal classes of gene expression during the *Chlamydia trachomatis* developmental cycle. Mol Microbiol 37:913–925

Shen L, Macnaughtan MA, Frohlich KM, Cong Y, Goodwin OY, Chou CW, LeCour L Jr, Krup K, Luo M, Worthylake DK (2015) Multipart chaperone-effector recognition in the type III secretion system of *Chlamydia trachomatis*. J Biol Chem 290:28141–28155

Silva-Herzog E, Joseph SS, Avery AK, Coba JA, Wolf K, Fields KA, Plano GV (2011) Scc1 (CP0432) and Scc4 (CP0033) function as a type III secretion chaperone for CopN of *Chlamydia pneumoniae*. J Bacteriol 193:3490–3496

Sixt BS, Siegl A, Muller C, Watzka M, Wultsch A, Tziotis D, Montanaro J, Richter A, Schmitt-Kopplin P, Horn M (2013) Metabolic features of Protochlamydia amoebophila elementary bodies–a link between activity and infectivity in Chlamydiae. PLoS Pathog 9: e1003553

Skipp P, Robinson J, O'Connor CD, Clarke IN (2005) Shotgun proteomic analysis of *Chlamydia trachomatis*. Proteomics 5:1558–1573

Skipp PJ, Hughes C, McKenna T, Edwards R, Langridge J, Thomson NR, Clarke IN (2016) Quantitative proteomics of the infectious and replicative forms of *Chlamydia trachomatis*. PLoS ONE 11:e0149011

Stephens RS, Kalman S, Lammel C, Fan J, Marathe R, Aravind L, Mitchell W, Olinger L, Tatusov RL, Zhao Q, Koonin EV, Davis RW (1998) Genome sequence of an obligate intracellular pathogen of humans: *Chlamydia trachomatis*. Science 282:754–755

Subbarayal P, Karunakaran K, Winkler AC, Rother M, Gonzalez E, Meyer TF, Rudel T (2015) EphrinA2 receptor (EphA2) is an invasion and intracellular signaling receptor for *Chlamydia trachomatis*. PLoS Pathog 11:e1004846

Subtil A, Delevoye C, Balañá ME, Tastevin L, Perrinet S, Dautry-Varsat A (2005) A directed screen for chlamydial proteins secreted by a type III mechanism identifies a translocated protein and numerous other new candidates. Mol Microbiol 56:1636–1647

Swanson KA, Taylor LD, Frank SD, Sturdevant GL, Fischer ER, Carlson JH, Whitmire WM, Caldwell HD (2009) *Chlamydia trachomatis* polymorphic membrane protein D is an oligomeric autotransporter with a higher-order structure. Infect Immun 77:508–516

Tamura A, Matsumoto A, Higashi N (1967) Purification and chemical composition of reticulate bodies of the meningopneumonitis organisms. J Bacteriol 93:2003–2008

Tamura A, Matsumoto A, Manire GP, Higashi N (1971) Electron microscopic observations on the structure of the envelopes of mature elementary bodies and developmental reticulate forms of *Chlamydia psittaci*. J Bacteriol 105:355–360

Tan C, Hsia RC, Shou H, Haggerty CL, Ness RB, Gaydos CA, Dean D, Scurlock AM, Wilson DP, Bavoil PM (2009) *Chlamydia trachomatis*-infected patients display variable antibody profiles against the nine-member polymorphic membrane protein family. Infect Immun 77:3218–3226

Tan C, Hsia RC, Shou H, Carrasco JA, Rank RG, Bavoil PM (2010) Variable expression of surface-exposed polymorphic membrane proteins in in vitro-grown *Chlamydia trachomatis*. Cell Microbiol 12:174–187

Tang L, Chen J, Zhou Z, Yu P, Yang Z, Zhong G (2015) *Chlamydia*-secreted protease CPAF degrades host antimicrobial peptides. Microbes Infect 17:402–408

Thalmann J, Janik K, May M, Sommer K, Ebeling J, Hofmann F, Genth H, Klos A (2010) Actin re-organization induced by *Chlamydia trachomatis* serovar D–evidence for a critical role of the effector protein CT166 targeting Rac. PLoS ONE 5:e9887

Thwaites T, Nogueira AT, Campeotto I, Silva AP, Grieshaber SS, Carabeo RA (2014) The *Chlamydia* effector TarP mimics the mammalian leucine-aspartic acid motif of paxillin to subvert the focal adhesion kinase during invasion. J Biol Chem 289:30426–30442

Thwaites TR, Pedrosa AT, Peacick TP, Carabeo RA (2015) Vinculin interacts with the Chlamydia effector TarP via a tripartite vinculin binding domain to mediate actin recruitment and assembly at the plasma membrane. Front Cell Inf Microbiol 5:88

Tipples G, McClarty G (1993) The obligate intracellular bacterium *Chlamydia trachomatis* is auxotrophic for three of the four ribonucleoside triphosphates. Mol Microbiol 8:1105–1114

Vandahl BB, Birkelund S, Demol H, Hoorelbeke B, Christiansen G, Vandekerckhove J, Gevaert K (2001) Proteome analysis of the *Chlamydia pneumoniae* elementary body. Electrophoresis 22:1204–1223

Vromman F, Laverriere M, Perrinet S, Dufour A, Subtil A (2014) Quantitative monitoring of the *Chlamydia trachomatis* developmental cycle using GFP-expressing bacteria, microscopy and flow cytometry. PLoS ONE 9:e99197

Weber MM, Bauler LD, Lam J, Hackstadt T (2015) Expression and localization of predicted inclusion membrane proteins in *Chlamydia trachomatis*. Infect Immun 83:4710–4718

Yasir M, Pachikara ND, Bao X, Pan Z, Fan H (2011) Regulation of chlamydial infection by host autophagy and vacuolar ATPase-bearing organelles. Infect Immun 79:4019–4028

Manipulation of the Host Cell Cytoskeleton by *Chlamydia*

Ana T. Nogueira, Antonio T. Pedrosa and Rey A. Carabeo

Abstract *Chlamydiae* are obligate intracellular pathogens. They undergo a biphasic developmental cycle differentiating between the infectious but metabolically quiescent elementary body and the vegetative, but non-infectious reticulate body. *Chlamydia* spends a significant portion of its development in the non-infectious stage, demanding an effective strategy of manipulating the host cells to ensure its intracellular survival and replication. A common target of all *Chlamydia* species studied so far is the host cell cytoskeleton, with past and recent findings revealing crucial roles in invasion, inclusion maintenance, nutrient acquisition, and egress. The molecular details of how *Chlamydia* co-opts the cytoskeleton is becoming clearer, with bacterial factors and their corresponding host cell targets identified.

Contents

A.T. Nogueira · A.T. Pedrosa · R.A. Carabeo (✉)
School of Molecular Biosciences, College of Veterinary Medicine,
Washington State University, Pullman, WA, USA
e-mail: rcarabeo@vetmed.wsu.edu

Current Topics in Microbiology and Immunology (2018) 412:59–80
DOI 10.1007/82_2016_10

Published Online: 20 May 2016

1 Cytoskeletal Dynamics in Epithelial Cells

1.1 Actin

The actin cytoskeleton is a dynamic structure that is composed of architecturally distinct complexes that take on a mesh-like dendritic arrangement or bundles of filamentous structures. Both are associated with distinct functions and are induced to form by locally driven stimuli that activate specific nucleation, polymerization, and remodeling machineries. Lamellipodia formation in motile cells is mediated by dendritic arrays of branched filaments at the leading edge, whereas linear actin bundles are formed in filopodia within lamellipodia. Actin remodeling is crucial to motility, nutrient acquisition, cell division, and organization of intracellular trafficking.

Actin dynamics is regulated by shifting the balance between monomeric globular actin (G-actin) and polymeric filamentous actin (F-actin) states. By having a pool of F-actin at steady states, the cell can respond quickly to immediate demands to remodel actin, with net assembly and disassembly at the opposite ends of the filaments, resulting in the polarized orientation of F-actin. Polymerization is generally favored at the barbed end than at the pointed end (Wanger and Wegner 1985; Pring et al. 1992), creating a net flux of actin subunits that result in a process called treadmilling (Schaus et al. 2007). Treadmilling is regulated through the control of availability of actin subunits by actin-binding proteins (ABP), or by increasing the rate-limiting step of actin depolymerization at the pointed end via the action of actin depolymerization factor ADF/cofilin, or by regulating the availability of barbed ends for polymerization by capping or destabilization (Koestler et al. 2013; Johnston et al. 2015).

Localized polymerization of actin is dependent on the spatial regulation of nucleation promoting factors (NPFs) of actin assembly. NPFs are found at lamellipodial protrusion, focal adhesions, podosomes, endosomal scission, and at sites of invasion by microbial pathogens (Yu et al. 2012; Grassart et al. 2014; Truong et al. 2014; Pizarro-Cerdá et al. 2015). NPFs, such as the WASP family of proteins, are activated in response to local stimuli and catalyze filament branching via their activation of the Arp2/3 complex. SCAR/WAVE and N-WASP generate branched and linear F-actin network found in lamellipodia (Nakagawa et al. 2001) and filopodia (Miki et al. 1998), respectively. N-WASP and WASH are also involved in vesicle scission and endocytosis (Benesch et al. 2005; Duleh and Welch 2010), while WHAMM/JMY functions to reorganize the Golgi apparatus (Campellone et al. 2008). NPF activation through interactions with upstream signaling-responsive effectors or phosphatidylinositol lipids reveals binding sites for actin and the Arp2/3 complex to create a complex to mediate localized actin polymerization (reviewed in Pizarro-Cerdá et al. 2015). These complexes are targets of a variety of bacterial pathogens to facilitate invasion, intracellular motility, egress, and dissemination.

1.2 Microtubules

Microtubules are highly dynamic polymeric structures composed of α and β tubulin proteins. They are nucleated at the microtubule organizing center (MTOC) and radiate toward the cell periphery. The MTOC is located near the nucleus and consists of the centrosome, γ-tubulin, and associated proteins to form a nucleating structure to which α and β tubulins are added. The formed microtubule displays polarity with the minus-end anchored at the MTOC and the plus-end oriented toward the plasma membrane. The dynamics at both ends are very different, with the minus-end-exhibiting restricted polymerization due to the capping activity of the γ-TuRC (Tubulin Ring Complex), while the plus-end being much more dynamic with constant growth and depolymerization, including catastrophe and rescue.

Microtubule dynamics are regulated by a number of factors, some intrinsic to the tubulin subunits, and others by binding to the ends and along the length of microtubules. Polymerization is dependent on guanoside triphosphate (GTP). GTP-bound tubulin is added at the plus-end, followed by the hydrolysis of GTP. However, there is a slight delay in GTP hydrolysis built into the system to create a cap-like structure composed of multiple subunits of newly incorporated GTP-tubulin subunits. When this structure is lost, the microtubule plus-end undergoes a catastrophe and rescue dynamics that is influenced by a number of plus-end tracking proteins (+TIPs). For example, the end-binding proteins associate with the plus-end, and along with a number of binding partners, including cytoplasmic linker proteins (CLIPs) and CLIP-associated proteins (CLASPs) suppress catastrophe events and/or induce rescue events (Komarova et al. 2005, 2009; Maiato et al. 2005; Honnappa et al. 2009; Al-Bassam et al. 2010). There are factors that bind to tubulin subunits to induce GTP hydrolysis (stathmin) (Belmont and Mitchison 1996; Howell et al. 1999; Larsson et al. 1999) or trigger catastrophe events (kinesin-13) (Newton et al. 2004; Mennella et al. 2005; Peris et al. 2009; Oguchi et al. 2011). A number of microtubule-associated proteins (MAPs) that bind along the length of the microtubules, including spastin, fidgetin, and katanin regulate stability. Thus, in addition to the inherent regulators, e.g. GTP-binding and hydrolysis, there are a number of MAPs whose activities are coordinated to ensure proper and timely modulation of stability, polymerization, and disassembly,

Tubulin subunits within the polymerized microtubles are also post-translationally modified via detyrosination, glutamylation, glycylation, and acetylation. These modifications are recognized by a number of MAPs, which then exert their stabilizing or destabilizing influence on the microtubule filament. For example, tyrosination is necessary for the binding of CLIP170 and p150Glued at the plus-end of microtubules (Peris 2006). This same post-translational modification decreases the association of depolymerizing machineries, such as kinesin-13, MCAK, or KIF2A (Peris et al. 2009). The net result is the accumulation of stable microtubule populations. Another post-translational modification, acetylation influences the ability of microtubules to interact with molecular motors, e.g. KIF5a, kinesin-1, and dynein motors (reviewed in de Forges et al. 2012). Acetylation also influences the interaction of organelles with microtubules, with mitochondria, but not endosomes displaying preference for acetylated microtubules (reviewed in de Forges et al. 2012).

Microtubules and associated proteins are essential in the intracellular organization and function of organelles. Microtubule poisons or depletion of microtubule-associated motors, such as dynein leads to the disorganization of the Golgi and the endoplasmic reticulum (ER) (Thyberg 1980; Wehland et al. 1983). In the absence of the microtubule network via treatment with nocodazole, the Golgi apparatus disperses into mini-stacks and fails to localize to the peri-nuclear region (Cole et al. 1996). Remarkably, nocodazole washout revealed the mini-stack migration along re-polymerized microtubules in a dynein-dependent manner (Ho et al. 1989).

There are numerous examples of bacterial pathogens engaging the microtubule network to facilitate invasion (reviewed in Radhakrishnan and Splitter 2012) or intracellular migration to the MTOC (Kim et al. 2001; Grieshaber et al. 2003).

1.3 Intermediate Filaments

The primary function of intermediate filaments is to provide tensile strength to cells to maintain their structure during compressing, twisting, and stretching. As such, they are crucial in preventing fracture of epithelial sheets and maintaining barrier function (Wagner et al. 2007). Filaments typically consist of alpha-helical rod-shaped subunits that polymerize to form protofilaments, which interact laterally to form a structure with high tensile strength. The staggered arrangement of the protofilaments also contributes to their elastic property (Traub et al. 1992; Geisler et al. 1992).

The dynamics of intermediate filaments lengthening is markedly different from those of actin and microtubules. Whereas these structures exist in dynamic equilibrium with a soluble pool of actin and microtubule subunits, respectively, their polymerization and depolymerization involves the addition and removal of subunits at the ends. Intermediate filaments do not display any polarity, and thus, subunit exchange, addition, and removal can occur anywhere along the lengths of protofilaments (Paramio et al. 1997). Through end-to-end annealing of these protofilaments, intermediate filaments are formed. Lateral interaction of the staggered annealed protofilaments promoted by cross-linking proteins increases the tensile strength (Steinböck et al. 2000).

The regulation of intermediate filament dynamics is not as well-characterized as those of actin and microtubule networks. For keratin, namely K8 and K18, a point of regulation is the phosphorylation at Ser431 and Ser52, respectively (Ku and Omary 1994, 1997). The effect is the increased solubility and altered polymerization. Another mechanism of regulation is the modulation of its attachment to structural complexes, including hemidesmosomes, intercellular junctions, and focal adhesions. For example, the focal adhesion has been reported to be the site of extensive keratin filament formation (Windoffer et al. 2006). Newly formed keratin filaments translocate continuously toward the cell center in a manner that depends on an intact local actin cytoskeleton. Vimentin filaments were also observed from the perinuclear region to interact with focal contacts at the cell edge (Tsuruta and Jones 2003). Thus, the interaction of intermediate filaments with other cytoskeletal networks indicates that coordination of function through co-regulation may be the norm.

2 The Host Cell Cytoskeleton and *Chlamydia* Invasion

2.1 Actin Recruitment During Invasion

In vitro, *Chlamydiae* display a high degree of promiscuity in regard to infection of cultured cells, possibly due to a ubiquitous receptor expressed in many cell types or the utilization of multiple adhesin-receptor interactions to facilitate entry. Regardless of the mechanism used, the assembly of filamentous actin at the base of the adhered chlamydial elementary body (EB) is observed (Majeed and Kihlström 1991; Carabeo et al. 2002, 2004; Clifton et al. 2004). Actin recruitment and F-actin assembly are essential to invasion (Majeed and Kihlström 1991; Schramm and Wyrick 1995; Boleti et al. 1999; Carabeo et al. 2002; Coombes and Mahony 2002). They are required for the formation of the actin-rich cell surface microvillar projections that surround the invading EB (Carabeo et al. 2002). The use of the actin-destabilizing drug, cytochalasin D and globular actin-sequestering compound latrunculin B led to the loss of the microvillar structures and markedly reduced invasion efficiencies (Majeed and Kihlström 1991; Schramm and Wyrick 1995; Boleti et al. 1999; Carabeo et al. 2002; Coombes and Mahony 2002). Interestingly, washout of cytochalasin D revealed the preferential re-establishment of the actin-rich cell surface microvillar-like projections at the sites of EB adhesion (Carabeo et al. 2002). Actin recruitment, as demonstrated by the use of EGFP-actin to track the spatial and temporal dynamics, is highly localized and transient (Carabeo et al. 2002, 2004). The origin of the signal that stimulates the host actin remodeling machinery may be the EB itself through the translocation of effectors to modulate host cell signaling at the site of invasion or the engagement of host cell receptors by adhesins on the *Chlamydia*. Additional evidence of a highly localized signaling during invasion is the phosphorylation of proteins at the sites of adhesion (Birkelund et al. 1994; Fawaz et al. 1997; Elwell et al. 2008).

2.2 Signaling to the Actin Remodeling Machinery

A genome-wide RNAi screen in Drosophila S2 cells identified the transmembrane tyrosine kinase platelet-derived growth factor receptor (PDGFR) and the fibroblast growth factor receptor (FGFR) as mediators of chlamydial invasion (Elwell et al. 2008) (Fig. 1). The latter was proposed to be involved in a tripartite interaction with the chlamydial EB through the bridging function of fibroblast growth factor 2 (FGF2) (Kim et al. 2011). In the former, Elwell et al. observed the PDGFR-dependent phosphorylation and activation of the Vav2 guanine nucleotide exchange factor (GEF) resulting in the switching on of the Rac GTPase. In addition, activating phosphorylation of two actin-nucleating factors, WAVE2 and cortactin were observed, with the former dependent on the Abelson kinase (c-Abl) (Elwell et al. 2008). These results were consistent with the report that implicated the Rac GTPase and the WAVE2 complex in chlamydial invasion (Carabeo et al. 2007).

Interestingly, a simultaneous publication by Lane et al. identified that the *Chlamydia trachomatis* type III effector TarP, when phosphorylated at specific tyrosine residues within the 50-amino-acid domain present in multiple copies (3–12 copies depending on the strain), was able to bind protein complexes that contain either Vav2 or Sos1, both modified by accessory proteins to function as GEFs of Rac1 (Lane et al. 2008). Furthermore, the association of Sos1 required the Abl-interactor 1 (Abi1), which may be linked to the binding and phosphorylation of TarP by c-Abl (Elwell et al. 2008). Thus, there may be cooperation between the PDGFR and TarP signaling, where Abl-phosphorylated TarP is the signaling scaffold to attract and concentrate host signaling molecules post-translationally activated by the PDGFR kinase activity.

The tyrosine-containing 50-amino-acid domain important for the signaling described above is unique to the *C. trachomatis* serovars (Clifton et al. 2004, 2005). Non-trachomatis species, including environmental and veterinary chlamydial pathogens do not harbor this domain in their respective TarP orthologs (Clifton et al. 2005). Yet, actin recruitment during invasion could be observed in the non-trachomatis strains tested, including *Chlamydia caviae* and *Chlamydia pneumoniae* (Boleti et al. 1999; Coombes and Mahony 2002; Subtil et al. 2004; Clifton et al. 2005). How is actin recruitment achieved in these species? As with

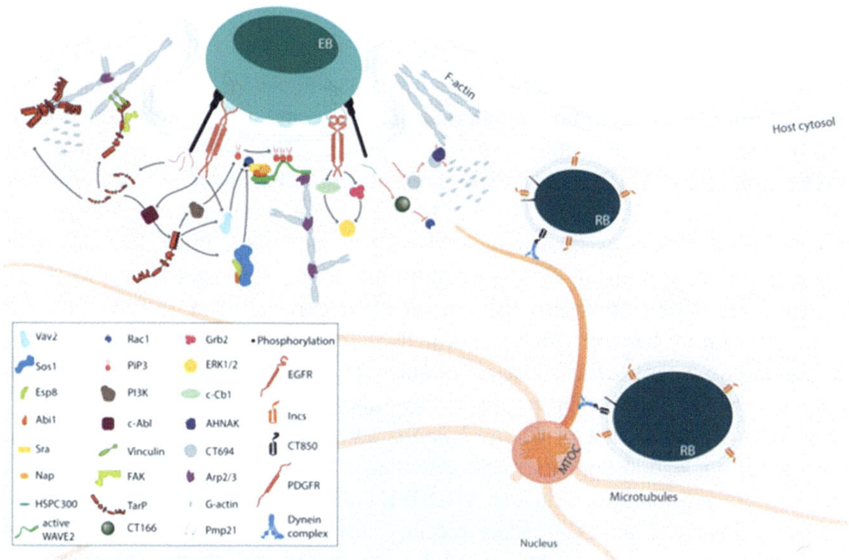

Fig. 1 A number of signaling pathways are induced during *Chlamydia* invasion to activate the actin remodeling machinery. The translocated type III effector TarP acts as a molecular scaffold to which host signaling is recruited and potentially cooperates with host cell receptors. The end result is the activation of the Arp2/3 actin-nucleating complex. TarP also functions as a bacterial nucleator of actin, forming filamentous actin structures, which could serve as docking sites for branched polymerization mediated by Arp2/3. Nascent *Chlamydia* inclusions engage the microtubule and hijack the dynein motor for translocation to the microtubule organizing center

C. trachomatis, the cooperation between host cell receptors and TarP appears to be involved (Kim et al. 2011). *C. pneumoniae* invasion requires the epidermal growth factor receptor (EGFR) and its interaction with the putative chlamydial adhesin Pmp21 (Mölleken et al. 2013). EGFR activation led to the recruitment of Grb2 and c-Cbl, and the activation of ERK1/2 (Mölleken et al. 2013). The specific localization of EGFR into a ring-like structure that surrounds *C. pneumoniae* EBs is suggestive of a role in invasion (Mölleken et al. 2013). It is possible that EGFR and TarP signaling pathways in *C. pneumoniae* may also cooperate to promote optimal signaling.

With regard to TarP function, we recently identified two conserved signaling motifs at the C-terminal half of TarP. The leucine-aspartic acid (LD) and vinculin-binding domain (VBD) specifically bound the focal adhesion kinase (FAK) and vinculin, respectively (Thwaites et al. 2014, 2015); and both interactions with TarP resulted in the recruitment of actin to the plasma membrane (Thwaites et al. 2014, 2015). Thus, a pseudo-focal adhesion complex at the base of the invading elementary body may form to mediate invasion signaling. Consistent with this notion is the recent report of *C. trachomatis* serovar E utilizing β-integrin as a receptor for invasion (Stallmann and Hegemann 2015).

2.3 Direct Actin Nucleation by TarP

In addition to its signaling scaffold role, TarP also nucleates actin polymerization directly through its actin-binding domains (ABD) and the proline-rich domain (PRD) (Jewett et al. 2006, 2010) (Fig. 1). The ABDs resemble the WAVE-homology 1 (WH1) domain present in NPFs, such as WAVE2 and N-WASp (Jewett et al. 2006). The ABDs of TarP are arranged in tandem and are present in either two or three copies (Jewett et al. 2010). PRD mediates TarP oligomerization to bring in close proximity the actin monomers bound to ABDs (Jewett et al. 2006) and raise the critical actin concentration to overcome the thermodynamic barrier that normally prevents the formation of nucleation-competent actin trimer or tetramer. However, in some cases, the PRD appears to be dispensable in the nucleating function of TarP orthologs harboring three ABDs, such as that of *C. trachomatis* serovar A (Jewett et al. 2010). The direct actin nucleation appears to be essential in invasion, as cells microinjected with monoclonal antibodies to the ABD/WH1 domain of TarP reduced invasion efficiency (Jewett et al. 2006). More recently, Jiwani et al. reported the functional cooperation between TarP and the Arp2/3 complex. When both were present, actin polymerization in in vitro reactions was quantitatively more robust than in the presence of TarP or the Arp2/3 complex alone (Jiwani et al. 2012). While the mechanism has yet to be characterized fully, it is likely that the TarP-nucleated actin filaments act as docking sites for the Arp2/3 complex to promote branched polymerization.

2.4 Disassembly of F-Actin at the Sites of Invasion

Actin recruitment is transient, and the disassembly of the formed F-actin network underneath the bacterium would be required. Otherwise, it poses a physical barrier that hinders the completion of internalization. It is not clear whether this disassembly process is controlled by *Chlamydia* or if it depends on host machinery, but a collection of evidence hints at the involvement of both. Reports point to roles of bacterial effectors in inhibiting actin cytoskeleton remodeling-related host cell signaling (Fig. 1). CT166 is proposed to inhibit Rac1 by glucosylation (Thalmann et al. 2010). In support of this mechanism of Rac1 inhibition, loss of glucosylation function of CT166 toward the related Ras GTPase was observed when the enzymatically important DXD motif was mutated (Thalmann et al. 2010; Bothe et al. 2015). Another potential mechanism is the regulation of the actin-binding AHNAK protein by CT694 (Bullock et al. 2012). Ectopic expression of CT694 led to the loss of actin stress fibers, and this activity required the interaction with AHNAK (Bullock et al. 2012). This suggests that the depolymerizing activity of the CT694-AHNAK complex may play a role in invasion. Actin depolymerizing factors have also been implicated indirectly. RNA interference screens identified cofilin to be necessary for chlamydial infection of Drosophila S2 cells, although it is not clear whether this requirement is during invasion or at later stages (Elwell et al. 2008).

2.5 *Microtubule and* Chlamydia *Invasion*

The role of microtubules in *Chlamydia* invasion remains unclear with very few reports describing the susceptibility of elementary body uptake to microtubule destabilizing drugs. Ward and Murray observed that *C. trachomatis* invasion was inhibited by vinblastine or vincristine, compounds that inhibit microtubule polymerization (Ward and Murray 1984). They also described the localization of microtubules to the newly endocytosed *Chlamydiae*, but the data did not distinguish between a direct role in uptake or simply a post-invasion localization to the newly endocytosed EB. The RNA interference screen studies conducted by Elwell et al. identified a number of host cell proteins that associate with or regulate the microtubule network, but the screen did not distinguish between effects on *Chlamydia* invasion or intracellular survival and replication (Elwell et al. 2008). It would not be surprising if microtubules were to be revealed as having an important role in invasion along with actin. Actin-microtubule interaction has been proposed for the invasion of a number of bacterial pathogens, including *Campylobacter jejuni* (Oelschlaeger et al. 1993; Biswas et al. 2000). This invasive pathogen utilizes actin- and microtubule-dependent mechanisms of entry, but the basis for this interaction has not been characterized. In the case of *Chlamydia*, actin and microtubules could cooperate to facilitate engulfment of the pathogen.

2.6 *Intermediate Filaments and* Chlamydia *Invasion*

The role of intermediate filaments on invasion has not been thoroughly investigated, but it would not be surprising because of the fundamental communication between the three major components of the cytoskeleton—filamentous actin, the microtubule network, and intermediate filaments (Chang and Goldman 2004). A potential involvement of intermediate filaments in invasion may be related to the FAK-dependent entry of *Chlamydia*, where pseudo-focal adhesion complexes are formed underneath the invading EB (Thwaites et al. 2014, 2015). Focal adhesions are sites of keratin filament assembly, with IF fragments relocating centripetally via interactions with the actin cytoskeleton (Windoffer et al. 2006; Leube et al. 2015). The significance of the intermediate filament association with focal adhesions is not completely clear, but may have a modulatory role in focal adhesion dynamics (Leube et al. 2015). Thus, the invasion-related pseudo-focal adhesion complexes may be subject to modulation by the colocalized intermediate filaments.

3 The Host Cell Cytoskeleton and the Vesicular Interactions and Structural Integrity of the Inclusion

3.1 *Early Observations of Nascent Inclusion Trafficking to the Microtubule Organizing Center*

Destabilization of the microtubule network leads to dramatic changes in the intracellular growth of *Chlamydia*. Dennis and Storz first reported that colchicine treatment of *Chlamydia psittaci*-infected mouse L cells led to larger inclusions (Dennis and Storz 1982). Campbell et al. observed microtubules surrounding the chlamydial inclusions and that the inclusions localized to the MTOC (Campbell et al. 1989a, b). Interestingly, when microtubules were allowed to re-polymerize after washout of nocodazole, rapid regeneration around the inclusions could be observed (Campbell et al. 1989b; Grieshaber et al. 2003). Studies by Schramm and Wyrick (1995) and Clausen et al. (1997) independently reported on additional changes to the intracellular growth of *Chlamydia* when the microtubule network was pharmacologically disrupted. The inclusions failed to translocate to the MTOC and multiple inclusions were observed (Schramm and Wyrick 1995; Clausen et al. 1997). For a number of chlamydial species, multiple nascent inclusions arising from high multiplicities of infection fuse to a single inclusion, and this homotypic fusion event is mediated by a functional microtubule network.

The association with the MTOC is a common feature of a number of chlamydial species, suggestive of an essential function (Clausen et al. 1997; Escalante-Ochoa et al. 1999). Because a number of nutrient-rich organelles concentrate around the MTOC by virtue of their association with the microtubule network, it is tempting to speculate a role for the MTOC localization that is related to nutrient acquisition. The chlamydial inclusion is known to transiently associate with multivesicular bodies (MVBs) (Beatty 2006, 2008; Robertson et al. 2009), lysosomes (Ouellette et al. 2011), autophagosomes (Al-Younes et al. 2004), the trans-Golgi network (TGN) (Hackstadt et al. 1995, 1996; Carabeo et al. 2003), the ER (Derré et al. 2011; Dumoux et al. 2012), and the endocytic recycling compartment (Ouellette et al. 2011) (Fig. 2). All of these compartments are potential sources of nutrients, including amino acids, lipids, cholesterol, and iron.

3.2 *Molecular Basis for MTOC Transport of Nascent Inclusions*

While the exact requirement for transport to the MTOC remains poorly defined, the molecular basis for this translocation process has become clearer (Fig. 2). Richards et al. determined that homotypic fusion is dependent on an intact microtubule network. Disruption of microtubule anchoring to the MTOC by expressing the EB1 mutant EB1.84 inhibited homotypic fusion (Richards et al. 2013). The role for an

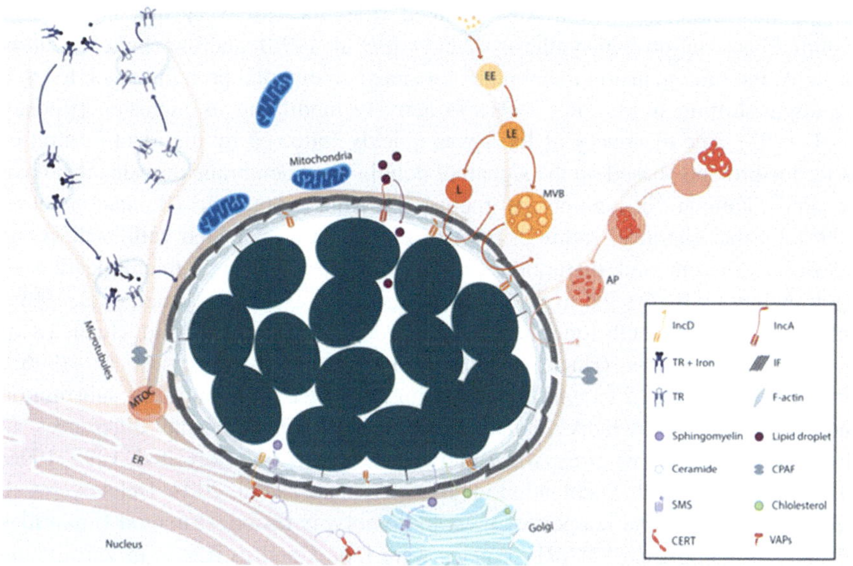

Fig. 2 The host cell cytoskeleton provides structural support for the growing inclusion and the maintenance of organelle distribution in its vicinity. A scaffold consisting of F-actin and cross-linked intermediate filaments (IF) are assembled around the inclusion. IF are remodeled by the chlamydial protease CPAF to accommodate the increase in size of the growing inclusion. The microtubule network surrounds the inclusion, and its post-translational detyrosination, as indicated by a different color facilitates the peri-inclusion localization of host cell organelles. *EE*—early endosomes; *LE*—late endosomes; *L*—lysosome; *MVB*—multivesicular body; *AP*—autophagosome; *TR*—transferrin receptor; *VAP*—vesicle-associated membrane protein-associated protein; *CERT*—ceramide transfer protein

intact microtubule is consistent with previous findings by Grieshaber et al. demonstrating a dynein-dependent directed transport of nascent inclusions along microtubule tracks to the MTOC (Grieshaber et al. 2003). Importantly, the process of transport to the MTOC was discovered to be directed by the pathogen, by substituting a pathogen-derived protein for the p50 dynamitin subunit (Grieshaber et al. 2003). Mittal et al. characterized the chlamydial protein CT850 and found it to interact with the dynein light chain DYNLT1; and as expected, DYNLT1 depletion led to the loss of MTOC-based aggregation of the nascent chlamydia-containing vacuoles (NCCVs) (Mital et al. 2015). Having a dedicated protein that interacts with the host dynein motor is indicative of an essential role in intracellular survival, and possibly in the development of disease. With the identification of the chlamydial factor, the biological relevance for MTOC localization can be characterized.

3.3 *Homotypic Fusion of* Chlamydia *Inclusions*

Once at the MTOC, the nascent inclusions are closely apposed to each other, possibly promoting inclusion fusion (Schramm and Wyrick 1995). Initial molecular insight into inclusion fusion was obtained from the discovery that the process required bacterial protein synthesis (Van Ooij et al. 1998), and the characterization of IncA, the first inclusion membrane-associated chlamydial protein, which led to a paradigm-shifting model of *Chlamydia* actively modifying its inclusion (Rockey et al. 1995). The discovery of IncA was quickly followed by the identification of other Inc proteins, based on the signature double-transmembrane domains that have become a hallmark of a number of inclusion membrane proteins (Bannantine et al. 1998). Further characterization of IncA revealed that it interacted with itself via its cytosolic domain; and disruption of this interaction through microinjection of neutralizing antibodies led to the loss of homotypic fusion (Hackstadt et al. 1999). Interestingly, this inclusion phenotype reproduced the multilobed character of *C. caviae* inclusions (Hackstadt et al. 1996, 1999; Rockey et al. 1996;). Examination of the *C. caviae* IncA ortholog identified an amino acid substitution that eliminated IncA-IncA interaction, possibly explaining the differences in inclusion morphologies of *C. caviae* and *C. trachomatis* (Rockey et al. 1995, 1996; Hackstadt et al. 1999; Suchland et al. 2000; Alzhanov et al. 2004; Delevoye et al. 2004, 2008). In further support of IncA in homotypic fusion, structural similarities of IncA to mammalian SNARE proteins were found, and its role in in vitro fusion assays confirmed (Delevoye et al. 2004, 2008; Paumet et al. 2009; Ronzone and Paumet 2013; Weber et al. 2016).

The role of inclusion fusion in *Chlamydia* biology is not known, but a potential biological relevance for inclusion fusion is that it enables genetic exchange between RBs. By fusing inclusions, RBs from different invasion events are placed in an optimal environment for lateral gene transfer and genetic recombination. However, being in the same inclusion is not an absolute requirement for genetic transfer (Suchland et al. 2009), but genetic exchange between RBs residing within the same inclusion would be more efficient when compared to interinclusion genetic transfer.

The working model that is emerging is that *Chlamydia* synthesizes CT850 to hijack the dynein motor complex and engage the microtubule network (Fig. 2). This leads to the transport of the nascent inclusion to the MTOC. IncA is synthesized by the inclusions, and based on the proposed SNARE-like structure, facilitates the homotypic fusion of multiple inclusions. Inclusion fusion could facilitate genetic exchange, although it is not required (Suchland et al. 2009). Positioning at the MTOC also could promote transient interactions with multiple nutrient-rich vesicles and organelles, providing an optimal environment for replication and production of infectious particles.

3.4 *Post-Translational Modification of Microtubules in* Chlamydia*-Infected Cells*

Post-translationally modified microtubules display changes to stability, with detyrosination associated with resistance to depolymerization or fragmentation. This process is achieved by the sequential removal of the original C-terminal tyrosine residue by a host tubulin carboxypeptidase from tubulin subunits within polymerized microtubules, followed by the re-addition of tyrosine by a tubulin tyrosine ligase. Despite the re-addition of a new tyrosine residue, the microtubule is classified as detyrosinated (reviewed in Song and Brady 2015). In *Chlamydia*-infected cells, detyrosinated microtubules (dtMT) were found at higher levels in infected cells at late times in infection, e.g. >24 h relative to uninfected cells (Al-Zeer et al. 2014) (Fig. 2). Interestingly, dtMTs were localized around inclusions and were relatively resistant to depolymerization induced by low-dose treatment with nocodazole (0.1 μM). A key observation was the inhibition of *Chlamydia* growth in the presence of parthenolide, a carboxypeptidase enzyme inhibitor. Parthenolide treatment also resulted in the loss of Golgi stacks that normally surrounded the inclusions (Al-Zeer et al. 2014). Thus, there might be a nutrition-related role for dtMTs in infected cells, and by stabilizing the subpopulation of microtubules that surrounds the inclusions, *Chlamydia* ensures that essential organelles, such as the Golgi apparatus remain juxtaposed to the inclusion. As mentioned above, the ER, mitochondria, and other organelles depend on microtubules for intracellular organization. Both are necessary for optimal chlamydial growth, and they localize specifically around the inclusion (Matsumoto et al. 1991; Derré et al. 2007, 2011; Dumoux et al. 2012). Thus, the inhibition of chlamydial growth arising from parthenolide treatment may not only affect the localization of the Golgi stack, but also of other organelles.

3.5 The Role of Actin and Intermediate Filaments in Inclusion Integrity

The role of actin in chlamydial inclusion biogenesis, maturation, and fusogenicity is relatively uncharacterized when compared to microtubules. While actin is robustly recruited during invasion, the F-actin network formed is rapidly disassembled. Based on live-cell imaging experiments, actin localization to nascent inclusions was not maintained, but instead re-established at later stages of inclusion maturation in the form of a scaffold that surrounds the mature inclusion (Campbell et al. 1989a; Kumar and Valdivia 2008; Chin et al. 2012) (Fig. 2). These structures are dynamic, with assembly being dependent on the RhoA GTPase, but independent of the Rho-associated protein kinase, ROCK (Kumar and Valdivia 2008). When disassembly was induced by latrunculin A, the inclusion exhibited weakened structural integrity (Kumar and Valdivia 2008). Thus, it appears that the actin network that surrounds the inclusion acts as a flexible scaffold that structurally support inclusion.

Intermediate filaments, specifically vimentin, cytokeratin-8, and cytokeratin-18 cooperated with the F-actin network to maintain the architectural integrity of the inclusion (Kumar and Valdivia 2008) (Fig. 2). Furthermore, the intermediate filaments were constantly remodeled by the chlamydial protease CPAF to accommodate the expanding inclusion (Dong et al. 2004; Kumar and Valdivia 2008; Savijoki et al. 2008). The specific cleavage of the head domain of vimentin by CPAF loosened, but did not completely disassemble the network (Kumar and Valdivia 2008). The cleavage of intermediate filaments reduced the lateral interactions of the protofilaments to provide sufficient flexibility to the scaffold during periods of rapid *Chlamydia* replication and inclusion growth (Kumar and Valdivia 2008). Given the importance of the actin-intermediate filament dynamics around the inclusion, it would not be surprising if there is a dedicated *Chlamydia*-driven machinery to recruit and remodel the cytoskeletal scaffold.

The actin localization around the inclusions was investigated further by Hybiske et al., and reported on the progressive actin recruitment at late times in infection in a manner that required a number of host signaling molecules, including N-WASP, myosin II, phosphatidylinositol 3-kinase, Rho GTPase, and ROCK among others (Hybiske and Stephens 2007; Chin et al. 2012) (Fig. 3). The recruitment of actin to the mature inclusion was also dependent on de novo chlamydial protein synthesis, but the specific protein(s) has not been identified (Chin et al. 2012). Were the actin structures observed by Hybiske et al. the same scaffold that Kumar and Valdivia described? The contrasting requirement for the RhoA kinase, ROCK, suggests that they might be distinct, but it remains possible that what Chin et al. observed may be the structure required for the extrusion of the inclusion, consistent with the timing of their observation e.g. >60 h post-infection (Chin et al. 2012). An intriguing possibility is that the actin/intermediate filament scaffold provides the structural foundation on which the extrusion machinery is assembled.

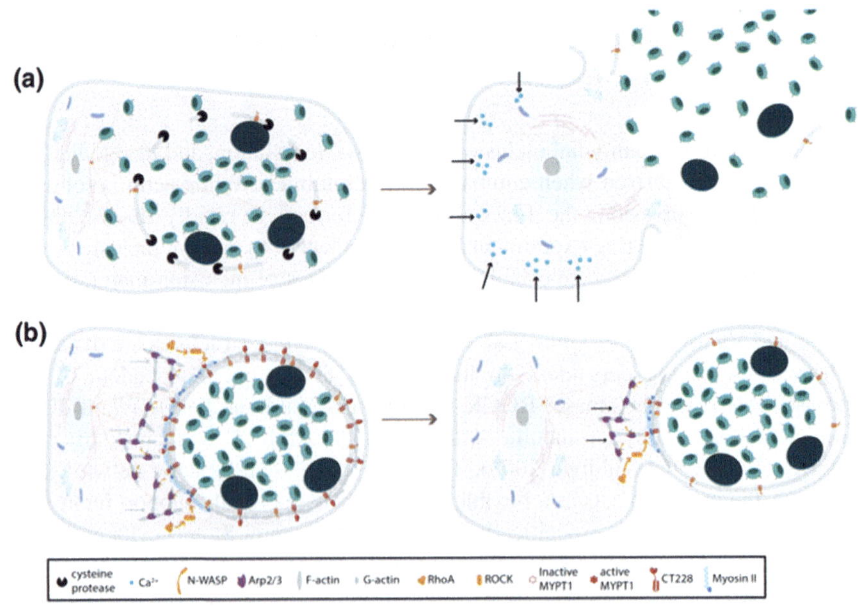

Fig. 3 *Chlamydia* egress can either be through host cell lysis or the extrusion of intact inclusions. Extrusion is dependent on host cell signaling that activates actin remodeling and the contractile function of myosin II

4 The Host Cell Cytoskeleton and *Chlamydia* Egress

4.1 Chlamydia *Egress by Extrusion of Intact Inclusions*

Chlamydia egress at the end-stage of infection is thought to occur via lysis, although there are hints from earlier reports that another mechanism that leaves the host cell intact, while infectious chlamydial particles are released (Todd and Caldwell 1985; Perfettini et al. 2003). Todd and Caldwell reported on the "scar" that remained at the plasma membrane after the presumed exocytosis of the chlamydial inclusion (Todd and Caldwell 1985). Hybiske and Stephens confirmed that a mechanism exists that extrudes intact inclusion (Fig. 3). They conducted a systematic investigation of potential host cell components involved in inclusion extrusion and identified the required host and bacterial factors, including actin, N-WASP, Rho GTPases, and myosin II in inclusion extrusion, cysteine proteases, and Ca^{2+} in host cell lysis-dependent egress (Hybiske and Stephens 2007). The activity of non-muscle myosin II was found to be indirectly modulated by *Chlamydia* via the inclusion membrane protein CT228 (Lutter et al. 2013). Lutter et al. discovered its interaction with the myosin phosphatase target 1 MYPT1, the regulatory subunit of protein phosphatase 1, leading to the sequestration of this negative regulator at the inclusion membrane. Interestingly, distinct domains within the inclusion were identified where either the active form of MYPT1 or the inactive form resided (Lutter et al. 2013). Active MYPT1 could be found around the inclusion, but the inactive form concentrated focally on a small microdomain that localized with active myosin light chain 2 (MLC2), myosin light chain kinase (MLCK), myosin IIA and myosin IIB (Lutter et al. 2013). The mechanical significance of this microdomain to inclusion extrusion remains to be elucidated. In addition, septins, which function as GTPases to regulate actin dynamics, was reported to be required for inclusion extrusion (Chin et al. 2012; Volceanov et al. 2014). Septins were found to organize in fibers around the inclusion and was speculated to serve as scaffolds for the assembly of the F-actin network essential for extrusion (Volceanov et al. 2014).

4.2 The Role of the Chlamydia *Plasmid in Extrusion Versus Lysis Decision*

A recent report by Yang et al. identified the role of the chlamydial plasmid in lytic exit (Yang et al. 2015). In plaquing assays, lytic *Chlamydiae* produce larger zones of cell death, while the plasmid-less L2R strain of *C. trachomatis* serovar L2 was inefficient in this process (Yang et al. 2015). Further investigations narrowed down the activity to the *Pgp4* open reading frame (Yang et al. 2015). How might the plasmid, and specifically Pgp4 be involved in favoring the lytic release of *Chlamydia*? The chlamydial plasmid is linked to virulence and regulation of genome-encoded genes (Carlson et al. 2008; Song et al. 2013), raising the possibility that the collection of chlamydial proteins involved in determining the means of egress is regulated by Pgp4.

From a pathogenesis perspective, while the plasmid-less strain is attenuated in in vivo infection models, the possibility exists that egress by extrusion is key to establishing chronic asymptomatic infection as proposed by Todd and Caldwell (Todd and Caldwell 1985). In addition, the protective immunity induced by the plasmid-less strain in the macaque model of ocular infection (Kari et al. 2011) may be due at least in part to the shift to the extrusion mode, raising the highly intriguing possibility that protective immunity may be enhanced by modulating the mechanism of *Chlamydia* egress from the host cell.

5 Summary

The cytoskeleton is a fundamental part of the host cell. Its involvement in a number of processes makes it an attractive target for subversion by microbial pathogens. For an obligate intracellular pathogen like *Chlamydia*, its ability to manipulate cytoskeleton-related host cell processes is paramount to its survival and replication. While the full mechanistic details of the subversion strategies remain unknown, the advent of genetic manipulation, including the creation of targeted mutants in *Chlamydia*, in conjunction with imaging and "-omics" techniques should substantially impact efforts to characterize *Chlamydia* basic biology, its virulence strategies, and important aspects of its interaction with the host.

References

Al-Bassam J, Kim H, Brouhard G et al (2010) CLASP promotes microtubule rescue by recruiting tubulin dimers to the microtubule. Dev Cell 19:245–258. doi:10.1016/j.devcel.2010.07.016

Al-Younes HM, Brinkmann V, Meyer TF (2004) Interaction of Chlamydia trachomatis serovar L2 with the host autophagic pathway. Infect Immun 72:4751–4762. doi:10.1128/IAI.72.8.4751-4762.2004

Al-Zeer MA, Al-Younes HM, Kerr M et al (2014) Chlamydia trachomatis remodels stable microtubules to coordinate Golgi stack recruitment to the chlamydial inclusion surface. Mol Microbiol 94:1285–1297. doi:10.1111/mmi.12829

Alzhanov D, Barnes J, Hruby DE, Rockey DD (2004) Chlamydial development is blocked in host cells transfected with Chlamydophila caviae incA. BMC Microbiol 4:24. doi:10.1186/1471-2180-4-24

Bannantine JP, Rockey DD, Hackstadt T (1998) Tandem genes of Chlamydia psittaci that encode proteins localized to the inclusion membrane. Mol Microbiol 28:1017–1026. doi:10.1046/j.1365-2958.1998.00867.x

Beatty WL (2006) Trafficking from CD63-positive late endocytic multivesicular bodies is essential for intracellular development of Chlamydia trachomatis. J Cell Sci 119:350–359. doi:10.1242/jcs.02733

Beatty WL (2008) Late endocytic multivesicular bodies intersect the chlamydial inclusion in the absence of CD63. Infect Immun 76:2872–2881. doi:10.1128/IAI.00129-08

Belmont LD, Mitchison TJ (1996) Identification of a protein that interacts with tubulin dimers and increases the catastrophe rate of microtubules. Cell 84:623–631. doi:10.1016/S0092-8674(00)81037-5

Benesch S, Polo S, Lai FPL et al (2005) N-WASP deficiency impairs EGF internalization and actin assembly at clathrin-coated pits. J Cell Sci 118:3103–3115. doi:10.1242/jcs.02444

Birkelund S, Johnsen H, Christiansen G (1994) Chlamydia trachomatis serovar L2 induces protein tyrosine phosphorylation during uptake by HeLa cells. Infect Immun 62:4900–4908

Biswas D, Itoh K, Sasakawa C (2000) Uptake pathways of clinical and healthy animal isolates of Campylobacter jejuni into INT-407 cells. FEMS Immunol Med Microbiol 29:203–211. doi:10.1111/j.1574-695X.2000.tb01524.x

Boleti H, Benmerah A, Ojcius DM, et al (1999) Chlamydia infection of epithelial cells expressing dynamin and Eps15 mutants: clathrin-independent entry into cells and dynamin-dependent productive growth. J Cell Sci 112 (Pt 1:1487–96)

Bothe M, Dutow P, Pich A et al (2015) DXD motif-dependent and -independent effects of the Chlamydia trachomatis cytotoxin CT166. Toxins (Basel) 7:621–637. doi:10.3390/toxins7020621

Bullock HD, Hower S, Fields KA (2012) Domain analyses reveal that Chlamydia trachomatis CT694 protein belongs to the membrane-localized family of type III effector proteins. J Biol Chem 287:28078–28086. doi:10.1074/jbc.M112.386904

Campbell S, Richmond SJ, Yates P (1989a) The development of Chlamydia trachomatis inclusions within the host eukaryotic cell during interphase and mitosis. J Gen Microbiol 135:1153–1165. doi:10.1099/00221287-135-5-1153

Campbell S, Richmond SJ, Yates PS (1989b) The effect of Chlamydia trachomatis infection on the host cell cytoskeleton and membrane compartments. J Gen Microbiol 135:2379–2386. doi:10.1099/00221287-135-9-2379

Campellone KG, Webb NJ, Znameroski EA, Welch MD (2008) WHAMM is an Arp2/3 complex activator that binds microtubules and functions in ER to Golgi transport. Cell 134:148–161. doi:10.1016/j.cell.2008.05.032

Carabeo RA, Grieshaber SS, Fischer E, Hackstadt T (2002) Chlamydia trachomatis induces remodeling of the actin cytoskeleton during attachment and entry into HeLa cells Chlamydia trachomatis induces remodeling of the actin cytoskeleton during attachment and entry into HeLa cells. 70:3793–3803. doi: 10.1128/IAI.70.7.3793

Carabeo RA, Mead DJ, Hackstadt T (2003) Golgi-dependent transport of cholesterol to the Chlamydia trachomatis inclusion. Proc Natl Acad Sci USA 100:6771–6776. doi:10.1073/pnas.1131289100

Carabeo RA, Grieshaber SS, Hasenkrug A et al (2004) Requirement for the Rac GTPase in Chlamydia trachomatis invasion of non-phagocytic cells. Traffic 5:418–425. doi:10.1111/j.1398-9219.2004.00184.x

Carabeo RA, Dooley CA, Grieshaber SS, Hackstadt T (2007) Rac interacts with Abi-1 and WAVE2 to promote an Arp2/3-dependent actin recruitment during chlamydial invasion. Cell Microbiol 9:2278–2288. doi:10.1111/j.1462-5822.2007.00958.x

Carlson JH, Whitmire WM, Crane DD et al (2008) The Chlamydia trachomatis plasmid is a transcriptional regulator of chromosomal genes and a virulence factor. Infect Immun 76:2273–2283. doi:10.1128/IAI.00102-08

Chang L, Goldman RD (2004) Intermediate filaments mediate cytoskeletal crosstalk. Nat Rev Mol Cell Biol 5:601–613. doi:10.1038/nrm1438

Chin E, Kirker K, Zuck M et al (2012) Actin recruitment to the Chlamydia inclusion is spatiotemporally regulated by a mechanism that requires host and bacterial factors. PLoS ONE 7:e46949. doi:10.1371/journal.pone.0046949

Clausen JD, Christiansen G, Holst HU, Birkelund S (1997) Chlamydia trachomatis utilizes the host cell microtubule network during early events of infection. Mol Microbiol 25:441–449. doi:10.1046/j.1365-2958.1997.4591832.x

Clifton DR, Fields KA, Grieshaber SS et al (2004) A chlamydial type III translocated protein is tyrosine-phosphorylated at the site of entry and associated with recruitment of actin. Proc Natl Acad Sci USA 101:10166–10171. doi:10.1073/pnas.0402829101

Clifton DR, Dooley CA, Grieshaber SS et al (2005) Tyrosine phosphorylation of the chlamydial effector protein tarp is species specific and not required for recruitment of actin. Infect Immun 73:3860–3868. doi:10.1128/IAI.73.7.3860-3868.2005

Cole NB, Sciaky N, Marotta A et al (1996) Golgi dispersal during microtubule disruption: regeneration of Golgi stacks at peripheral endoplasmic reticulum exit sites. Mol Biol Cell 7:631–650

Coombes BK, Mahony JB (2002) Identification of MEK- and phosphoinositide 3-kinase-dependent signalling as essential events during Chlamydia pneumoniae invasion of HEp2 cells. Cell Microbiol 4:447–460. doi:10.1046/j.1462-5822.2002.00203.x

de Forges H, Bouissou A, Perez F (2012) Interplay between microtubule dynamics and intracellular organization. Int J Biochem Cell Biol 44:266–274. doi:10.1016/j.biocel.2011.11.009

Delevoye C, Nilges M, Dautry-Varsat A, Subtil A (2004) Conservation of the biochemical properties of IncA from Chlamydia trachomatis and Chlamydia caviae: oligomerization of IncA mediates interaction between facing membranes. J Biol Chem 279:46896–46906. doi:10.1074/jbc.M407227200

Delevoye C, Nilges M, Dehoux P et al (2008) SNARE protein mimicry by an intracellular bacterium. PLoS Pathog 4:e1000022. doi:10.1371/journal.ppat.1000022

Dennis MW, Storz J (1982) Infectivity of Chlamydia psittaci of bovine and ovine origins for cultured cells. Am J Vet Res 43:1897–1902

Derré I, Pypaert M, Dautry-Varsat A, Agaisse H (2007) RNAi screen in Drosophila cells reveals the involvement of the Tom complex in Chlamydia infection. PLoS Pathog 3:1446–1458. doi:10.1371/journal.ppat.0030155

Derré I, Swiss R, Agaisse H (2011) The lipid transfer protein CERT interacts with the Chlamydia inclusion protein IncD and participates to ER-Chlamydia inclusion membrane contact sites. PLoS Pathog 7:e1002092. doi:10.1371/journal.ppat.1002092

Dong F, Su H, Huang Y et al (2004) Cleavage of host keratin 8 by a Chlamydia-secreted protease. Infect Immun 72:3863–3868. doi:10.1128/IAI.72.7.3863-3868.2004

Duleh SN, Welch MD (2010) WASH and the Arp2/3 complex regulate endosome shape and trafficking. Cytoskelet (Hoboken) 67:193–206. doi:10.1002/cm.20437

Dumoux M, Clare DK, Saibil HR, Hayward RD (2012) Chlamydiae assemble a pathogen synapse to hijack the host endoplasmic reticulum. Traffic 13:1612–1627. doi:10.1111/tra.12002

Elwell CA, Ceesay A, Kim JH et al (2008) RNA interference screen identifies Abl kinase and PDGFR signaling in Chlamydia trachomatis entry. PLoS Pathog 4:e1000021. doi:10.1371/journal.ppat.1000021

Escalante-Ochoa C, Ducatelle R, Charlier G et al (1999) Significance of host cell kinesin in the development of Chlamydia psittaci. Infect Immun 67:5441–5446

Fawaz FS, van Ooij C, Homola E et al (1997) Infection with Chlamydia trachomatis alters the tyrosine phosphorylation and/or localization of several host cell proteins including cortactin. Infect Immun 65:5301–5308

Geisler N, Schünemann J, Weber K (1992) Chemical cross-linking indicates a staggered and antiparallel protofilament of desmin intermediate filaments and characterizes one higher-level complex between protofilaments. Eur J Biochem 206:841–852

Grassart A, Cheng AT, Hong SH et al (2014) Actin and dynamin2 dynamics and interplay during clathrin-mediated endocytosis. J Cell Biol 205:721–735. doi:10.1083/jcb.201403041

Grieshaber SS, Grieshaber NA, Hackstadt T (2003) Chlamydia trachomatis uses host cell dynein to traffic to the microtubule-organizing center in a p50 dynamitin-independent process. J Cell Sci 116:3793–3802. doi:10.1242/jcs.00695

Hackstadt T, Scidmore MA, Rockey DD (1995) Lipid metabolism in Chlamydia trachomatis-infected cells: directed trafficking of Golgi-derived sphingolipids to the chlamydial inclusion. Proc Natl Acad Sci USA 92:4877–4881

Hackstadt T, Rockey DD, Heinzen RA, Scidmore MA (1996) Chlamydia trachomatis interrupts an exocytic pathway to acquire endogenously synthesized sphingomyelin in transit from the Golgi apparatus to the plasma membrane. EMBO J 15:964–977

Hackstadt T, Scidmore-Carlson MA, Shaw EI, Fischer ER (1999) The Chlamydia trachomatis IncA protein is required for homotypic vesicle fusion. Cell Microbiol 1:119–130. doi:10.1046/j.1462-5822.1999.00012.x

Ho WC, Allan VJ, van Meer G et al (1989) Reclustering of scattered Golgi elements occurs along microtubules. Eur J Cell Biol 48:250–263

Honnappa S, Gouveia SM, Weisbrich A et al (2009) An EB1-binding motif acts as a microtubule tip localization signal. Cell 138:366–376. doi:10.1016/j.cell.2009.04.065

Howell B, Larsson N, Gullberg M, Cassimeris L (1999) Dissociation of the tubulin-sequestering and microtubule catastrophe-promoting activities of oncoprotein 18/stathmin. Mol Biol Cell 10:105–118

Hybiske K, Stephens RS (2007) Mechanisms of host cell exit by the intracellular bacterium Chlamydia. Proc Natl Acad Sci USA 104:11430–11435. doi:10.1073/pnas.0703218104

Jewett TJ, Fischer ER, Mead DJ, Hackstadt T (2006) Chlamydial TARP is a bacterial nucleator of actin. Proc Natl Acad Sci USA 103:15599–15604. doi:10.1073/pnas.0603044103

Jewett TJ, Miller NJ, Dooley CA, Hackstadt T (2010) The conserved Tarp actin binding domain is important for chlamydial invasion. PLoS Pathog 6:e1000997. doi:10.1371/journal.ppat.1000997

Jiwani S, Ohr RJ, Fischer ER et al (2012) Chlamydia trachomatis Tarp cooperates with the Arp2/3 complex to increase the rate of actin polymerization. Biochem Biophys Res Commun 420:816–821. doi:10.1016/j.bbrc.2012.03.080

Johnston AB, Collins A, Goode BL (2015) High-speed depolymerization at actin filament ends jointly catalysed by Twinfilin and Srv2/CAP. Nat Cell Biol 17:1504–1511. doi:10.1038/ncb3252

Kari L, Whitmire WM, Olivares-Zavaleta N et al (2011) A live-attenuated chlamydial vaccine protects against trachoma in nonhuman primates. J Exp Med 208:2217–2223. doi:10.1084/jem.20111266

Kim SW, Ihn KS, Han SH et al (2001) Microtubule- and dynein-mediated movement of Orientia tsutsugamushi to the microtubule organizing center. Infect Immun 69:494–500. doi:10.1128/IAI.69.1.494-500.2001

Kim JH, Jiang S, Elwell CA, Engel JN (2011) Chlamydia trachomatis co-opts the FGF2 signaling pathway to enhance infection. PLoS Pathog 7:e1002285. doi:10.1371/journal.ppat.1002285

Koestler SA, Steffen A, Nemethova M et al (2013) Arp2/3 complex is essential for actin network treadmilling as well as for targeting of capping protein and cofilin. Mol Biol Cell 24:2861–2875. doi:10.1091/mbc.E12-12-0857

Komarova Y, Lansbergen G, Galjart N et al (2005) EB1 and EB3 control CLIP dissociation from the ends of growing microtubules. Mol Biol Cell 16:5334–5345. doi:10.1091/mbc.E05-07-0614

Komarova Y, De Groot CO, Grigoriev I et al (2009) Mammalian end binding proteins control persistent microtubule growth. J Cell Biol 184:691–706. doi:10.1083/jcb.200807179

Ku NO, Omary MB (1994) Identification of the major physiologic phosphorylation site of human keratin 18: potential kinases and a role in filament reorganization. J Cell Biol 127:161–171

Ku NO, Omary MB (1997) Phosphorylation of human keratin 8 in vivo at conserved head domain serine 23 and at epidermal growth factor-stimulated tail domain serine 431. J Biol Chem 272:7556–7564

Kumar Y, Valdivia RH (2008) Actin and intermediate filaments stabilize the Chlamydia trachomatis vacuole by forming dynamic structural scaffolds. Cell Host Microbe 4:159–169. doi:10.1016/j.chom.2008.05.018

Lane BJ, Mutchler C, Al Khodor S et al (2008) Chlamydial entry involves TARP binding of guanine nucleotide exchange factors. PLoS Pathog 4:e1000014

Larsson N, Segerman B, Gradin HM et al (1999) Mutations of oncoprotein 18/stathmin identify tubulin-directed regulatory activities distinct from tubulin association. Mol Cell Biol 19:2242–2250

Leube RE, Moch M, Windoffer R (2015) Intermediate filaments and the regulation of focal adhesion. Curr Opin Cell Biol 32:13–20. doi:10.1016/j.ceb.2014.09.011

Lutter EI, Barger AC, Nair V, Hackstadt T (2013) Chlamydia trachomatis inclusion membrane protein CT228 recruits elements of the myosin phosphatase pathway to regulate release mechanisms. Cell Rep 3:1921–1931. doi:10.1016/j.celrep.2013.04.027

Maiato H, Khodjakov A, Rieder CL (2005) Drosophila CLASP is required for the incorporation of microtubule subunits into fluxing kinetochore fibres. Nat Cell Biol 7:42–47. doi:10.1038/ncb1207

Majeed M, Kihlström E (1991) Mobilization of F-actin and clathrin during redistribution of Chlamydia trachomatis to an intracellular site in eucaryotic cells. Infect Immun 59:4465–4472

Matsumoto A, Bessho H, Uehira K, Suda T (1991) Morphological studies of the association of mitochondria with chlamydial inclusions and the fusion of chlamydial inclusions. J Electron Microsc (Tokyo) 40:356–363

Mennella V, Rogers GC, Rogers SL et al (2005) Functionally distinct kinesin-13 family members cooperate to regulate microtubule dynamics during interphase. Nat Cell Biol 7:235–245. doi:10.1038/ncb1222

Miki H, Sasaki T, Takai Y, Takenawa T (1998) Induction of filopodium formation by a WASP-related actin-depolymerizing protein N-WASP. Nature 391:93–96. doi:10.1038/34208

Mital J, Lutter EI, Barger AC et al (2015) Chlamydia trachomatis inclusion membrane protein CT850 interacts with the dynein light chain DYNLT1 (Tctex1). Biochem Biophys Res Commun 462:165–170. doi:10.1016/j.bbrc.2015.04.116

Mölleken K, Becker E, Hegemann JH (2013) The Chlamydia pneumoniae invasin protein Pmp21 recruits the EGF receptor for host cell entry. PLoS Pathog 9:e1003325. doi:10.1371/journal.ppat.1003325

Nakagawa H, Miki H, Ito M et al (2001) N-WASP, WAVE and Mena play different roles in the organization of actin cytoskeleton in lamellipodia. J Cell Sci 114:1555–1565

Newton CN, Wagenbach M, Ovechkina Y et al (2004) MCAK, a Kin I kinesin, increases the catastrophe frequency of steady-state HeLa cell microtubules in an ATP-dependent manner in vitro. FEBS Lett 572:80–84. doi:10.1016/j.febslet.2004.06.093

Oelschlaeger TA, Guerry P, Kopecko DJ (1993) Unusual microtubule-dependent endocytosis mechanisms triggered by Campylobacter jejuni and Citrobacter freundii. Proc Natl Acad Sci USA 90:6884–6888

Oguchi Y, Uchimura S, Ohki T et al (2011) The bidirectional depolymerizer MCAK generates force by disassembling both microtubule ends. Nat Cell Biol 13:846–852. doi:10.1038/ncb2256

Ouellette SP, Dorsey FC, Moshiach S et al (2011) Chlamydia species-dependent differences in the growth requirement for lysosomes. PLoS ONE 6:e16783. doi:10.1371/journal.pone.0016783

Paramio JM, Casanova ML, Alonso A, Jorcano JL (1997) Keratin intermediate filament dynamics in cell heterokaryons reveals diverse behaviour of different keratins. J Cell Sci 110 (Pt 9:1099–111)

Paumet F, Wesolowski J, Garcia-Diaz A et al (2009) Intracellular bacteria encode inhibitory SNARE-like proteins. PLoS ONE 4:e7375. doi:10.1371/journal.pone.0007375

Perfettini J-L, Hospital V, Stahl L et al (2003) Cell death and inflammation during infection with the obligate intracellular pathogen, Chlamydia. Biochimie 85:763–769

Peris L (2006) Tubulin tyrosination is a major factor affecting the recruitment of CAP-Gly proteins at microtubule plus ends. J Cell Biol 174:839–849. doi:10.1083/jcb.200512058

Peris L, Wagenbach M, Lafanechère L et al (2009) Motor-dependent microtubule disassembly driven by tubulin tyrosination. J Cell Biol 185:1159–1166. doi:10.1083/jcb.200902142

Pizarro-Cerdá J, Kühbacher A, Cossart P (2015) Phosphoinositides and host-pathogen interactions. Biochim Biophys Acta 1851:911–918. doi:10.1016/j.bbalip.2014.09.011

Pring M, Weber A, Bubb MR (1992) Profilin-actin complexes directly elongate actin filaments at the barbed end. Biochemistry 31:1827–1836

Radhakrishnan GK, Splitter GA (2012) Modulation of host microtubule dynamics by pathogenic bacteria. Biomol Concepts. 3:571–580

Richards TS, Knowlton AE, Grieshaber SS (2013) Chlamydia trachomatis homotypic inclusion fusion is promoted by host microtubule trafficking. BMC Microbiol 13:185. doi:10.1186/1471-2180-13-185

Robertson DK, Gu L, Rowe RK, Beatty WL (2009) Inclusion biogenesis and reactivation of persistent Chlamydia trachomatis requires host cell sphingolipid biosynthesis. PLoS Pathog 5: e1000664. doi:10.1371/journal.ppat.1000664

Rockey DD, Heinzen RA, Hackstadt T (1995) Cloning and characterization of a Chlamydia psittaci gene coding for a protein localized in the inclusion membrane of infected cells. Mol Microbiol 15:617–626. doi:10.1111/j.1365-2958.1995.tb02371.x

Rockey DD, Fischer ER, Hackstadt T (1996) Temporal analysis of the developing Chlamydia psittaci inclusion by use of fluorescence and electron microscopy. Infect Immun 64:4269–4278

Ronzone E, Paumet F (2013) Two coiled-coil domains of Chlamydia trachomatis IncA affect membrane fusion events during infection. PLoS ONE 8:e69769. doi:10.1371/journal.pone.0069769

Savijoki K, Alvesalo J, Vuorela P et al (2008) Proteomic analysis of Chlamydia pneumoniae-infected HL cells reveals extensive degradation of cytoskeletal proteins. FEMS Immunol Med Microbiol 54:375–384. doi:10.1111/j.1574-695X.2008.00488.x

Schaus TE, Taylor EW, Borisy GG (2007) Self-organization of actin filament orientation in the dendritic-nucleation/array-treadmilling model. Proc Natl Acad Sci USA 104:7086–7091. doi:10.1073/pnas.0701943104

Schramm N, Wyrick PB (1995) Cytoskeletal requirements in Chlamydia trachomatis infection of host cells. Infect Immun 63:324–332

Song Y, Brady ST (2015) Post-translational modifications of tubulin: pathways to functional diversity of microtubules. Trends Cell Biol 25:125–136. doi:10.1016/j.tcb.2014.10.004

Song L, Carlson JH, Whitmire WM et al (2013) Chlamydia trachomatis plasmid-encoded Pgp4 is a transcriptional regulator of virulence-associated genes. Infect Immun 81:636–644. doi:10.1128/IAI.01305-12

Stallmann S, Hegemann JH (2015) The Chlamydia trachomatis Ctad1 invasin exploits the human integrin β1 receptor for host cell entry. Cell Microbiol. doi:10.1111/cmi.12549

Steinböck FA, Nikolic B, Coulombe PA, et al (2000) Dose-dependent linkage, assembly inhibition and disassembly of vimentin and cytokeratin 5/14 filaments through plectin's intermediate filament-binding domain. J Cell Sci 113 (Pt 3:483–491)

Subtil A, Wyplosz B, Balañá ME, Dautry-Varsat A (2004) Analysis of Chlamydia caviae entry sites and involvement of Cdc42 and Rac activity. J Cell Sci 117:3923–3933. doi:10.1242/jcs.01247

Suchland RJ, Rockey DD, Bannantine JP, Stamm WE (2000) Isolates of Chlamydia trachomatis that occupy nonfusogenic inclusions lack IncA, a protein localized to the inclusion membrane. Infect Immun 68:360–367

Suchland RJ, Sandoz KM, Jeffrey BM et al (2009) Horizontal transfer of tetracycline resistance among Chlamydia spp. in vitro. Antimicrob Agents Chemother 53:4604–4611. doi:10.1128/AAC.00477-09

Thalmann J, Janik K, May M et al (2010) Actin re-organization induced by Chlamydia trachomatis serovar D–evidence for a critical role of the effector protein CT166 targeting Rac. PLoS ONE 5:e9887. doi:10.1371/journal.pone.0009887

Thwaites T, Nogueira AT, Campeotto I et al (2014) The Chlamydia effector TarP mimics the mammalian leucine-aspartic acid motif of paxillin to subvert the focal adhesion kinase during invasion. J Biol Chem 289:30426–30442. doi:10.1074/jbc.M114.604876

Thwaites TR, Pedrosa AT, Peacock TP, Carabeo RA (2015) Vinculin interacts with the Chlamydia effector TarP Via a tripartite vinculin binding domain to mediate actin recruitment and assembly at the plasma membrane. Front Cell Infect Microbiol 5:88. doi:10.3389/fcimb.2015.00088

Thyberg J (1980) Internalization of cationized ferritin into the Golgi complex of cultured mouse peritoneal macrophages. Effects of colchicine and cytochalasin B. Eur J Cell Biol 23:95–103

Todd WJ, Caldwell HD (1985) The interaction of Chlamydia trachomatis with host cells: ultrastructural studies of the mechanism of release of a biovar II strain from HeLa 229 cells. J Infect Dis 151:1037–1044

Traub P, Scherbarth A, Wiegers W, Shoeman RL (1992) Salt-stable interaction of the amino-terminal head region of vimentin with the alpha-helical rod domain of cytoplasmic intermediate filament proteins and its relevance to protofilament structure and filament formation and stability. J Cell Sci 101 (Pt 2:363–381)

Truong D, Copeland JW, Brumell JH (2014) Bacterial subversion of host cytoskeletal machinery: hijacking formins and the Arp2/3 complex. BioEssays 36:687–696. doi:10.1002/bies.201400038

Tsuruta D, Jones JCR (2003) The vimentin cytoskeleton regulates focal contact size and adhesion of endothelial cells subjected to shear stress. J Cell Sci 116:4977–4984. doi:10.1242/jcs.00823

Van Ooij C, Homola E, Kincaid E, Engel J (1998) Fusion of Chlamydia trachomatis-containing inclusions is inhibited at low temperatures and requires bacterial protein synthesis. Infect Immun 66:5364–5371

Volceanov L, Herbst K, Biniossek M et al (2014) Septins arrange F-actin-containing fibers on the Chlamydia trachomatis inclusion and are required for normal release of the inclusion by extrusion. MBio 5:e01802–e01814. doi:10.1128/mBio.01802-14

Wanger M, Wegner A (1985) Equilibrium constant for binding of an actin filament capping protein to the barbed end of actin filaments. Biochemistry 24:1035–1040

Wagner OI, Rammensee S, Korde N et al (2007) Softness, strength and self-repair in intermediate filament networks. Exp Cell Res 313:2228–2235. doi:10.1016/j.yexcr.2007.04.025

Ward ME, Murray A (1984) Control mechanisms governing the infectivity of Chlamydia trachomatis for HeLa cells: mechanisms of endocytosis. J Gen Microbiol 130:1765–1780. doi:10.1099/00221287-130-7-1765

Weber MM, Noriea NF, Bauler LD et al (2016) A functional core of IncA is required for Chlamydia trachomatis inclusion fusion. J Bacteriol. doi:10.1128/JB.00933-15

Wehland J, Henkart M, Klausner R, Sandoval IV (1983) Role of microtubules in the distribution of the Golgi apparatus: effect of taxol and microinjected anti-alpha-tubulin antibodies. Proc Natl Acad Sci USA 80:4286–4290

Windoffer R, Kölsch A, Wöll S, Leube RE (2006) Focal adhesions are hotspots for keratin filament precursor formation. J Cell Biol 173:341–348. doi:10.1083/jcb.200511124

Yang C, Starr T, Song L et al (2015) Chlamydial lytic exit from host cells is plasmid regulated. MBio 6:e01648–e01615. doi:10.1128/mBio.01648-15

Yu X, Zech T, McDonald L et al (2012) N-WASP coordinates the delivery and F-actin-mediated capture of MT1-MMP at invasive pseudopods. J Cell Biol 199:527–544. doi:10.1083/jcb.201203025

Subversion of Cell-Autonomous Host Defense by *Chlamydia* Infection

Annette Fischer and Thomas Rudel

Abstract Obligate intracellular bacteria entirely depend on the metabolites of their host cell for survival and generation of progeny. Due to their lifestyle inside a eukaryotic cell and the lack of any extracellular niche, they have to perfectly adapt to compartmentalized intracellular environment of the host cell and counteract the numerous defense strategies intrinsically present in all eukaryotic cells. This so-called cell-autonomous defense is present in all cell types encountering *Chlamydia* infection and is in addition closely linked to the cellular innate immune defense of the mammalian host. Cell type and chlamydial species-restricted mechanisms point a long-term evolutionary adaptation that builds the basis of the currently observed host and cell-type tropism among different *Chlamydia* species. This review will summarize the current knowledge on the strategies pathogenic *Chlamydia* species have developed to subvert and overcome the multiple mechanisms by which eukaryotic cells defend themselves against intracellular pathogens.

Abbreviations

DAMP	Danger-associated molecular pattern
GBP	Guanylate-binding protein
IDO	2,3-indoleamine dioxygenase
IRG	Immunity-related GTPase
ISG	Interferon-stimulated gene
NLR	NOD-like receptor
PAMP	Pathogen-associated molecular pattern
PRR	Pattern recognition receptor
RNS	Reactive nitrogen species
ROS	Reactive oxygen species

A. Fischer · T. Rudel (✉)
Department of Microbiology and Biocenter, University of Würzburg,
Am Hubland, 97074 Wuerzburg, Germany
e-mail: thomas.rudel@biozentrum.uni-wuerzburg.de

A. Fischer
e-mail: annette.fischer@uni-wuerzburg.de

Current Topics in Microbiology and Immunology (2018) 412:81–106
DOI 10.1007/82_2016_13

Published Online: 13 May 2016

T3SS Type 3 secretion system
T4SS Type 4 secretion system
TLR Toll-like receptor
ULK Uncoordinated 51-like kinase

Contents

1 Introduction

The family Chlamydiaceae consists of environmental and pathogenic *Chlamydia* species with the most relevant human pathogenic species *Chlamydia trachomatis* (*Ctr*) and *Chlamydia pneumoniae* (*Cpn*). *Ctr* is the most common sexually transmitted pathogen and causes infections of the urogenital tract resulting in pelvic inflammatory disease (Bebear and de Barbeyrac 2009; Bartlett et al. 2013) and infertility (Baud and Greub 2011) or severe eye infections called trachoma (Wright et al. 2008). On the contrary, *Cpn* cause infections of the upper respiratory tract leading to community-acquired pneumonia, bronchitis (Grayston et al. 1993; Hahn 1998), or asthma (Hahn 1998) and are discussed to be associated with atherosclerotic cardiovascular disease (Boman and Hammerschlag 2002), Alzheimer's disease, and multiple sclerosis (Stratton and Sriram 2003). Besides the two major human pathogenic *Chlamydia* species, *Chlamydia psittaci* (*Cps*) can be transmitted from birds to humans, thereby causing severe pneumonia called psittacosis (Knittler and Sachse 2015). *Simkania negevensis* (*Sn*) was thought to be an environmental bacterium; however, recent work shows that *Sn* can infect several human cell lines and is discussed to be associated with lung infections in humans (Friedman et al. 2003; Greenberg et al. 2003).

All *Chlamydia* are obligate intracellular pathogens that replicate inside their host cell and undergo a biphasic life cycle (Moulder 1991). The infectious but non-replicating form of *Chlamydia* is called elementary body (EB) which differentiates after host cell entry into the replicative form called reticulate body (RB). RBs multiply by binary fission, redifferentiate into EBs at the end of the developmental cycle, and are then released by host cell lysis or extrusion. If *Chlamydia*-infected cells are challenged with antibiotics, interferon (IFN) γ, or face nutrition starvation, RBs differentiate into a persistence form called aberrant body (AB) (Beatty et al. 1994b). ABs do not multiply and are like RBs not able to infect cells. Since RBs and ABs are non-infectious, premature host cell death would cause the complete loss of infectious progeny. Therefore, *Chlamydia* established multiple mechanisms to prevent host cell death induced either by intracellular stress signals or by the immune system (Sharma and Rudel 2009; Bastidas et al. 2013). All *Chlamydia* species are able to inhibit apoptosis by the block of mitochondrial Cytochrome *c* release and inhibition of Caspase-3 activation, whereas apoptosis signaling via Caspase-8 activation is permitted (Fan et al. 1998; Fischer et al. 2004). However, the detailed molecular mechanisms underlying the inhibition of apoptosis vary between each *Chlamydia* species and will be discussed in detail below.

Chlamydia preferably infect epithelial cells and thereby induce the secretion of pro-inflammatory cytokines and recruitment of leukocytes to the site of infection. Induction of an inflammatory response by infected epithelial cells as well as inflammatory leukocytes causes direct damage to the surrounding tissue (Rasmussen et al. 1997). Reinfection by *Chlamydia* is frequently observed (Burstein et al. 1998; Molano et al. 2005) inducing repeated inflammation, severe tissue damage, and scarring, which are the main symptoms and causes of pathogenesis during *Chlamydia* infections (Darville and Hiltke 2010). It was shown that IFNγ secretion by T cells is important for the clearance of *Chlamydia* infections (Perry et al. 1997; Cotter et al. 1997). In cell culture experiments, low doses of INFγ induce persistence in *Chlamydia* (Beatty et al. 1993, 1994b). However, IFNγ-induced persistence in vivo has not been shown yet. During each round of the developmental cycle, *Chlamydia* produce hundreds of infectious progeny which would cause a rapid spread and progression of the infection. Nevertheless, clinical *Chlamydia* infections tend to remain asymptomatic and slowly progressing, in line with frequent persistence and reactivation phases and non-continuous chlamydial replication in the patient (Beatty et al. 1994b; Phillips Campbell et al. 2012).

2 Innate Immunity Against Intracellular Bacteria

2.1 The Innate Immune System

The innate immune system is conserved in all plant and animal species and uses unspecific but efficient mechanisms to inhibit pathogen entry and replication inside the host. Human pathogens have to enter their host via the dermis or mucosa, which represent a natural barrier for invading pathogens. These tissues are covered with cilia, mucus, or saliva containing antimicrobial peptides or enzymes, such as defensins or lysozyme. Furthermore, after successful invasion of the host, the bacteria are combatted by the cellular arm of the innate immune system represented by professional phagocytes such as macrophages, monocytes, neutrophils, and dendritic cells. Pathogenic bacteria are phagocytized by immune cells and end up mostly in phagosomes. Fusion of the phagosome with lysosomes results in the acidification as well as accumulation of hydrolytic enzymes, antimicrobial peptides, and the production of reactive oxygen species (ROS) to finally inactivate and destroy the pathogen (Kumar et al. 2011; Gordon and Read 2002).

The innate immune system identifies pathogens by highly conserved microbial structures, the so-called pathogen-associated molecular patterns (PAMPs). PAMPs, e.g., lipopolysaccharide, peptidoglycan, or flagellin, are recognized by pattern recognition receptors (PRRs) which initiate an immune response upon ligand binding. PRRs expressed on the cell surface sense extracellular pathogens. They include Toll-like receptors (TLRs), C-type lectin receptors (CLRs), and scavenger receptors. Alternatively, NOD-like receptors (NLRs) and RIG-I-like receptors (RLRs) represent intracellular PRRs which are able to sense intracellular bacteria, their effector proteins or toxins (Kumar et al. 2009, 2011). In general, PRR ligand binding activates NF-κB and MAPK signaling cascades, leading to the expression and secretion of pro-inflammatory cytokines, chemokines, type I IFNs, and antimicrobial peptides. PAMP recognition by TLRs induces complex formation of the adaptor protein MyD88 with IRAK and TRAF6, which triggers phosphorylation and subsequent degradation of IκB. Destruction of IκB activates the transcription regulator NF-κB, which translocates into the nucleus to induce gene expression of multiple pro-inflammatory genes, such as the pro-inflammatory cytokines interleukin (IL)-1β, IL-6, tumor necrosis factor (TNF) α, and type I IFNs (Takeuchi and Akira 2010; Kawai and Akira 2006). These cytokines are sensed by the surrounding cells and induce an inflammatory response including enhanced vascular endothelial permeability, recruitment of effector immune cells to the site of infection, production of acute-phase proteins, and cell death of inflamed tissue.

2.2 Cell-autonomous Immunity

To evade the recognition by the innate immune system, some bacteria acquired the ability to invade and replicate inside cells (Kumar and Valdivia 2009). However, all cells of the body are armed with cell-autonomous defense mechanism to restrict intracellular bacterial survival and replication independent of the immune system (MacMicking 2012). These cell-autonomous defense mechanisms include targeting the pathogen to phagolysosomes or autophagosomes, NF-κB- and IFN-dependent expression of cytokines and antimicrobial effectors, the activation of the inflammasome and IL-1β secretion, and the induction of host cell death. The recognition and destruction of the pathogen by these inherent mechanisms usually leads to the activation of the innate immune system. Neighboring cells are alerted by cytokine signaling, enhancing also the efficiency of cell-autonomous defense mechanisms against invading bacteria (Gomes and Dikic 2014; Meunier and Broz 2015; Shimada et al. 2012). Cell-autonomous defense mechanisms and the innate immune system, in particular the activation of professional phagocytes, are closely connected in their fight against pathogenic microbes and rely to some extent on the same mechanisms.

Some bacteria acquired the ability to invade and replicate in cells to avoid recognition by the complement system or patrolling immune cells. Most bacteria enter their host cell by induced phagocytosis and thereby end up in phagosomes, which then fuse with lysosomes leading to the destruction of the bacteria. One possibility to evade lysosomal destruction is the phagosomal escape of the bacteria into the cytosol. However, cytosolic bacteria or their secreted effector proteins and toxins are sensed by intracellular PRRs, e.g., NLRs or RLRs, which activate inflammatory response mechanisms or infection-induced host cell death (Akira et al. 2006; Broz and Monack 2011, 2013; Meunier and Broz 2015). Furthermore, cytosolic bacteria can be recognized by the autophagy system and be destroyed in autophagosomes in a process called xenophagy (Randow and Youle 2014; Deretic et al. 2013). Only some bacteria, such as *Listeria monocytogenes*, *Francisella novicida,* and *Shigella flexneri,* are able to replicate in the host cell cytosol and avoid xenophagy and induction of inflammation (Asrat et al. 2014; Kumar and Valdivia 2009; Yang et al. 2015). For instance, *L. monocytogenes* expresses the virulence factor listeriolysin O to lyse the phagosome and enable cytosolic replication (Joseph and Goebel 2007). Other intracellular bacteria, e.g., *Ctr, Salmonella typhimurium, Legionella pneumophila,* and *Mycobacterium tuberculosis,* have developed mechanisms to block fusion of the phagosome with lysosomes and are thereby able to replicate inside a so-called pathogen containing vacuole (PCV) (Simon and Hilbi 2015; Creasey and Isberg 2014). Inside the PCV, the bacteria are protected from detection by the immune system. However, the bacteria have to actively maintain the PCV, block fusion with lysosomes, and manipulate host cell signaling to establish its intracellular replication niche. Intracellular bacteria accomplish this through the secretion of effector proteins by their type 3 (T3SS) and type 4 secretion systems (T4SS). Mutation or inactivation of effector proteins or their delivery machines most often results in the breakdown of the PCV, recognition of the bacteria by the autophagy machinery, and induction of an innate immune response which leads to a rapid clearance of infection (Beuzon et al. 2000; Creasey and Isberg 2012; Vergne et al. 2004).

Nevertheless, vacuolar replicating bacteria are not completely protected from the recognition of the innate immune system. Secreted effector proteins as well as components of their secretion machinery are recognized by intracellular NLRs and thereby induce assembly of a multiprotein complex called inflammasome (Lamkanfi and Dixit 2011). Dependent on the N-terminal domain of NLRs, which is important for the interaction with the adaptor protein ASC, they are categorized into NLRPs containing a PYR domain or NLRCs with a CARD domain (Oviedo-Boyso et al. 2014; Schroder and Tschopp 2010). Upon ligand binding or sensing of intracellular stress signals—so-called danger-associated molecular patterns (DAMPs)—NLRs associate with the adaptor protein ASC and induce autocatalytic cleavage of pro-Caspase-1 to form an active inflammasome (Lamkanfi et al. 2007). Inflammasomes are involved in the activation and secretion of the pro-inflammatory cytokines IL-1β and IL-18 or induction of cell death called pyroptosis, accompanied by DNA fragmentation, perforation of the plasma membrane, cell swelling, and finally cell lysis (Lamkanfi and Dixit 2014).

One major class of cytokines involved in defense of intracellular pathogens is interferon which is classified into three families: the type I, type II, and type III IFNs. Type I IFNs include among others IFNα and IFNβ, which are expressed and secreted upon PRR activation (Ivashkiv and Donlin 2014; Schneider et al. 2014; Platanias 2005). In contrast, the class of type II interferon comprises only IFNγ, which is released by activated T lymphocytes and natural killer cells (Schneider et al. 2014; Sadler and Williams 2008; Nathan et al. 1983). Type I and type II IFNs promote the expression of over 2000 IFN-stimulated genes (ISGs), which enhance pathogen detection and restrict intracellular replication of viruses and bacteria by inducing the production of ROS and reactive nitrogen species (RNS), destabilizing membranes of the PCV to induce autophagy, as well as limiting availability of intracellular cations (MacMicking 2012; Coccia and Battistini 2015).

Xenophagy, a selective form of autophagy, represents a cell-autonomous defense mechanism to eliminate invading microorganisms directly upon phagocytosis or after release of the bacteria into the cytosol (Gomes and Dikic 2014). Upon induction of autophagy, the uncoordinated 51-like kinase (ULK) complex initiates autophagosome biogenesis. Subsequently, ATG12- and LC3-conjugation systems are assembled that promote autophagosome elongation and engulfment of the material into double-membraned autophagosomes, which are targeted for lysosomal destruction (Deretic et al. 2013). Ubiquitination of free bacteria, as reported for cytosolic *Salmonella* (van Wijk et al. 2012), is a common "eat-me" signal for selective autophagy. The ubiquitin moieties are recognized by specific autophagy receptors, such as p62, NDP52, or optineurin (OPNT), which recruit the autophagy machinery via LC3 interaction to induce autolysosomal degradation of the pathogen (Gomes and Dikic 2014). Furthermore, phagolysosomal destruction of phagocytosed microorganisms is enhanced by a mechanism called LC3-associated phagocytosis (LAP), which is induced by TLR signaling. During LAP, the phagosomal membrane is directly modified with LC3 by the LC3-conjugation system of the autophagy machinery, which enhances maturation to phagolysosomes (Sanjuan et al. 2007, 2009).

3 Subversion of Host Innate Defense by *Chlamydia*

3.1 *Interference with IFN-Signaling and Autophagy*

Chlamydia are able to infect multiple cell types including epithelial and endothelial cells and macrophages. The ability for intracellular survival and replication in these cells varies tremendously between different *Chlamydia* species (Herweg and Rudel 2015; Beagley et al. 2009). All *Chlamydia* prefer non-immune cells for intracellular replication. However, EBs released from the host cell can be phagocytosed by macrophages patrolling in tissues. If *Chlamydia* are able to prevent maturation of the phagolysosome, they can survive, persist, or even replicate in macrophages. *Cpn* and *Sn* are able to multiply in macrophages and produce infectious progeny, whereas *Ctr* and *Cps* fail to replicate in these immune cells (Beagley et al. 2009). *Ctr* and *Cps* are directed to autolysosomes, since their inclusions are positive for the well-known autophagy and lysosomal markers such as LC3 and Rab7, respectively (Sun et al. 2012; Al-Zeer et al. 2013).

Each *Chlamydia* species is well-adapted to the immune system of their respective host but is susceptible to defense mechanisms of divergent host species. These differences in the response to infection can be explained by the differences in IFN-signaling between human and murine cells. For instance, challenging a mouse with the human pathogenic strain *Ctr* results in an attenuated infection, which is rapidly cleared compared to infections with the murine adapted *Cmu* strain MoPn (McClarty et al. 2007; Nelson et al. 2005). IFN-signaling is an important element in the defense of intracellular pathogens. In particular, IFNγ is a major mediator of antimicrobial defense against *Chlamydia* (Rottenberg et al. 2002; Carlin and Weller 1995) and plays a role in the species-dependent clearance of *Chlamydia* infections (McClarty et al. 2007; Nelson et al. 2005; Roshick et al. 2006). It was shown that *Chlamydia* infection of INFγ-challenged human cells induces 2,3-indoleamine dioxygenase (IDO) expression, which catalyzes degradation of tryptophan pools important for chlamydial intracellular growth (Beatty et al. 1994a). *Ctr* but not *Cmu* express a functional tryptophan synthase enzyme *trp*RBA and are thereby able to overcome IFNγ-induced tryptophan starvation (Caldwell et al. 2003). However, *Ctr* infection of murine cells in the presence of IFNγ does not induce IDO but IFNγ-stimulated genes (ISGs) expression. The superfamily of ISGs includes guanylate-binding proteins (GBPs) and the immunity-related GTPases (IRGs), further divided into GKS and immunity-related GTPase family M (Irgm) proteins. Both families of GTPases are involved in the restriction of intracellular bacteria by targeting phagosomes to induce lysis and infection clearance by autophagy (MacMicking 2012; Meunier and Broz 2015). During *Ctr* infection in murine cells, the inclusion membrane is targeted by Irga6, Irgb10, GBP1, and GBP2 upon IFNγ treatment (Bernstein-Hanley et al. 2006; Coers et al. 2008; Al-Zeer et al. 2009; Haldar et al. 2013). MEFs depleted for Irgb10 are not able to restrict *Ctr* growth upon IFNγ treatment, whereas the participation of Irga6 in restricting *Ctr* replication is controversially discussed. Coers and co-workers showed that the depletion of Irga6 did not affect the control of *Ctr* infection in IFNγ-treated mouse cells (Coers et al. 2008), whereas other groups reported a major participation of Irga6 in restricting *Ctr* infection (Nelson et al. 2005; Al-Zeer et al. 2009). Irgm proteins represent intrinsic regulators of IRGs and also participate in *Ctr* defense in mice (Al-Zeer et al. 2009; Coers et al. 2008; Haldar et al. 2013; MacMicking 2012). Altogether, the mechanism underlying clearance of *Ctr* infections in IFNγ-stimulated mouse cells is dependent on autophagy and involves ISG, which mark the PCV for autophagy and autolysosomal degradation (Al-Zeer et al. 2009; Haldar et al. 2014, 2015). Induction of autophagy in the absence of IFNγ-signaling does not result in restriction of *Ctr* growth in MEFs underlining the important role of ISGs to mark the chlamydial inclusion for recognition by the autophagy system (Pachikara et al. 2009). It has been proposed that rodent adapted *Cmu* prevent IFNγ-induced autophagolysosomal destruction of the inclusion by secretion of the protein TC438. This effector exhibits homologies to the cysteine protease domain of YopT of *Yersinia pestis* and the UDP-glycosyltransferase domain of the large clostridial toxin (LCT) which both inactivate GTPases by removal of lipid modification. *Cmu* may secrete TC438 to inactivate IRGs and thereby prevent targeting of the inclusion to the autolysosomal system (Fig. 1) (Read et al. 2000; Belland et al. 2001; Nelson et al. 2005).

The work of Al-Younes describes an alternative function of LC3 for *Ctr* infection. They report a recruitment of LC3 and its known interaction partner MAP1 (microtubule-associated protein 1) to the *Ctr* inclusion upon 18-h post-infection (hpi). Depletion of LC3 or MAP1 results in reduced chlamydial growth and infectivity. By recruitment of LC3 and thereby also MAP1 *Ctr* may interact with the microtubule network to get access to vesicles transporting lipids and other nutrients, which could be crucial for its survival (Al-Younes et al. 2004, 2011).

3.2 Interference with Inflammasome Activation and Inflammation

Infection of epithelial cells, the preferred host cell type of *Chlamydia*, induces chemokine and cytokine secretion resulting in the recruitment of leukocytes and an augmented cellular inflammatory response (Rasmussen et al. 1997). *Chlamydia* recognition by the host is predominantly mediated by TLR2 and to a minor extent by TLR4 (Shimada et al. 2012; Prebeck et al. 2001; Darville et al. 2003; O'Connell et al. 2006). TLR2 activation of epithelial cells induces the expression of chemokines such as IL-6, IL-8, and GM-CSF via NF-κB signaling, which recruits macrophages, dendritic cells, and natural killer cells to the site of infection (Darville and Hiltke 2010). Recruited leukocytes then produce high amounts of TNFα, IL-1β, and IFNγ causing a local inflammation and tissue damage, what finally results in the pathology of *Chlamydia* infections (Darville and Hiltke 2010). Infection of epithelial and immune cells by *Chlamydia* induces the formation of the inflammasome by stimulation of

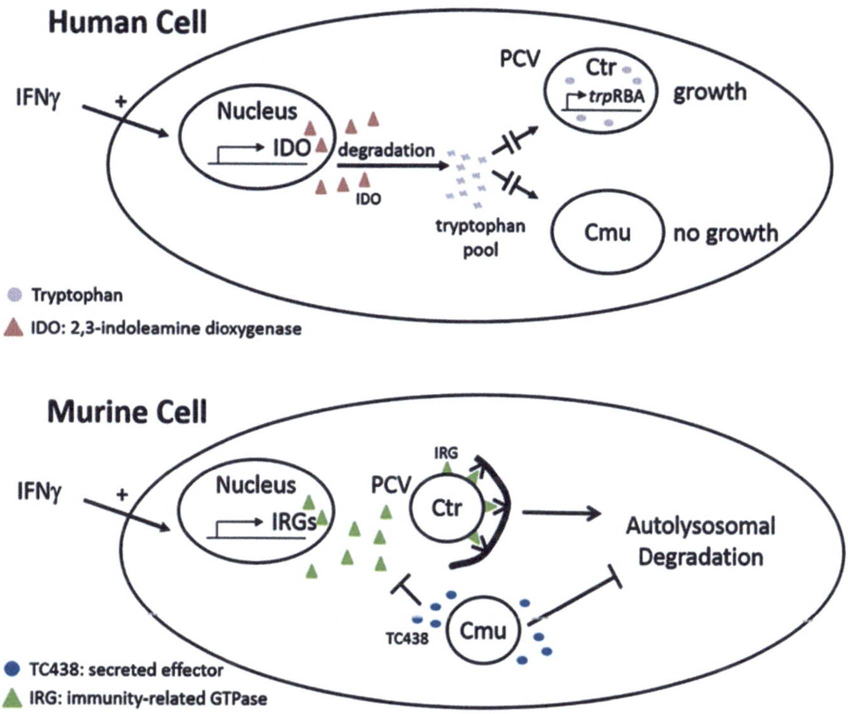

Fig. 1 Host cell adaptation of *Chlamydia* upon IFNγ treatment. IFNγ stimulation of *Chlamydia*-infected human epithelial cells results in the upregulation of IDO which catalyzes the degradation of cellular tryptophan pools. *Ctr* express a functional tryptophan synthase, whereas the *trp*RBA operon of *Cmu* is mutated. Therefore, *Cmu* growth is limited upon IFNγ stimulation resulting in tryptophan starvation. In murine cells, IFNγ stimulation results in the expression of immunity-related GTPases which mark the inclusion for autophagosomal degradation. *Cmu* but not *Ctr* secrete the effector TC438 which inactivates IRGs and through it the detection by the autophagy machinery

intracellular NLRs (He et al. 2010; Nagarajan et al. 2012; Abdul-Sater et al. 2009, 2010a). Pathogen recognition together with intracellular stress stimuli then triggers inflammasome activation by autocatalytic activation of Caspase-1. Two inflammasomes have been extensively studied: the NLRP3 and the NLRC4 inflammasomes. NLRP3 inflammasome assembly has been shown to be induced by bacterial structures, but also by cell inherent stress signals related to mitochondrial integrity and functionality (Shin and Brodsky 2015). However, final NLRP3 inflammasome activation requires potassium efflux and mitochondrial ROS (Kahlenberg and Dubyak 2004; Petrilli et al. 2007; Zhou et al. 2011; Munoz-Planillo et al. 2013). On the contrary, NLRC4 exclusively sense bacterial flagellin or structurally related proteins from the T3SS (Zhao et al. 2011; Miao et al. 2010). Activation of inflammasomes results either in the processing and secretion of the pro-inflammatory cytokines IL-1β and IL-18 or in the initiation of cell death by pyroptosis.

Infection of epithelial cells with *Ctr* stimulates formation of the NLRP3 inflammasome. Moreover, active replication and secretion of type 3 effector proteins into the host cell cytosol trigger potassium efflux and ROS production which contribute to NLRP3 inflammasome activation by Caspase-1 processing. Depletion of NLRP3 or ASC by RNA interference (RNAi) prevents Caspase-1 activation in *Ctr*-infected cells (Abdul-Sater et al. 2009, 2010a). However, *Ctr*-triggered activation of Caspase-1 does not induce IL-1β secretion but seems to be essential for optimal chlamydial growth in epithelial cells, since the chemical inhibition of Caspase-1 massively interferes with bacterial replication and infectivity. In general, Caspase-1 activity is mainly linked to IL-1β processing, although recent studies identified additional substrates (Shao et al. 2007; Gurcel et al. 2006) and Abdul-Sater et al. proposed a participation of Caspase-1 in chlamydial lipid acquisition, which is essential for their survival (Fig. 2) (Abdul-Sater et al. 2009, 2010a).

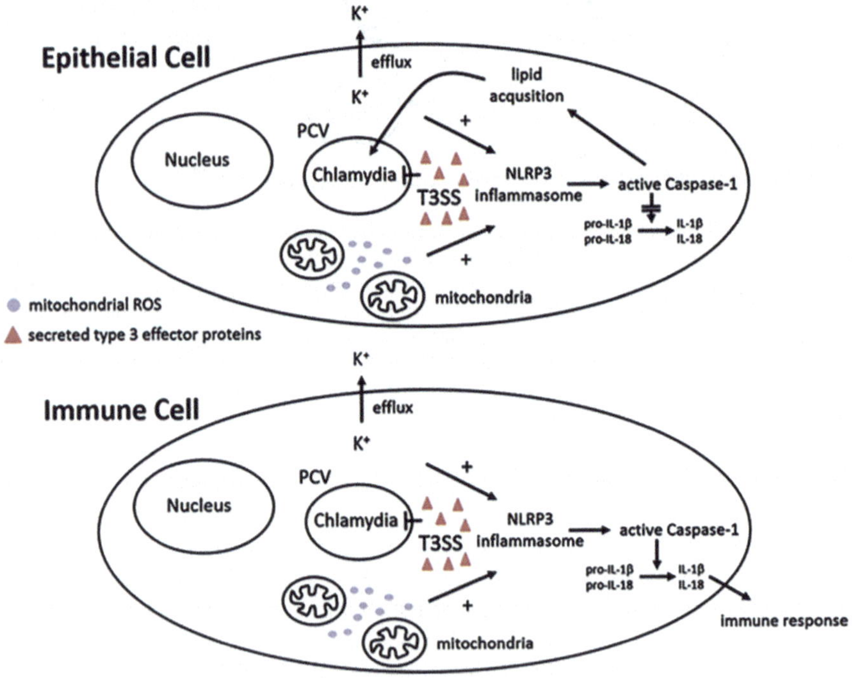

Fig. 2 *Chlamydia*-triggered NLRP3 inflammasome activation. Intracellular replicating *Chlamydia* as well as the components of the T3SS induce the formation of the NLRP3 inflammasome. Final activation of the NLRP3 and autocatalytic processing of Caspase-1 is triggered by infection-induced K^+ efflux and production of mitochondrial ROS. In epithelial cells, Caspase-1 activation does not induce IL-1β and IL-18 processing but is essential for chlamydial lipid acquisition and growth. In leukocytes, *Chlamydia*-stimulated NLRP3 and Caspase-1 activation result in IL-1β and IL-18 processing

In contrast to epithelial cells, infection of macrophages, monocytes, or dendritic cells with *Chlamydia* induces IL-1β and IL-18 secretion (He et al. 2010; Flego et al. 2013; Abdul-Sater et al. 2010b). In immune cells, Caspase-1 activation is mediated by the same pathway described in epithelial cells: TLR2 signaling induces pro-IL-1β expression and potassium efflux and ROS trigger Caspase-1 autocatalytic activation crucial for IL-1β processing and secretion (Fig. 2) (Flego et al. 2013; He et al. 2010; Itoh et al. 2014; Abdul-Sater et al. 2010b). Besides potassium efflux and ROS as the two major inducers of NLRP3 and Caspase-1, a participation of the protein kinase Syk (spleen tyrosine kinase) was described (Abdul-Sater et al. 2010b). Syk is reported to be involved in the NLRP3 activation in response to fungal infection (Gross et al. 2009; Said-Sadier et al. 2010). Furthermore, Syk phosphorylates the chlamydial type 3 secreted protein TARP upon transmission into the host cytosol (Mehlitz et al. 2008). Depletion of Syk in human monocytes by RNAi resulted in reduced Caspase-1 activation and thereby minor IL-1β secretion compared to control cells. At least in human monocytes, the activation of NLRP3 is controlled by two alternative routes; however, both routes activate Caspase-1 and induce IL-1β secretion (Abdul-Sater et al. 2010b).

The importance of IL-1 signaling became clear during *Cpn* and *Cmu* infection studies in mice deficient in the inflammasome or IL-1 signaling. Pulmonary infection with *Cpn* in Casp-1$^{-/-}$ mice resulted in delayed cytokine secretion, impaired infection clearance and thereby increased mortality in response to *Cpn* infection. The same phenotype was obtained by pharmacological inhibition of IL-1 receptor signaling (Shimada et al. 2011). Furthermore, IL-1β secretion was dependent on the activation of the NLRP3/ASC inflammasome (Shimada et al. 2011). IL-1 signaling and inflammasome activation has also been shown to be important for the control of *Cmu* infection. Depletion of IL-1β or IL-1 receptor caused increased *Cmu* growth and delayed clearance but less tissue damage (Nagarajan et al. 2012). However, secretion of IL-1β in mice upon *Cmu* infection seems to be independent from ASC inflammasomes in their model. Although the activation of the inflammasome is important for restriction of chlamydial growth, ASC$^{-/-}$ or NLRP3$^{-/-}$ mice showed no reduction in IL-1β levels during mid-phase and late phase of infection. Only the initial IL-1β and overall IL-18 secretion is dependent on inflammasome formation. Therefore, other so far unknown IL-1β activating mechanisms must occur during mid-phase and late phase of *Cmu* infection (Nagarajan et al. 2012).

Besides the secretion of IL-1β, infection-mediated activation of the inflammasome can also induce pyroptotic cell death. IRGs and GBPs mediate PCV lysis, causing PAMP spillage into the cytosol and stimulation of the inflammasome via the canonical and non-canonical pathway to Caspase-1 and Caspase-11 activation (Pilla et al. 2014; Shenoy et al. 2012). Similar results were reported for *Cmu* infections in macrophages during which GBPs promote Caspase-11 and NLRP3/Caspase-1 inflammasome activation and pyroptosis (Finethy et al. 2015). However, GBPs do not directly interact with the inclusion nor are chlamydial particles released into the cytosol in IFNγ-treated macrophages. Therefore, a direct activation of Caspase-11 and NLRP3 inflammasomes by GBPs without preceding lysis of the PCV has been postulated (Finethy et al. 2015).

4 Inhibition of Host Cell Death

The induction of host cell death due to an infection is one form of cell-autonomous defense (MacMicking 2012). There exist multiple forms of programed cell death which are activated by various stimuli and mainly differ in the property to induce an inflammatory response or not (Galluzzi et al. 2016; Bergsbaken et al. 2009). As already described, pyroptosis is a form of programed cell death triggered by infection-stimulated activation of the inflammasome. Pyroptosis is characterized by cell lysis and a release of immunogenic cytosolic material into the extracellular space which amplifies the inflammatory response (Lamkanfi and Dixit 2014; Bergsbaken et al. 2009). In contrast, apoptosis is not directly linked to infection-induced cell death but is a mechanism to remove damaged or old cells from the body without induction of inflammation. Common signals for apoptosis induction are DNA damage, ER-stress, ROS, nutrition limitation, or lack of survival signals (Green et al. 2014). Intracellular replication of bacteria commonly causes DNA damage, ER-stress, or ROS production, which in turn induces apoptosis pathways (Gao and Kwaik 2000; Ashida et al. 2011). Obligate intracellular bacteria such as *Chlamydia, Coxiella,* or *Rickettsia* depend on their host cell and therefore, prevent apoptosis initiation by various mechanisms (Ashida et al. 2011; Rudel et al. 2010; Bohme and Rudel 2009). Controversially, induction of non-apoptotic cell death following *Chlamydia* infection was reported, too (Ying et al. 2006). However, multiple studies have confirmed that *Chlamydia* predominantly blocks apoptosis induction in epithelial cells and that the reported infection-induced cell death might be linked to severe cell damage instead of specific apoptosis induction (Sharma and Rudel 2009). But, *Chlamydia* are able to induce cell death in immune cells which contribute to immune evasion. For instance, *Cpn*-infected activated T lymphocytes die by activation of apoptotic and pyroptotic pathways (Olivares-Zavaleta et al. 2011) or by TNFα secreted by neighboring *Ctr*-infected macrophages (Jendro et al. 2004).

Apoptosis-inducing extracellular (extrinsic) or intracellular (intrinsic) stimuli trigger a signaling cascade resulting in the mitochondrial outer membrane permeabilization (MOMP), release of Cytochrome *c,* and subsequent activation of Caspases. MOMP is regulated by the Bcl-2 family members (Moldoveanu et al. 2014) and Caspase activation can be opposed by inhibitor of apoptosis proteins (IAPs) (Kocab and Duckett 2015). Furthermore, the transcription of multiple pro-survival and anti-apoptotic genes is regulated by the transcription factor NF-κB (Luo et al. 2005). The checkpoints regulating MOMP as well as NF-κB activity represent the major targets of bacterial manipulation of apoptosis signaling (Bohme and Rudel 2009). Moreover, the activation of pro-survival signaling pathways, e.g., PI3K/AKT or MEK/ERK, promotes cell survival and reduced sensitivity toward stress stimuli and is also a common strategy to ensure host cell survival (Bohme and Rudel 2009).

4.1 Manipulation of Survival Signaling Pathways

Directly upon host cell adhesion and entry, *Chlamydia* activate the PI3K/AKT and MEK/ERK pathways (Rajalingam et al. 2008; Verbeke et al. 2006; Buchholz and Stephens 2007; Chen et al. 2010). In general, PI3K/AKT signaling is important for cell proliferation, survival, and migration as well as inhibition of apoptosis. AKT as direct substrate of PI3K stimulates HDM2-mediated p53 depletion, NF-κB-dependent expression of pro-survival and anti-apoptotic genes, and inhibition of GSK-3 to enable cell proliferation (Thorpe et al. 2015). Also the MEK/ERK signaling pathway regulates cell survival, proliferation, and differentiation as well as the inhibition of apoptosis by the activation of multiple transcription factors such as NF-κB or c-Myc. Furthermore, ERK catalyzes the phosphorylation of BIM or Bad as pro-apoptotic proteins to induce their degradation (Mebratu and Tesfaigzi 2009; McCubrey et al. 2007).

During *Ctr* infection, two activation waves for PI3K/AKT signaling are described: bacterial adhesion and invasion triggers initial activation which recedes after 60-min post-infection. This initial PI3K/AKT signaling is essential to establish the infection. The second activation boost starts 8 hpi and is maintained till late phase of infection (Rajalingam et al. 2008). It was recently shown that EphA2 functions as adhesion and invasion receptor for *Ctr*. Binding of EBs to EphA2 activates the receptor and induces its internalization. Furthermore, active EphA2 then recruits and activates PI3K to trigger first PI3K/AKT signaling wave. After internalization, EphA2 is enriched at the inclusion membrane where it again recruits and activates PI3K signaling (Subbarayal et al. 2015). *Sn*-mediated apoptosis resistance also depends partially on the activation of the PI3K/AKT signaling (Karunakaran et al. 2011) and for *Cpn* the infection-induced activation of MEK/ERK and PI3K/AKT signaling was reported to be involved in the invasion process (Coombes and Mahony 2002). Another pathway to AKT activation and chlamydial development depends on the EGF receptor signaling (Patel et al. 2014), highlighting the crucial role of PI3K/AKT signaling for *Chlamydia* infection. Temporal ERK signaling characteristics are comparable to PI3K/AKT signaling and are important for chlamydial nutrition acquisition (Su et al. 2004) as well as expression of anti-apoptotic proteins (Rajalingam et al. 2008). Further, *Ctr* development depends on the transcriptional activity of AP-1, a heterodimeric transcription factor that regulates the expression of a large range of host genes related to inflammation, stress, and cell survival (Olive et al. 2014).

The hypoxia-induced factor-1α (HIF-1α), which controls gene expression of glycolytic enzymes, VEGF, and several anti-apoptotic proteins, is stabilized during a short period of the infection cycle (Rupp et al. 2007). The stabilization of the transcription factor between 12 and 20 hpi is dependent on ERK signaling since the inhibition of ERK by the specific inhibitor UO126 decreases HIF-1α accumulation (Sharma et al. 2011). Furthermore, shedding of TNFR1 from the cell surface of infected cells is dependent on ERK signaling. *Ctr*-infected cells exhibit reduced amounts of TNFR1 on the cell surface but increased total protein in the cell. High amounts of TNFR1 and TNFR2 are accumulated in the cell in the Golgi or around the inclusion, but this enrichment is independent from EKR signaling. However, MEK/ERK signaling activates the metalloprotease TACE which removes specifically TNFR1 but not TNFR2 from the cell surface and thereby reduces the susceptibility of the infected cell toward TNFα-induced apoptosis (Paland et al. 2008).

4.2 Enrichment of Anti-apoptotic Proteins

Apoptosis initiation by MOMP is tightly regulated by the pro- and anti-apoptotic proteins of the Bcl-2 family. Pro- and anti-apoptotic Bcl-2 proteins form dimers and are thereby inactive. The binding affinities are altered upon stress stimuli, which cause degradation of anti-apoptotic proteins and thereby the release and activation of pro-apoptotic Bcl-2 proteins, among them the main effectors Bax and Bak. Bax and Bak oligomerize upon activation to form pores in the mitochondrial outer membrane causing Cytochrome *c* release. Hence, the ratio of pro- and anti-apoptotic proteins controls apoptosis initiation or cell survival (Shamas-Din et al. 2013). Furthermore, members of the IAP family regulate cell survival, proliferation, and differentiation primarily by modulation of multiple signaling pathways such as NF-κB, MAPK, TLR, or NOD. Due to their impact on NF-κB and MAPK signaling, IAPs are also involved in the modulation of immune signaling (Beug et al. 2012). It was also reported that IAPs are able to inhibit Caspase activity and that the overexpression of IAPs promotes apoptosis resistance (LaCasse et al. 1998; Gyrd-Hansen and Meier 2010).

Depending on the *Chlamydia* species, several anti-apoptotic proteins are upregulated or stabilized. Upon 16 h of *Ctr* infection, the Bcl-2 protein family member Mcl-1 is massively enriched by increased gene expression as well as stabilization on protein level (Rajalingam et al. 2008). Inhibition of the MEK/ERK or PI3K/AKT pathway results in reduced Mcl-1 accumulation since MEK/ERK signaling regulates *mcl1* gene expression and PI3K/AKT signaling interferes in Mcl-1 ubiquitination and degradation (Thomas et al. 2010). Depletion of Mcl-1 by RNAi in cells infected with actively replicating or persistent *Ctr* significantly sensitized the infected cells for apoptosis indicating that Mcl-1 is a regulator of *Ctr*-mediated apoptosis resistance (Rajalingam et al. 2008; Sharma et al. 2011; Rodel et al. 2012). Besides Mcl-1, two other anti-apoptotic proteins belonging to the inhibitor of apoptosis protein family are enriched during *Ctr* infection: cIAP-2 and Survivin. Of these, only cIAP-2 shows an increased gene transcription in a time-dependent manner, whereas the transcription of the Survivin gene exhibits no infection-mediated upregulation. However, both anti-apoptotic proteins are stabilized on protein level (Rajalingam et al. 2006). The anti-apoptotic function of cIAP-2 during *Ctr* infection depends on the formation of heterodimer complexes with cIAP-1 or XIAP. Depletion of one of these proteins prevents complex formation sensitizing *Ctr*-infected cells for apoptosis. So far, the function of Survivin during *Ctr* infection is unknown since the depletion of this protein does not interfere with infection-induced apoptosis resistance (Rajalingam et al. 2006). Also, the anti-apoptotic mechanisms that rely on cIAP-2 during active *Ctr* infection do not occur during persistent *Ctr* infection since cIAP-2 is less stabilized and its depletion during IFNγ-induced persistence does not alter apoptosis resistance (Rodel et al. 2012). *Cpn*-mediated apoptosis resistance depends on cIAP-1 and cIAP-2 as well as on the activation and translocation of the transcription factor NF-κB. During *Cpn* infection, cIAP-2 but not cIAP-1 is enriched depending on NF-κB activity. However, depletion or inactivation of one of these factors significantly sensitizes *Cpn*-infected cells for apoptosis (Paland et al. 2006). The apoptosis resistance in *Sn* infection also depends on the stabilization of cIAP-1 and cIAP-2 (Karunakaran et al. 2011). The stabilization of cIAP-2 might be an evolutionary conserved mechanism within the order *Chlamydiales* to prevent host cell apoptosis. Nevertheless, each species has adopted further individual resistance mechanisms. For cIAP-1, an additional role in the regulation of innate immune signaling during *Cpn* infection was described because *Cpn* lung infection of cIAP-1$^{-/-}$ mice showed increased infection but less inflammation compared to wild-type mice. As already mentioned, IAPs are important regulators of immune signaling via the NF-κB pathway and depletion of cIAP-1 might interfere with cytokine signaling upon infection (Prakash et al. 2009). Furthermore, *Chlamydia* appears to engage in addition other mechanisms of mediating apoptosis resistance. For instance, the PI3K/AKT pathway is not strongly activated in mouse fibroblasts (Siegl et al. 2014) and resistance toward apoptosis induction has been shown in this cell type to be independent of IAPs and Mcl-1 (Ying et al. 2008).

During infection, *Ctr* express and secrete multiple proteins by their T3SS. One family of secreted proteins is the inclusion proteins (Incs) which are anchored by their transmembrane domain in the inclusion membrane. It was shown that Incs can specifically interact with transport vesicles through interaction with Rab and Syntaxin proteins (Damiani et al. 2014). Furthermore, a specific interaction of IncG with the host cell protein 14-3-3β was shown (Scidmore and Hackstadt 2001). PI3K signaling leads to the phosphorylation of the pro-apoptotic BH3-only protein Bad which specifically binds to 14-3-3β in the phosphorylated state. Therefore, *Ctr* but not *Cpn* are able to sequester pro-apoptotic phosphorylated Bad to the inclusion by 14-3-3β and IncG complex formation to impede with apoptosis induction (Verbeke et al. 2006). Cpn1027 is an Inc protein of *Cpn* which sequesters Caprin2 to the inclusion. Caprin2 and GSK3 form the β-catenin destruction complex to induce β-catenin degradation. Thereby, spatial segregation of Caprin2 and GSK3 from β-catenin enables β-catenin-dependent gene expression of multiple anti-apoptotic proteins such as Bcl-2 which mediates apoptosis resistance of *Cpn*-infected cells (Flores and Zhong 2015).

4.3 Depletion of P53

Intracellular replication of bacteria induces DNA damage, ROS production, and other cellular stresses which may eventually induce apoptosis in the host cell. *Chlamydia* infection elicits ROS production since moderate levels of ROS appear to be essential for the initiation of the infection. As a consequence, host cell DNA is severely damaged (Chumduri et al. 2013; Prusty et al. 2013). ROS induce Caspase-1 activation which is not only involved in the processing of pro-inflammatory cytokines but also in lipid metabolism. The acquisition of lipids such as ceramide and sphingolipids from the host cell is essential for chlamydial replication (Chumduri et al. 2013; Padberg et al. 2013; Abdul-Sater et al. 2010a).

However, for productive replication, *Chlamydia* have to prevent DNA damage response accompanied by p53 activation and induction of apoptosis (Siegl and Rudel 2015). Genomic instability or DNA damage is sensed by the tumor suppressor protein p53 which consequently induces cell cycle arrest, activation of DNA repair mechanisms, or apoptosis. Under normal conditions, p53 level is permanently marked for proteasomal degradation by the E3 ubiquitin ligase HDM2 which gets activated by PI3K/AKT survival signaling. However, upon cellular stress p53 gets stabilized to activate DNA repair and block cellular metabolism by the inhibition of glycolysis and the pentose phosphate pathway (PPP). Dependent on the degree of damage, p53 also induces apoptosis by the stimulation of Bax and Bak oligomerization as well as increased gene expression of multiple pro-apoptotic proteins such as Bax, Puma, or Noxa (Siegl and Rudel 2015). *Chlamydia* actively deplete p53 levels during infection and enriched p53 levels in the cell interfere with chlamydial inclusion formation and replication (Siegl et al. 2014; Gonzalez et al. 2014). Eradication of p53 was shown to depend on PI3K/AKT signaling and HDM2-mediated p53 ubiquitination and proteasomal degradation. Gonzalez et al. showed that p53 depletion is, at least to some extent, important for chlamydial apoptosis resistance (Gonzalez et al. 2014). Moreover, Siegl and co-workers described an additional role of p53 during *Chlamy*dia infection related to the host cell metabolism. P53 is known to inhibit the PPP which is important for the production of NADPH and nucleotide precursors (Jiang et al. 2011). All *Chlamydia* depend on the host cell pool of NADPH (Prusty et al. 2012) and nucleotide precursors and therefore p53-mediated shutdown of the PPP results in block of bacterial growth (Siegl et al. 2014). Glucose-6-phosphate dehydrogenase (G6PD) is the first enzyme in the PPP and the major target of p53. Ectopically overexpressed G6PD completely restores p53-induced growth arrest of *Chlamydia* which reveals the underlying mechanism of p53-mediated chlamydial growth inhibition by limitation of metabolites. Depletion of p53 during *Chlamydia* infection, therefore, not only blocks host cell death, but is also necessary for productive replication of RBs by provision of essential metabolites.

5 Concluding Remarks

The obligate intracellular lifestyle forces *Chlamydia* to deal with numerous defense strategies cells have evolved to defeat invading bacteria. It is therefore not surprising that *Chlamydia* counteracts cell intrinsic anti-bacterial pathways that respond to the recognition of PAMPs, general cell stress, and infection-induced cell damage. However, although cross-species infections are found among the Chlamydiales, the long-term evolution-driven adaptation of chlamydial species has shaped a pathogen-specific defense. It is noteworthy that such closely related species as *Ctr* and *Cmu* are facing entirely different responses to IFNγ exposure and consequently have evolved efficient counterstriking activities. Rather surprisingly, species selection does not appear to mainly depend on different host cell surfaces, e.g., specific receptors mediating bacterial binding and uptake since different *Chlamydia* species infect a broad range of cell species and cell types. It is rather the mode of intracellular accommodation that permits more or less productive replication or persistence. The mechanisms how the innate immune system, the cell-autonomous defense, and host cell death affect chlamydial infection have gained significant attention over the past years and many of the central signaling pathways have meanwhile been elucidated. It is currently unclear if and, when indicated, how all these central lines of defense against intracellular pathogens are connected to the metabolic status of the cell (Eisenreich et al. 2013). This connection may be particularly relevant in the case of an obligate intracellular pathogen such as *Chlamydia* that is—in its dependence—closely connected to the host metabolism.

References

Abdul-Sater AA, Koo E, Hacker G, Ojcius DM (2009) Inflammasome-dependent caspase-1 activation in cervical epithelial cells stimulates growth of the intracellular pathogen *Chlamydia trachomatis*. J Biol Chem 284(39):26789–26796. doi:10.1074/jbc.M109.026823

Abdul-Sater AA, Said-Sadier N, Lam VM, Singh B, Pettengill MA, Soares F, Tattoli I, Lipinski S, Girardin SE, Rosenstiel P, Ojcius DM (2010a) Enhancement of reactive oxygen species production and chlamydial infection by the mitochondrial Nod-like family member NLRX1. J Biol Chem 285(53):41637–41645. doi:10.1074/jbc.M110.137885

Abdul-Sater AA, Said-Sadier N, Padilla EV, Ojcius DM (2010b) Chlamydial infection of monocytes stimulates IL-1beta secretion through activation of the NLRP3 inflammasome. Microbes Infect 12(8–9):652–661. doi:10.1016/j.micinf.2010.04.008

Akira S, Uematsu S, Takeuchi O (2006) Pathogen recognition and innate immunity. Cell 124 (4):783–801. doi:10.1016/j.cell.2006.02.015

Al-Younes HM, Brinkmann V, Meyer TF (2004) Interaction of *Chlamydia trachomatis* serovar L2 with the host autophagic pathway. Infect Immun 72(8):4751–4762. doi:10.1128/IAI.72.8.4751-4762.2004

Al-Younes HM, Al-Zeer MA, Khalil H, Gussmann J, Karlas A, Machuy N, Brinkmann V, Braun PR, Meyer TF (2011) Autophagy-independent function of MAP-LC3 during intracellular propagation of *Chlamydia trachomatis*. Autophagy 7(8):814–828

Al-Zeer MA, Al-Younes HM, Braun PR, Zerrahn J, Meyer TF (2009) IFN-gamma-inducible Irga6 mediates host resistance against *Chlamydia trachomatis* via autophagy. PLoS ONE 4(2):e4588. doi:10.1371/journal.pone.0004588

Al-Zeer MA, Al-Younes HM, Lauster D, Abu Lubad M, Meyer TF (2013) Autophagy restricts *Chlamydia trachomatis* growth in human macrophages via IFNG-inducible guanylate binding proteins. Autophagy 9(1):50–62. doi:10.4161/auto.22482

Ashida H, Mimuro H, Ogawa M, Kobayashi T, Sanada T, Kim M, Sasakawa C (2011) Cell death and infection: a double-edged sword for host and pathogen survival. J Cell Biol 195(6):931–942. doi:10.1083/jcb.201108081

Asrat S, de Jesus DA, Hempstead AD, Ramabhadran V, Isberg RR (2014) Bacterial pathogen manipulation of host membrane trafficking. Annu Rev Cell Dev Biol 30:79–109. doi:10.1146/annurev-cellbio-100913-013439

Bartlett EC, Levison WB, Munday PE (2013) Pelvic inflammatory disease. BMJ 346:f3189. doi:10.1136/bmj.f3189

Bastidas RJ, Elwell CA, Engel JN, Valdivia RH (2013) Chlamydial intracellular survival strategies. Cold Spring Harb Perspect Med 3(5):a010256. doi:10.1101/cshperspect.a010256

Baud D, Greub G (2011) Intracellular bacteria and adverse pregnancy outcomes. Clin Microbiol Infect 17(9):1312–1322. doi:10.1111/j.1469-0691.2011.03604.x

Beagley KW, Huston WM, Hansbro PM, Timms P (2009) Chlamydial infection of immune cells: altered function and implications for disease. Crit Rev Immunol 29(4):275–305

Beatty WL, Byrne GI, Morrison RP (1993) Morphologic and antigenic characterization of interferon gamma-mediated persistent *Chlamydia trachomatis* infection in vitro. Proc Natl Acad Sci U S A 90(9):3998–4002

Beatty WL, Belanger TA, Desai AA, Morrison RP, Byrne GI (1994a) Tryptophan depletion as a mechanism of gamma interferon-mediated chlamydial persistence. Infect Immun 62(9): 3705–3711

Beatty WL, Morrison RP, Byrne GI (1994b) Persistent chlamydiae: from cell culture to a paradigm for chlamydial pathogenesis. Microbiol Rev 58(4):686–699

Bebear C, de Barbeyrac B (2009) Genital *Chlamydia trachomatis* infections. Clin Microbiol Infect 15(1):4–10. doi:10.1111/j.1469-0691.2008.02647.x

Belland RJ, Scidmore MA, Crane DD, Hogan DM, Whitmire W, McClarty G, Caldwell HD (2001) *Chlamydia trachomatis* cytotoxicity associated with complete and partial cytotoxin genes. Proc Natl Acad Sci U S A 98(24):13984–13989. doi:10.1073/pnas.241377698

Bergsbaken T, Fink SL, Cookson BT (2009) Pyroptosis: host cell death and inflammation. Nat Rev Microbiol 7(2):99–109. doi:10.1038/nrmicro2070

Bernstein-Hanley I, Coers J, Balsara ZR, Taylor GA, Starnbach MN, Dietrich WF (2006) The p47 GTPases Igtp and Irgb10 map to the *Chlamydia trachomatis* susceptibility locus Ctrq-3 and mediate cellular resistance in mice. Proc Natl Acad Sci U S A 103(38):14092–14097. doi:10.1073/pnas.0603338103

Beug ST, Cheung HH, LaCasse EC, Korneluk RG (2012) Modulation of immune signalling by inhibitors of apoptosis. Trends Immunol 33(11):535–545. doi:10.1016/j.it.2012.06.004

Beuzon CR, Meresse S, Unsworth KE, Ruiz-Albert J, Garvis S, Waterman SR, Ryder TA, Boucrot E, Holden DW (2000) Salmonella maintains the integrity of its intracellular vacuole through the action of SifA. EMBO J 19(13):3235–3249. doi:10.1093/emboj/19.13.3235

Bohme L, Rudel T (2009) Host cell death machinery as a target for bacterial pathogens. Microbes Infect 11(13):1063–1070. doi:10.1016/j.micinf.2009.08.014

Boman J, Hammerschlag MR (2002) *Chlamydia pneumoniae* and atherosclerosis: critical assessment of diagnostic methods and relevance to treatment studies. Clin Microbiol Rev 15 (1):1–20

Broz P, Monack DM (2011) Molecular mechanisms of inflammasome activation during microbial infections. Immunol Rev 243(1):174–190. doi:10.1111/j.1600-065X.2011.01041.x

Broz P, Monack DM (2013) Newly described pattern recognition receptors team up against intracellular pathogens. Nat Rev Immunol 13(8):551–565. doi:10.1038/nri3479

Buchholz KR, Stephens RS (2007) The extracellular signal-regulated kinase/mitogen-activated protein kinase pathway induces the inflammatory factor interleukin-8 following *Chlamydia trachomatis* infection. Infect Immun 75(12):5924–5929. doi:10.1128/IAI.01029-07

Burstein GR, Gaydos CA, Diener-West M, Howell MR, Zenilman JM, Quinn TC (1998) Incident *Chlamydia trachomatis* infections among inner-city adolescent females. JAMA 280(6): 521–526

Caldwell HD, Wood H, Crane D, Bailey R, Jones RB, Mabey D, Maclean I, Mohammed Z, Peeling R, Roshick C, Schachter J, Solomon AW, Stamm WE, Suchland RJ, Taylor L, West SK, Quinn TC, Belland RJ, McClarty G (2003) Polymorphisms in *Chlamydia trachomatis* tryptophan synthase genes differentiate between genital and ocular isolates. J Clin Invest 111(11):1757–1769. doi:10.1172/JCI17993

Carlin JM, Weller JB (1995) Potentiation of interferon-mediated inhibition of Chlamydia infection by interleukin-1 in human macrophage cultures. Infect Immun 63(5):1870–1875

Chen F, Cheng W, Zhang S, Zhong G, Yu P (2010) [Induction of IL-8 by *Chlamydia trachomatis* through MAPK pathway rather than NF-kappaB pathway]. Zhong nan da xue xue bao Yi xue ban. J Central South Univ Med Sci 35(4):307–313. doi:10.3969/j.issn.1672-7347.2010.04.005

Chumduri C, Gurumurthy RK, Zadora PK, Mi Y, Meyer TF (2013) Chlamydia infection promotes host DNA damage and proliferation but impairs the DNA damage response. Cell Host Microbe 13(6):746–758. doi:10.1016/j.chom.2013.05.010

Coccia EM, Battistini A (2015) Early IFN type I response: Learning from microbial evasion strategies. Semin Immunol 27(2):85–101. doi:10.1016/j.smim.2015.03.005

Coers J, Bernstein-Hanley I, Grotsky D, Parvanova I, Howard JC, Taylor GA, Dietrich WF, Starnbach MN (2008) Chlamydia muridarum evades growth restriction by the IFN gamma-inducible host resistance factor Irgb10. J Immunol 180(9):6237–6245

Coombes BK, Mahony JB (2002) Identification of MEK- and phosphoinositide 3-kinase-dependent signalling as essential events during *Chlamydia pneumoniae* invasion of HEp2 cells. Cell Microbiol 4(7):447–460

Cotter TW, Ramsey KH, Miranpuri GS, Poulsen CE, Byrne GI (1997) Dissemination of *Chlamydia trachomatis* chronic genital tract infection in gamma interferon gene knockout mice. Infect Immun 65(6):2145–2152

Creasey EA, Isberg RR (2012) The protein SdhA maintains the integrity of the legionella-containing vacuole. Proc Natl Acad Sci U S A 109(9):3481–3486. doi:10.1073/pnas.1121286109

Creasey EA, Isberg RR (2014) Maintenance of vacuole integrity by bacterial pathogens. Curr Opin Microbiol 17:46–52. doi:10.1016/j.mib.2013.11.005

Damiani MT, Gambarte Tudela J, Capmany A (2014) Targeting eukaryotic Rab proteins: a smart strategy for chlamydial survival and replication. Cell Microbiol 16(9):1329–1338. doi:10.1111/cmi.12325

Darville T, Hiltke TJ (2010) Pathogenesis of genital tract disease due to *Chlamydia trachomatis*. J Infect Dis 201(Suppl 2):S114–S125

Darville T, O'Neill JM, Andrews CW Jr, Nagarajan UM, Stahl L, Ojcius DM (2003) Toll-like receptor-2, but not Toll-like receptor-4, is essential for development of oviduct pathology in chlamydial genital tract infection. J Immunol 171(11):6187–6197

Deretic V, Saitoh T, Akira S (2013) Autophagy in infection, inflammation and immunity. Nat Rev Immunol 13(10):722–737. doi:10.1038/nri3532

Eisenreich W, Heesemann J, Rudel T, Goebel W (2013) Metabolic host responses to infection by intracellular bacterial pathogens. Front Cellul Infect Microbiol 3:24. doi:10.3389/fcimb.2013.00024

Fan T, Lu H, Hu H, Shi L, McClarty GA, Nance DM, Greenberg AH, Zhong G (1998) Inhibition of apoptosis in chlamydia-infected cells: blockade of mitochondrial cytochrome c release and caspase activation. J Exp Med 187(4):487–496

Finethy R, Jorgensen I, Haldar AK, de Zoete MR, Strowig T, Flavell RA, Yamamoto M, Nagarajan UM, Miao EA, Coers J (2015) Guanylate binding proteins enable rapid activation of canonical and noncanonical inflammasomes in chlamydia-infected macrophages. Infect Immun 83(12):4740–4749. doi:10.1128/IAI.00856-15

Fischer SF, Harlander T, Vier J, Hacker G (2004) Protection against CD95-induced apoptosis by chlamydial infection at a mitochondrial step. Infect Immun 72(2):1107–1115

Flego D, Bianco M, Quattrini A, Mancini F, Carollo M, Schiavoni I, Ciervo A, Ausiello CM, Fedele G (2013) *Chlamydia pneumoniae* modulates human monocyte-derived dendritic cells functions driving the induction of a Type 1/Type 17 inflammatory response. Microbes Infect 15 (2):105–114. doi:10.1016/j.micinf.2012.11.004

Flores R, Zhong G (2015) The *Chlamydia pneumoniae* inclusion membrane protein Cpn 1027 interacts with host cell Wnt signaling pathway regulator cytoplasmic activation/proliferation-associated protein 2 (Caprin2). PLoS ONE 10(5):e0127909. doi:10.1371/journal.pone.0127909

Friedman MG, Dvoskin B, Kahane S (2003) Infections with the chlamydia-like microorganism *Simkania negevensis*, a possible emerging pathogen. Microbes Infect 5(11):1013–1021

Galluzzi L, Lopez-Soto A, Kumar S, Kroemer G (2016) Caspases connect cell-death signaling to organismal homeostasis. Immunity 44(2):221–231. doi:10.1016/j.immuni.2016.01.020

Gao LY, Kwaik YA (2000) The modulation of host cell apoptosis by intracellular bacterial pathogens. Trends Microbiol 8(7):306–313

Gomes LC, Dikic I (2014) Autophagy in antimicrobial immunity. Mol Cell 54(2):224–233. doi:10.1016/j.molcel.2014.03.009

Gonzalez E, Rother M, Kerr MC, Al-Zeer MA, Abu-Lubad M, Kessler M, Brinkmann V, Loewer A, Meyer TF (2014) Chlamydia infection depends on a functional MDM2-p53 axis. Nat Commun 5:5201. doi:10.1038/ncomms6201

Gordon SB, Read RC (2002) Macrophage defences against respiratory tract infections. Br Med Bull 61:45–61

Grayston JT, Aldous MB, Easton A, Wang SP, Kuo CC, Campbell LA, Altman J (1993) Evidence that *Chlamydia pneumoniae* causes pneumonia and bronchitis. J Infect Dis 168(5):1231–1235

Green DR, Galluzzi L, Kroemer G (2014) Cell biology. Metabolic control of cell death. Science 345(6203):1250256. doi:10.1126/science.1250256

Greenberg D, Banerji A, Friedman MG, Chiu CH, Kahane S (2003) High rate of Simkania negevensis among Canadian inuit infants hospitalized with lower respiratory tract infections. Scand J Infect Dis 35(8):506–508. doi:10.1080/00365540310014648

Gross O, Poeck H, Bscheider M, Dostert C, Hannesschlager N, Endres S, Hartmann G, Tardivel A, Schweighoffer E, Tybulewicz V, Mocsai A, Tschopp J, Ruland J (2009) Syk kinase signalling couples to the Nlrp3 inflammasome for anti-fungal host defence. Nature 459(7245):433–436. doi:10.1038/nature07965

Gurcel L, Abrami L, Girardin S, Tschopp J, van der Goot FG (2006) Caspase-1 activation of lipid metabolic pathways in response to bacterial pore-forming toxins promotes cell survival. Cell 126(6):1135–1145. doi:10.1016/j.cell.2006.07.033

Gyrd-Hansen M, Meier P (2010) IAPs: from caspase inhibitors to modulators of NF-kappaB, inflammation and cancer. Nat Rev Cancer 10(8):561–574. doi:10.1038/nrc2889

Hahn DL (1998) *Chlamydia pneumoniae* and asthma. Thorax 53(12):1095–1096

Haldar AK, Saka HA, Piro AS, Dunn JD, Henry SC, Taylor GA, Frickel EM, Valdivia RH, Coers J (2013) IRG and GBP host resistance factors target aberrant, "non-self" vacuoles characterized by the missing of "self" IRGM proteins. PLoS Pathog 9(6):e1003414. doi:10.1371/journal.ppat.1003414

Haldar AK, Piro AS, Pilla DM, Yamamoto M, Coers J (2014) The E2-like conjugation enzyme Atg3 promotes binding of IRG and Gbp proteins to Chlamydia- and Toxoplasma-containing vacuoles and host resistance. PLoS ONE 9(1):e86684. doi:10.1371/journal.pone.0086684

Haldar AK, Foltz C, Finethy R, Piro AS, Feeley EM, Pilla-Moffett DM, Komatsu M, Frickel EM, Coers J (2015) Ubiquitin systems mark pathogen-containing vacuoles as targets for host defense by guanylate binding proteins. Proc Natl Acad Sci U S A 112(41):E5628–E5637. doi:10.1073/pnas.1515966112

He X, Mekasha S, Mavrogiorgos N, Fitzgerald KA, Lien E, Ingalls RR (2010) Inflammation and fibrosis during *Chlamydia pneumoniae* infection is regulated by IL-1 and the NLRP3/ASC inflammasome. J Immunol 184(10):5743–5754. doi:10.4049/jimmunol.0903937

Herweg JA, Rudel T (2015) Interaction of Chlamydiae with human macrophages. FEBS J. doi:10.1111/febs.13609

Itoh R, Murakami I, Chou B, Ishii K, Soejima T, Suzuki T, Hiromatsu K (2014) *Chlamydia pneumoniae* harness host NLRP3 inflammasome-mediated caspase-1 activation for optimal intracellular growth in murine macrophages. Biochem Biophys Res Commun 452(3):689–694. doi:10.1016/j.bbrc.2014.08.128

Ivashkiv LB, Donlin LT (2014) Regulation of type I interferon responses. Nat Rev Immunol 14(1):36–49. doi:10.1038/nri3581

Jendro MC, Fingerle F, Deutsch T, Liese A, Kohler L, Kuipers JG, Raum E, Martin M, Zeidler H (2004) *Chlamydia trachomatis*-infected macrophages induce apoptosis of activated T cells by secretion of tumor necrosis factor-alpha in vitro. Med Microbiol Immunol 193(1):45–52. doi:10.1007/s00430-003-0182-1

Jiang P, Du W, Wang X, Mancuso A, Gao X, Wu M, Yang X (2011) p53 regulates biosynthesis through direct inactivation of glucose-6-phosphate dehydrogenase. Nat Cell Biol 13(3):310–316. doi:10.1038/ncb2172

Joseph B, Goebel W (2007) Life of Listeria monocytogenes in the host cells' cytosol. Microbes Infect 9(10):1188–1195. doi:10.1016/j.micinf.2007.05.006

Kahlenberg JM, Dubyak GR (2004) Mechanisms of caspase-1 activation by P2X7 receptor-mediated K+ release. Am J Physiol Cell Physiol 286(5):C1100–C1108. doi:10.1152/ajpcell.00494.2003

Karunakaran K, Mehlitz A, Rudel T (2011) Evolutionary conservation of infection-induced cell death inhibition among Chlamydiales. PLoS ONE 6(7):e22528. doi:10.1371/journal.pone.0022528

Kawai T, Akira S (2006) TLR signaling. Cell Death Differ 13(5):816–825. doi:10.1038/sj.cdd.4401850

Knittler MR, Sachse K (2015) Chlamydia psittaci: update on an underestimated zoonotic agent. Pathogens and disease 73(1):1–15. doi:10.1093/femspd/ftu007

Kocab AJ, Duckett CS (2015) Inhibitor of apoptosis proteins as intracellular signaling intermediates. FEBS J. doi:10.1111/febs.13554

Kumar Y, Valdivia RH (2009) Leading a sheltered life: intracellular pathogens and maintenance of vacuolar compartments. Cell Host Microbe 5(6):593–601. doi:10.1016/j.chom.2009.05.014

Kumar H, Kawai T, Akira S (2009) Toll-like receptors and innate immunity. Biochem Biophys Res Commun 388(4):621–625. doi:10.1016/j.bbrc.2009.08.062

Kumar H, Kawai T, Akira S (2011) Pathogen recognition by the innate immune system. Int Rev Immunol 30(1):16–34. doi:10.3109/08830185.2010.529976

LaCasse EC, Baird S, Korneluk RG, MacKenzie AE (1998) The inhibitors of apoptosis (IAPs) and their emerging role in cancer. Oncogene 17(25):3247–3259. doi:10.1038/sj.onc.1202569

Lamkanfi M, Dixit VM (2011) Modulation of inflammasome pathways by bacterial and viral pathogens. J Immunol 187(2):597–602. doi:10.4049/jimmunol.1100229

Lamkanfi M, Dixit VM (2014) Mechanisms and functions of inflammasomes. Cell 157(5):1013–1022. doi:10.1016/j.cell.2014.04.007

Lamkanfi M, Kanneganti TD, Franchi L, Nunez G (2007) Caspase-1 inflammasomes in infection and inflammation. J Leukoc Biol 82(2):220–225. doi:10.1189/jlb.1206756

Luo JL, Kamata H, Karin M (2005) The anti-death machinery in IKK/NF-kappaB signaling. J Clin Immunol 25(6):541–550. doi:10.1007/s10875-005-8217-6

MacMicking JD (2012) Interferon-inducible effector mechanisms in cell-autonomous immunity. Nat Rev Immunol 12(5):367–382. doi:10.1038/nri3210

McClarty G, Caldwell HD, Nelson DE (2007) Chlamydial interferon gamma immune evasion influences infection tropism. Curr Opin Microbiol 10(1):47–51. doi:10.1016/j.mib.2006.12.003

McCubrey JA, Steelman LS, Chappell WH, Abrams SL, Wong EW, Chang F, Lehmann B, Terrian DM, Milella M, Tafuri A, Stivala F, Libra M, Basecke J, Evangelisti C, Martelli AM, Franklin RA (2007) Roles of the Raf/MEK/ERK pathway in cell growth, malignant transformation and drug resistance. Biochim Biophys Acta 1773(8):1263–1284. doi:10.1016/j.bbamcr.2006.10.001

Mebratu Y, Tesfaigzi Y (2009) How ERK1/2 activation controls cell proliferation and cell death: is subcellular localization the answer? Cell Cycle 8(8):1168–1175

Mehlitz A, Banhart S, Hess S, Selbach M, Meyer TF (2008) Complex kinase requirements for *Chlamydia trachomatis* Tarp phosphorylation. FEMS Microbiol Lett 289(2):233–240. doi:10.1111/j.1574-6968.2008.01390.x

Meunier E, Broz P (2015) Interferon-inducible GTPases in cell autonomous and innate immunity. Cell Microbiol. doi:10.1111/cmi.12546

Miao EA, Mao DP, Yudkovsky N, Bonneau R, Lorang CG, Warren SE, Leaf IA, Aderem A (2010) Innate immune detection of the type III secretion apparatus through the NLRC4 inflammasome. Proc Natl Acad Sci U S A 107(7):3076–3080. doi:10.1073/pnas.0913087107

Molano M, Meijer CJ, Weiderpass E, Arslan A, Posso H, Franceschi S, Ronderos M, Munoz N, van den Brule AJ (2005) The natural course of *Chlamydia trachomatis* infection in asymptomatic Colombian women: a 5-year follow-up study. J Infect Dis 191(6):907–916. doi:10.1086/428287

Moldoveanu T, Follis AV, Kriwacki RW, Green DR (2014) Many players in BCL-2 family affairs. Trends Biochem Sci 39(3):101–111. doi:10.1016/j.tibs.2013.12.006

Moulder JW (1991) Interaction of chlamydiae and host cells in vitro. Microbiol Rev 55(1): 143–190

Munoz-Planillo R, Kuffa P, Martinez-Colon G, Smith BL, Rajendiran TM, Nunez G (2013) K(+) efflux is the common trigger of NLRP3 inflammasome activation by bacterial toxins and particulate matter. Immunity 38(6):1142–1153. doi:10.1016/j.immuni.2013.05.016

Nagarajan UM, Sikes JD, Yeruva L, Prantner D (2012) Significant role of IL-1 signaling, but limited role of inflammasome activation, in oviduct pathology during Chlamydia muridarum genital infection. J Immunol 188(6):2866–2875. doi:10.4049/jimmunol.1103461

Nathan CF, Murray HW, Wiebe ME, Rubin BY (1983) Identification of interferon-gamma as the lymphokine that activates human macrophage oxidative metabolism and antimicrobial activity. J Exp Med 158(3):670–689

Nelson DE, Virok DP, Wood H, Roshick C, Johnson RM, Whitmire WM, Crane DD, Steele-Mortimer O, Kari L, McClarty G, Caldwell HD (2005) Chlamydial IFN-gamma immune evasion is linked to host infection tropism. Proc Natl Acad Sci U S A 102(30):10658–10663. doi:10.1073/pnas.0504198102

O'Connell CM, Ionova IA, Quayle AJ, Visintin A, Ingalls RR (2006) Localization of TLR2 and MyD88 to *Chlamydia trachomatis* inclusions. Evidence for signaling by intracellular TLR2 during infection with an obligate intracellular pathogen. J Biol Chem 281(3):1652–1659. doi:10.1074/jbc.M510182200

Olivares-Zavaleta N, Carmody A, Messer R, Whitmire WM, Caldwell HD (2011) *Chlamydia pneumoniae* inhibits activated human T lymphocyte proliferation by the induction of apoptotic and pyroptotic pathways. J Immunol 186(12):7120–7126. doi:10.4049/jimmunol.1100393

Olive AJ, Haff MG, Emanuele MJ, Sack LM, Barker JR, Elledge SJ, Starnbach MN (2014) *Chlamydia trachomatis*-induced alterations in the host cell proteome are required for intracellular growth. Cell Host Microbe 15(1):113–124. doi:10.1016/j.chom.2013.12.009

Oviedo-Boyso J, Bravo-Patino A, Baizabal-Aguirre VM (2014) Collaborative action of Toll-like and NOD-like receptors as modulators of the inflammatory response to pathogenic bacteria. Mediators Inflamm 2014:432785. doi:10.1155/2014/432785

Pachikara N, Zhang H, Pan Z, Jin S, Fan H (2009) Productive *Chlamydia trachomatis* lymphogranuloma venereum 434 infection in cells with augmented or inactivated autophagic activities. FEMS Microbiol Lett 292(2):240–249. doi:10.1111/j.1574-6968.2009.01494.x

Padberg I, Janssen S, Meyer TF (2013) *Chlamydia trachomatis* inhibits telomeric DNA damage signaling via transient hTERT upregulation. Int J Med Microbiol 303(8):463–474. doi:10.1016/j.ijmm.2013.06.001

Paland N, Rajalingam K, Machuy N, Szczepek A, Wehrl W, Rudel T (2006) NF-kappaB and inhibitor of apoptosis proteins are required for apoptosis resistance of epithelial cells persistently infected with Chlamydophila pneumoniae. Cell Microbiol 8(10):1643–1655. doi:10.1111/j.1462-5822.2006.00739.x

Paland N, Bohme L, Gurumurthy RK, Maurer A, Szczepek AJ, Rudel T (2008) Reduced display of tumor necrosis factor receptor I at the host cell surface supports infection with *Chlamydia trachomatis*. J Biol Chem 283(10):6438–6448. doi:10.1074/jbc.M708422200

Patel AL, Chen X, Wood ST, Stuart ES, Arcaro KF, Molina DP, Petrovic S, Furdui CM, Tsang AW (2014) Activation of epidermal growth factor receptor is required for *Chlamydia trachomatis* development. BMC Microbiol 14:277. doi:10.1186/s12866-014-0277-4

Perry LL, Feilzer K, Caldwell HD (1997) Immunity to *Chlamydia trachomatis* is mediated by T helper 1 cells through IFN-gamma-dependent and -independent pathways. J Immunol 158 (7):3344–3352

Petrilli V, Papin S, Dostert C, Mayor A, Martinon F, Tschopp J (2007) Activation of the NALP3 inflammasome is triggered by low intracellular potassium concentration. Cell Death Differ 14 (9):1583–1589. doi:10.1038/sj.cdd.4402195

Phillips Campbell R, Kintner J, Whittimore J, Schoborg RV (2012) Chlamydia muridarum enters a viable but non-infectious state in amoxicillin-treated BALB/c mice. Microbes Infect 14 (13):1177–1185. doi:10.1016/j.micinf.2012.07.017

Pilla DM, Hagar JA, Haldar AK, Mason AK, Degrandi D, Pfeffer K, Ernst RK, Yamamoto M, Miao EA, Coers J (2014) Guanylate binding proteins promote caspase-11-dependent pyroptosis in response to cytoplasmic LPS. Proc Natl Acad Sci U S A 111(16):6046–6051. doi:10.1073/pnas.1321700111

Platanias LC (2005) Mechanisms of type-I- and type-II-interferon-mediated signalling. Nat Rev Immunol 5(5):375–386. doi:10.1038/nri1604

Prakash H, Becker D, Bohme L, Albert L, Witzenrath M, Rosseau S, Meyer TF, Rudel T (2009) cIAP 1 controls innate immunity to C. pneumoniae pulmonary infection. PLoS ONE 4(8): e6519. doi:10.1371/journal.pone.0006519

Prebeck S, Kirschning C, Durr S, da Costa C, Donath B, Brand K, Redecke V, Wagner H, Miethke T (2001) Predominant role of toll-like receptor 2 versus 4 in *Chlamydia pneumoniae*-induced activation of dendritic cells. J Immunol 167(6):3316–3323

Prusty BK, Bohme L, Bergmann B, Siegl C, Krause E, Mehlitz A, Rudel T (2012) Imbalanced oxidative stress causes chlamydial persistence during non-productive human herpes virus co-infection. PLoS ONE 7(10):e47427. doi:10.1371/journal.pone.0047427

Prusty BK, Krohne G, Rudel T (2013) Reactivation of chromosomally integrated human herpesvirus-6 by telomeric circle formation. PLoS Genet 9(12):e1004033. doi:10.1371/journal.pgen.1004033

Rajalingam K, Sharma M, Paland N, Hurwitz R, Thieck O, Oswald M, Machuy N, Rudel T (2006) IAP-IAP complexes required for apoptosis resistance of C. trachomatis-infected cells. PLoS Pathog 2(10):e114. doi:10.1371/journal.ppat.0020114

Rajalingam K, Sharma M, Lohmann C, Oswald M, Thieck O, Froelich CJ, Rudel T (2008) Mcl-1 is a key regulator of apoptosis resistance in *Chlamydia trachomatis*-infected cells. PLoS ONE 3(9):e3102. doi:10.1371/journal.pone.0003102

Randow F, Youle RJ (2014) Self and nonself: how autophagy targets mitochondria and bacteria. Cell Host Microbe 15(4):403–411. doi:10.1016/j.chom.2014.03.012

Rasmussen SJ, Eckmann L, Quayle AJ, Shen L, Zhang YX, Anderson DJ, Fierer J, Stephens RS, Kagnoff MF (1997) Secretion of proinflammatory cytokines by epithelial cells in response to Chlamydia infection suggests a central role for epithelial cells in chlamydial pathogenesis. J Clin Invest 99(1):77–87. doi:10.1172/JCI119136

Read TD, Brunham RC, Shen C, Gill SR, Heidelberg JF, White O, Hickey EK, Peterson J, Utterback T, Berry K, Bass S, Linher K, Weidman J, Khouri H, Craven B, Bowman C, Dodson R, Gwinn M, Nelson W, DeBoy R, Kolonay J, McClarty G, Salzberg SL, Eisen J, Fraser CM (2000) Genome sequences of *Chlamydia trachomatis* MoPn and *Chlamydia pneumoniae* AR39. Nucleic Acids Res 28(6):1397–1406

Rodel J, Grosse C, Yu H, Wolf K, Otto GP, Liebler-Tenorio E, Forsbach-Birk V, Straube E (2012) Persistent *Chlamydia trachomatis* infection of HeLa cells mediates apoptosis resistance through a Chlamydia protease-like activity factor-independent mechanism and induces high mobility group box 1 release. Infect Immun 80(1):195–205. doi:10.1128/IAI.05619-11

Roshick C, Wood H, Caldwell HD, McClarty G (2006) Comparison of gamma interferon-mediated antichlamydial defense mechanisms in human and mouse cells. Infect Immun 74(1):225–238. doi:10.1128/IAI.74.1.225-238.2006

Rottenberg ME, Gigliotti-Rothfuchs A, Wigzell H (2002) The role of IFN-gamma in the outcome of chlamydial infection. Curr Opin Immunol 14(4):444–451

Rudel T, Kepp O, Kozjak-Pavlovic V (2010) Interactions between bacterial pathogens and mitochondrial cell death pathways. Nat Rev Microbiol 8(10):693–705. doi:10.1038/nrmicro2421

Rupp J, Gieffers J, Klinger M, van Zandbergen G, Wrase R, Maass M, Solbach W, Deiwick J, Hellwig-Burgel T (2007) *Chlamydia pneumoniae* directly interferes with HIF-1alpha stabilization in human host cells. Cell Microbiol 9(9):2181–2191. doi:10.1111/j.1462-5822.2007.00948.x

Sadler AJ, Williams BR (2008) Interferon-inducible antiviral effectors. Nat Rev Immunol 8 (7):559–568. doi:10.1038/nri2314

Said-Sadier N, Padilla E, Langsley G, Ojcius DM (2010) Aspergillus fumigatus stimulates the NLRP3 inflammasome through a pathway requiring ROS production and the Syk tyrosine kinase. PLoS ONE 5(4):e10008. doi:10.1371/journal.pone.0010008

Sanjuan MA, Dillon CP, Tait SW, Moshiach S, Dorsey F, Connell S, Komatsu M, Tanaka K, Cleveland JL, Withoff S, Green DR (2007) Toll-like receptor signalling in macrophages links the autophagy pathway to phagocytosis. Nature 450(7173):1253–1257. doi:10.1038/nature06421

Sanjuan MA, Milasta S, Green DR (2009) Toll-like receptor signaling in the lysosomal pathways. Immunol Rev 227(1):203–220. doi:10.1111/j.1600-065X.2008.00732.x

Schneider WM, Chevillotte MD, Rice CM (2014) Interferon-stimulated genes: a complex web of host defenses. Annu Rev Immunol 32:513–545. doi:10.1146/annurev-immunol-032713-120231

Schroder K, Tschopp J (2010) The inflammasomes. Cell 140(6):821–832. doi:10.1016/j.cell.2010.01.040

Scidmore MA, Hackstadt T (2001) Mammalian 14-3-3beta associates with the *Chlamydia trachomatis* inclusion membrane via its interaction with IncG. Mol Microbiol 39(6):1638–1650

Shamas-Din A, Kale J, Leber B, Andrews DW (2013) Mechanisms of action of Bcl-2 family proteins. Cold Spring Harb Perspect Biol 5(4):a008714. doi:10.1101/cshperspect.a008714

Shao W, Yeretssian G, Doiron K, Hussain SN, Saleh M (2007) The caspase-1 digestome identifies the glycolysis pathway as a target during infection and septic shock. J Biol Chem 282 (50):36321–36329. doi:10.1074/jbc.M708182200

Sharma M, Rudel T (2009) Apoptosis resistance in Chlamydia-infected cells: a fate worse than death? FEMS Immunol Med Microbiol 55(2):154–161. doi:10.1111/j.1574-695X.2008.00515.x

Sharma M, Machuy N, Bohme L, Karunakaran K, Maurer AP, Meyer TF, Rudel T (2011) HIF-1alpha is involved in mediating apoptosis resistance to *Chlamydia trachomatis*-infected cells. Cell Microbiol 13(10):1573–1585. doi:10.1111/j.1462-5822.2011.01642.x

Shenoy AR, Wellington DA, Kumar P, Kassa H, Booth CJ, Cresswell P, MacMicking JD (2012) GBP5 promotes NLRP3 inflammasome assembly and immunity in mammals. Science 336 (6080):481–485. doi:10.1126/science.1217141

Shimada K, Crother TR, Karlin J, Chen S, Chiba N, Ramanujan VK, Vergnes L, Ojcius DM, Arditi M (2011) Caspase-1 dependent IL-1beta secretion is critical for host defense in a mouse model of *Chlamydia pneumoniae* lung infection. PLoS ONE 6(6):e21477. doi:10.1371/journal.pone.0021477

Shimada K, Crother TR, Arditi M (2012) Innate immune responses to *Chlamydia pneumoniae* infection: role of TLRs, NLRs, and the inflammasome. Microbes Infect 14(14):1301–1307. doi:10.1016/j.micinf.2012.08.004

Shin S, Brodsky IE (2015) The inflammasome: Learning from bacterial evasion strategies. Semin Immunol 27(2):102–110. doi:10.1016/j.smim.2015.03.006

Siegl C, Rudel T (2015) Modulation of p53 during bacterial infections. Nat Rev Microbiol 13 (12):741–748. doi:10.1038/nrmicro3537

Siegl C, Prusty BK, Karunakaran K, Wischhusen J, Rudel T (2014) Tumor suppressor p53 alters host cell metabolism to limit *Chlamydia trachomatis* infection. Cell Rep 9(3):918–929. doi:10.1016/j.celrep.2014.10.004

Simon S, Hilbi H (2015) Subversion of cell-autonomous immunity and cell migration by *Legionella pneumophila* effectors. Front Immunol 6:447. doi:10.3389/fimmu.2015.00447

Stratton CW, Sriram S (2003) Association of *Chlamydia pneumoniae* with central nervous system disease. Microbes Infect 5(13):1249–1253

Su H, McClarty G, Dong F, Hatch GM, Pan ZK, Zhong G (2004) Activation of Raf/MEK/ERK/cPLA2 signaling pathway is essential for chlamydial acquisition of host glycerophospholipids. J Biol Chem 279(10):9409–9416. doi:10.1074/jbc.M312008200

Subbarayal P, Karunakaran K, Winkler AC, Rother M, Gonzalez E, Meyer TF, Rudel T (2015) EphrinA2 receptor (EphA2) is an invasion and intracellular signaling receptor for *Chlamydia trachomatis*. PLoS Pathog 11(4):e1004846. doi:10.1371/journal.ppat.1004846

Sun HS, Eng EW, Jeganathan S, Sin AT, Patel PC, Gracey E, Inman RD, Terebiznik MR, Harrison RE (2012) *Chlamydia trachomatis* vacuole maturation in infected macrophages. J Leukoc Biol 92(4):815–827. doi:10.1189/jlb.0711336

Takeuchi O, Akira S (2010) Pattern recognition receptors and inflammation. Cell 140(6):805–820. doi:10.1016/j.cell.2010.01.022

Thomas LW, Lam C, Edwards SW (2010) Mcl 1; the molecular regulation of protein function. FEBS Lett 584(14):2981–2989. doi:10.1016/j.febslet.2010.05.061

Thorpe LM, Yuzugullu H, Zhao JJ (2015) PI3K in cancer: divergent roles of isoforms, modes of activation and therapeutic targeting. Nat Rev Cancer 15(1):7–24. doi:10.1038/nrc3860

van Wijk SJ, Fiskin E, Putyrski M, Pampaloni F, Hou J, Wild P, Kensche T, Grecco HE, Bastiaens P, Dikic I (2012) Fluorescence-based sensors to monitor localization and functions of linear and K63-linked ubiquitin chains in cells. Mol Cell 47(5):797–809. doi:10.1016/j.molcel.2012.06.017

Verbeke P, Welter-Stahl L, Ying S, Hansen J, Hacker G, Darville T, Ojcius DM (2006) Recruitment of BAD by the *Chlamydia trachomatis* vacuole correlates with host-cell survival. PLoS Pathog 2(5):e45. doi:10.1371/journal.ppat.0020045

Vergne I, Chua J, Singh SB, Deretic V (2004) Cell biology of mycobacterium tuberculosis phagosome. Annu Rev Cell Dev Biol 20:367–394. doi:10.1146/annurev.cellbio.20.010403.114015

Wright HR, Turner A, Taylor HR (2008) Trachoma. Lancet 371(9628):1945–1954. doi:10.1016/S0140-6736(08)60836-3

Yang SC, Hung CF, Aljuffali IA, Fang JY (2015) The roles of the virulence factor IpaB in Shigella spp. in the escape from immune cells and invasion of epithelial cells. Microbiol Res 181:43–51. doi:10.1016/j.micres.2015.08.006

Ying S, Fischer SF, Pettengill M, Conte D, Paschen SA, Ojcius DM, Hacker G (2006) Characterization of host cell death induced by *Chlamydia trachomatis*. Infect Immun 74 (11):6057–6066. doi:10.1128/IAI.00760-06

Ying S, Christian JG, Paschen SA, Hacker G (2008) *Chlamydia trachomatis* can protect host cells against apoptosis in the absence of cellular Inhibitor of Apoptosis Proteins and Mcl-1. Microbes Infect 10(1):97–101. doi:10.1016/j.micinf.2007.10.005

Zhao Y, Yang J, Shi J, Gong YN, Lu Q, Xu H, Liu L, Shao F (2011) The NLRC4 inflammasome receptors for bacterial flagellin and type III secretion apparatus. Nature 477(7366):596–600. doi:10.1038/nature10510

Zhou R, Yazdi AS, Menu P, Tschopp J (2011) A role for mitochondria in NLRP3 inflammasome activation. Nature 469(7329):221–225. doi:10.1038/nature09663

The Hidden Genomics of *Chlamydia trachomatis*

James Hadfield, Angèle Bénard, Daryl Domman and Nicholas Thomson

Abstract The application of whole-genome sequencing has moved us on from sequencing single genomes to defining unravelling population structures in different niches, and at the -species, -serotype or even -genus level, and in local, national and global settings. This has been instrumental in cataloguing and revealing a huge a range of diversity in this bacterium, when at first we thought there was little. Genomics has challenged assumptions, added insight, as well as confusion and glimpses of truths. What is clear is that at a time when we start to realise the extent and nature of the diversity contained within a genus or a species like this, the huge depth of knowledge communities have developed, through cell biology, as well as the new found molecular approaches will be more precious than ever to link genotype to phenotype. Here we detail the technological developments and insights we have seen during the relatively short time since we began to see the hidden genome of *Chlamydia trachomatis*.

Contents

J. Hadfield · A. Bénard · D. Domman · N. Thomson
Wellcome Trust Sanger Institute, Wellcome Genome Campus, Hinxton CB10 1SA, UK

N. Thomson (✉)
London School of Hygiene and Tropical Medicine, London WC1E 7HT, UK
e-mail: nrt@sanger.ac.uk

Current Topics in Microbiology and Immunology (2018) 412:107–132
DOI 10.1007/82_2017_39

Published Online: 26 October 2017

1 Introduction

Chlamydia trachomatis infections, including their sequelae, are a major public health concern globally resulting in significant morbidity and healthcare costs. It has been estimated that *C. trachomatis* is the most common bacterial sexually transmitted infection (STI) worldwide with 131 million cases amongst adults annually (2014; Newman et al. 2015). In the UK alone chlamydia treatment is estimated to cost the National Health System up to 100 million pounds every year (www.chlamydiascreening.nhs.uk). However, *C. trachomatis* is perhaps less well known for its ability to cause the severe ocular disease, trachoma or infectious blindness, from which an estimated 232 million people are at risk worldwide (WHO-report 2014).

The German radiologist Ludwig Halberstädter and the Austrian zoologist Stanislaus von Prowazek set out in 1903 for the island of Java to identify the causative agent of syphilis. In 1907, while in the city of Jakarta, they examined scrapings from an eye infection, which showed an infected stained conjunctival epithelial cell with "intracytoplasmic vacuoles" containing small and large particles. When these inclusions were examined further with Giemsa-staining, they observed small, condensed particles that appeared to surround the nucleus of the infected cells. Halberstädter and von Prowazek initially thought these organisms were protozoa and were given the name "Chlamydozoa" after the Greek word "chlamys", or cloak-like mantle, for their appearance to "cloak" the nucleus of the infected cells. It was not until the 1960s that these organisms were finally identified as bacteria, after a brief classification as viruses due to their intracellular lifestyle, but they still retained the provenance of "chlamy" (Al-Rifai 1988; Schachter and Caldwell 1980). Today, the causative agent of blinding trachoma is known as *C. trachomatis*.

C. trachomatis belongs to a phylum of obligate, intracellular bacteria called the *Chlamydiae*, whose members span incredible phylogenetic and host diversity (Fig. 1). Related members of the family *Chlamydiaceae* contain many other important animal and human pathogens. For example, *Chlamydia pneumoniae* is a causative agent of pneumonia in humans, but also infects a diverse set of mammals,

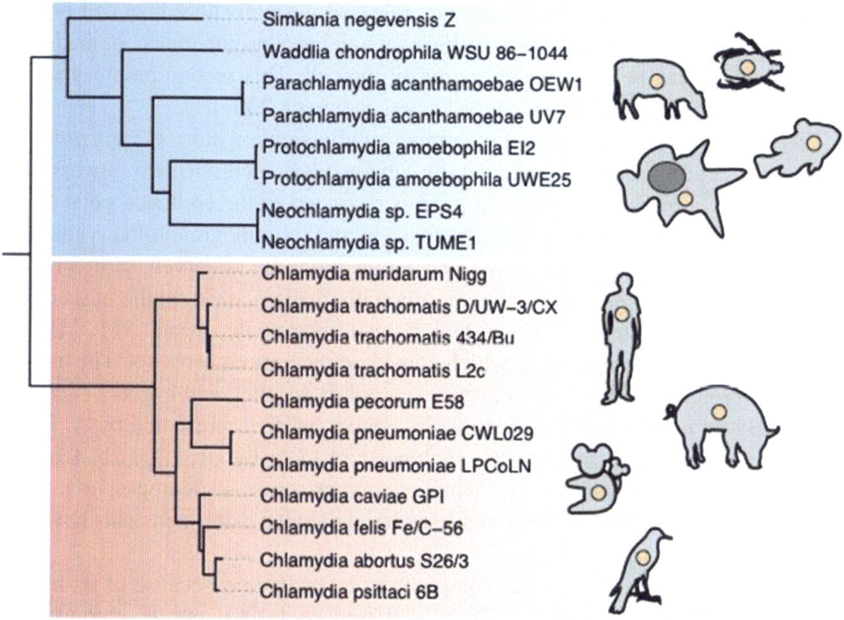

Fig. 1 Phylogeny of the Chlamydiae, with *Chlamydia* species shaded in *red*. Phylogeny constructed from 32 phylogenetic marker proteins taken from (Domman et al. 2014)

marsupials, amphibians and reptiles (Horn et al. 2004; Taylor-Brown et al. 2015). *Chlamydophila abortus* is responsible for fatal abortion within cattle, horses, rabbits and mice, while the avian and mammalian infecting *Chlamydophila psittaci* causes potentially lethal psittacosis in humans (Longbottom and Coulter 2003). Other members of the chlamydial phylum outside of the family *Chlamydiaceae* were discovered to reside within single-celled protists suggesting that this may represent a major novel reservoir for chlamydial organisms (Amann et al. 1997) There are currently seven described chlamydial families that are colloquially termed "environmental chlamydia" that are associated with a dizzying array of hosts ranging from amoeba, insects, fish, arthropods and marine worms (Horn 2008; Taylor-Brown et al. 2015). A recent study suggests there may be over 350 chlamydial families (Lagkouvardos et al. 2014), highlighting the extensive diversity seen within this phylum.

Despite the diversity in host range and phylogenetic distance, all chlamydiae are obligate, intracellular parasites that share a unique bi-phasic developmental cycle. The *C. trachomatis* developmental cycle begins when the extracellular, non-replicative form, termed elementary bodies (EBs), binds to a host cell and enters via endocytosis. The EBs differentiate into the fully metabolically active and replicative form, termed reticulate bodies (RBs) within an inclusion membrane. The RBs divide within the inclusion while scavenging host-derived ATP and nucleotides. Via a still unknown mechanism, at around 48 h post-infection, RBs begin to differentiate back into EBs, which are then released through either host cell lysis or extrusion which is a distinct exit pathway whereby a protuberance or inclusion membrane bleb can be seen extending out of the cell. This second pathway leaves the host cell intact (Ward 1983; Hybiske and Stephens 2007).

There are also considerable taxonomic subdivisions within *C. trachomatis*: based on infection profile, *C. trachomatis* can be subdivided into two biovars. The first is the trachoma biovar whose tropism is restricted to the epithelial cells of the eye and of the genital tract. The second is the lymphogranuloma venereum (LGV) biovar that is more invasive and while normally observed as a STI can spread systemically. These biovars were originally distinguished on the basis of the variation of the immuno-dominant major outer membrane protein (MOMP) by using microimmunofluorescence, which helped define various serovars. This is now done genotypically using the sequence variation in the *ompA* gene encoding MOMP. Based on this classification, ocular genotypes are represented by A, B and C genotypes, urogenital by D to K genotypes and LGV by L1, L2, L2b, L2c and L3. Globally the most common urogenital genotypes across all demographics are E, F and D, whereas LGV currently tends to be associated with men who have sex with men (MSM).

C. trachomatis has led the way for genomic investigation because of its impact in human health. However, during this time there have been major developments in our understanding of the wider diversity of this phylum.

Despite knowing about some of the unique biology of this organism in exquisite detail, until recently very little was known about the natural history and evolution of this organism. This area has been most recently explored through whole-genome sequencing (WGS). The size and type of questions that have been answered by WGS have, like for other bacterial pathogens, changed as the technologies have developed and the cost of sequencing has fallen while access to high-throughput machines has increased. This has also been facilitated by the development of approaches and protocols that have allowed direct sequencing without the need to culture this bacterium. This chapter will focus on *C. trachomatis* and the advances in our understanding that have been unravelled through unlocking the hidden details of the genome.

2 Next Generation Sequencing Techniques

The first chlamydial genomes were generated using the chain-termination method relying on the selective incorporation of one of the four possible dideoxynucleotides, originally radioactively labelled and more recently fluorescently labelled, which when incorporated into the growing DNA chain terminate DNA strand elongation. When the DNA strand resulting from the terminated reactions is separately run on an acrylamide gel, the fluorescent signal detected on the end of the terminated fragments could be used to determine the order of the bases and therefore the sequence. This method, referred to as Sanger sequencing, was able to generate "reads" of over 1 kb in length, but typically generating around 700 bps of accurate sequence in what was called a single sequence read. A sequencing read (referred to as a read from now on) is the sequential sequence of one sample at the end of the sequencing run. This technique, which was first automated by Applied Biosystems and formed the mainstay of the human genome project, was used to produce the first *C. trachomatis* genome of trachoma strain *C. trachomatis*, Har-13 (serovar A) in 1998 (Stephens et al. 1998). The output of this type of approach was measured in megabases, an impressive metric at the time, and while the sequence was accurate, the costs and output made sequencing genomes, even small bacterial genomes, an expensive endeavour.

More recently, Sanger sequencing has been supplanted by next generation sequencing (NGS) for genome-scale analysis. The most commonly used platform is the Illumina short-read sequencing platform. "Illumina sequencing", like Sanger sequencing, relies on the principle of incorporating modified fluorescently labelled bases into growing DNA chains. However, the gain in throughput comes from being able to sequence millions of short DNA segments simultaneously on a single small microscope slide-sized glass flow cell, massively parallelising the whole process.

2.1 Culture-Based Versus Culture-Independent Sequencing

Next generation sequencing has been developed for sequencing purified target DNA. For the most commonly sequenced bacteria, which can grow axenically, this is not a problem. However, for intracellular bacteria such as *Chlamydia,* this was one of the major barriers to sequencing with the first *C. trachomatis* genomes being generated from isolates propagated in multiple tissue culture flasks, over multiple passages, in order to obtain enough material for sequencing (O'Neill et al. 2013; Thomson et al. 2008). In addition to this being slow and costly, some strains may be recalcitrant to culture. In the UK, like many other countries, there has been a tendency to a move away from live collections of diagnostic samples and culture-based diagnosis towards molecular methods that collect samples in lysis buffer, thereby limiting the number of live isolates available to research. For these reasons, alternative DNA sequencing methods have been developed and applied to *Chlamydia* that bypassed the need for culture (O'Neill et al. 2013; Seth-Smith et al. 2013a, b). These can be summarised as non-targeted and targeted approaches. Non-targeted approaches include simply deep sequencing of a clinical sample (Andersson et al. 2013). However, when applied as a method to sequence a specific genome, it is expensive and the contaminating human DNA and other microbial DNA effectively mask the target DNA. This can be improved by DNA enrichment approaches, which aim to deplete the host DNA in clinical samples such as MolYsis Molzym (for more detail see Horz et al. 2010). While these enrich for microbial DNA by removing the methylated host DNA, it is difficult to generate highly accurate genome sequences, for a specific bacterium, from a complex clinical sample in a scalable manner.

Recently more targeted approaches have been used to sequence the genomes from single bacterial cells isolated by micromanipulation, microfluidics or flow cytometry (reviewed in Lasken 2012; Yilmaz and Singh 2012). While they are increasingly useful for some applications, such as comparing the variation between individual cells of the same species within a complex mix, these techniques are also highly time and resource consuming. Hence, more targeted and scalable approaches have been developed and applied to *Chlamydia*, as described below.

2.2 Immuno-magnetic Separation and Multiple Displacement Amplification (IMS-MDA)

Whole-genome amplification (WGA), in particular multiple displacement amplification (MDA), can be used on very low concentrations of starting material to generate the quantities of DNA required for sequencing (Blanco et al. 1989). MDA essentially amplifies high molecular weight DNA using Φ29 polymerase and random hexamer primers (Dean et al. 2001; Hosono et al. 2003). When combined with immuno-magnetic separation (IMS), this provided the ability to enrich or extract bacterial cells of interest before purifying the DNA and then amplifying their genomes by MDA. IMS uses antibodies tagged to magnetic beads to bind surface proteins on intact target cells which are then isolated magnetically. The necessary amount of (pre-amplification) DNA for whole-genome reconstruction was found to be ~5000 genome copies (Seth-Smith et al. 2013a, b) The sequence data produced by genome amplification methods can suffer from a more variable depth of coverage across the genome compared to culture-based methods. This can present a problem for many bioinformatic tools, which assume relatively even coverage. Thankfully, the advancements in single-cell sequencing have been accompanied by bioinformatics improvements, which mitigate this variability. It should also be noted that this technique also results in the sequencing of other bacteria, albeit at lower depth than the target. This may be seen by analysing the contigs from assembly and is easily removed by using a reference genome as a scaffold. This approach has been successfully applied to a range of bacteria including *C. trachomatis* reducing the time involved in generating a genome from weeks to hours (Putman et al. 2013; Seth-Smith et al. 2013a, b).

2.3 Target DNA Pull-Down

One of the main limitations of IMS-MDA (and culture) is a requirement for intact bacterial cells to which the antibodies can bind, in order to enrich for the genomic

DNA of interest. As mentioned above, in recent years, swabs from many commercial diagnostic companies have been collected directly into lysis buffer, and thus the possibility of obtaining live/intact cells has dramatically decreased. This stimulated the development of other targeted approaches that enrich for specific bacterial DNA from complex samples prior to sequencing. One such approach that has been applied to several *Chlamydia* species as well as to viruses and human exome sequencing is the target enrichment system called SureSelect™ (Agilent) (Chilamakuri et al. 2014; Christiansen et al. 2014; Garcia-Garcia et al. 2016; Joseph et al. 2014). By building a library of RNA oligonucleotides, called baits (typically 120-mers), from known sequence data, sheared target DNA may be hybridized and purified for sequencing. Importantly, the RNA baits cannot be sequenced and so are not represented in the final sequence data. A limitation of this approach is that novel regions of DNA will not be pulled down. This is of particular significance to bacteria as phenotypically important traits such as antimicrobial resistance are frequently acquired horizontally and will not be detected unless this is present in the bait design. *C. trachomatis* genomic variation tends to be much subtler than seen in free-living bacteria, and so this may not appear as such an important consideration (see below).

3 *C. trachomatis* in the Genomic Era: Genome Content

The first genome of *C. trachomatis* appeared in 1998 as one of the first bacterial species to be sequenced (Stephens et al. 1998). For chlamydial research, it was particularly significant because "the continuing inability to perform basic laboratory genetic manipulations is a feature of this organism" (Bavoil and Wyrick 2006). The full sequence of a genotype D urogenital strain (D/UW3) revealed a 1.04 Mb chromosome containing 894 protein-coding genes and GC percentage of 41%, together with a 7.4 kb plasmid. Such a small genome is consistent with genomic streamlining due to their intracellular lifestyle and parasitism of host metabolites.

The completed genome even with its small size provided many surprises including a pathway for peptidoglycan biosynthesis, the presence of which, despite this bacteria natural sensitivity to penicillin, was not detected experimentally in the cell wall until 2014 (Liechti et al. 2014). Many possible virulence factors were observed including a type III secretion system and nine paralogous polymorphic membrane protein genes (*pmp*). Many pathways that were considered to be essential in bacteria were missing, including those needed to synthesize some essential amino acids and nucleotides, the cell division protein *ftsZ* previously thought to be essential, DNA oxidative damage repair proteins as well as genes involved in transformation and competency.

It took another 10 years for the complete set of chlamydia pathotypes to be sequenced. In addition to D/UW3, these included the trachoma strain *C. trachomatis*, Har-13 (serovar A) and a classical LGV strain (serovar L2) as well as a LGV proctitis strain (genotype L2b) (Carlson et al. 2005; Stephens et al. 1998;

Thomson et al. 2008). Subsequently, the research focus moved onto comparative genomics, beginning with comparing synteny (in bacteria considered to be the conservation in gene order and orientation).

3.1 Comparative Genomics and Genome Synteny

A quick glance at the aligned genomes is sufficient to highlight the high degree of synteny between *C. trachomatis* with almost no disruptions nor evidence for rearrangements; this is very different from most free-living bacterial genomes (Fig. 2). This simple observation has become a challenge for genomics: how could we explain the seemingly clear and significant differences in tropism, disease outcome and growth differences between the ocular, urogenital and LGV biovars in the absence of obvious major differences in their genome content?

From these analyses, it was clear that over 90% of all genes are common to all isolates from the different biovars (Thomson et al. 2008) with very little or no recent horizontally acquired DNA.

The region showing the highest degree of variation between chlamydial genomes is the plasticity zone or PZ, which includes virulence genes as well as the tryptophan synthesis operon (Read et al. 2003, 2013; Taylor et al. 2010; Thomson et al. 2008). Indeed, the PZ is the only region showing signs of recent reductive evolution such as pseudogenisation and gene loss. This is consistent with *C. trachomatis* being a highly adapted obligate intracellular pathogen (Horn et al. 2004; Joseph et al. 2012).

Initial work focused on elucidating the differences between strains that cause the three different tropisms. Despite the high synteny and homology between isolates, it became clear that isolates causing different tropisms were genetically distinct and carried many non-synonymous mutations as well as pseudogenes and gene gain/loss albeit to a lesser degree. Comparison between a LGV and urogenital isolates

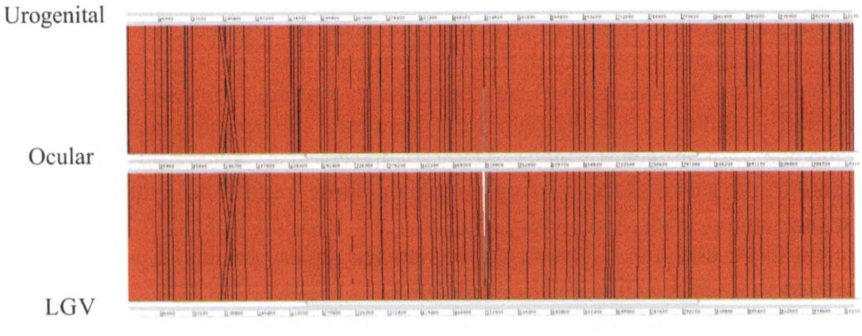

Fig. 2 Genomic synteny between three reference strains of *C. trachomatis*. *Red* blocks joining genomes indicate sequence similarity. Reference genomes used included D/UW3 (urogenital), A/Har13 (ocular) and L2/434/BU (LGV)

concluded that no additional genes could account for the differences in disease outcome, indicating that the genetic basis for tropism is more subtle than may have been expected (Thomson et al. 2008).

4 The Link Between Tryptophan and Ocular Isolates

Interferon gamma (IFN-γ) is a key component of the innate immune response to chlamydial infections. One of the mechanisms of action results in the degradation of available tryptophan, which has been shown to prevent the growth and development of RBs (Fehlner-Gardiner et al. 2002). Sequencing of the genome revealed a limited tryptophan synthesis pathway, encoded by *trpRBA*, which can convert indole into tryptophan (Carlson et al. 2005; Stephens et al. 1998). Comparison between ocular and urogenital isolates revealed that ocular strains have a non-functional tryptophan synthesis pathway, implying that this is not an essential function for ocular isolates (Carlson et al. 2005). While this could be the beginning of further genome reduction, it has been postulated that this is one of the most important differences between ocular and urogenital isolates whereby urogenital strains use the ability to convert the indole excreted as a waste product by surrounding microbiota in the genital tract to make tryptophan and elude host immune response (Fehlner-Gardiner et al. 2002). The significance being that indole is widely available in the genital tract but is not present in the eye (Caldwell et al. 2003).

5 Species Phylogeny

Prior to the genomics age, the species was divided into three groups based on tropism (ocular/urogenital/LGV) associated with serotype. Based on the sequencing of certain genomic regions, in particular the serotype-determining gene *ompA*, it became clear that the evolutionary history of genomic regions was not concordant with the three-division hypothesis (Brunelle and Sensabaugh 2006; Gomes et al. 2006). As we entered the genomics age, studies began to increase in size, considering up to 52 whole genomes (Gomes et al. 2006; Harris et al. 2012; Joseph et al. 2011, 2012; Putman et al. 2013). The principal finding from these studies is a species phylogeny comprising four distinct lineages denoted Trachoma 1 (T1) and Trachoma 2 (T2), the classical ocular lineage and the LGV lineage as shown in Fig. 3.

The species phylogeny comprises two lineages representing the two biovars (LGV and trachoma) separated by around 5000 vertically acquired base differences or single nucleotide polymorphisms (SNPs; long red branch, Fig. 3) (Harris et al. 2012). The trachoma biovar comprises three monophylies in this phylogeny, two of which consist of isolates collected form urogenital STI samples, and one that

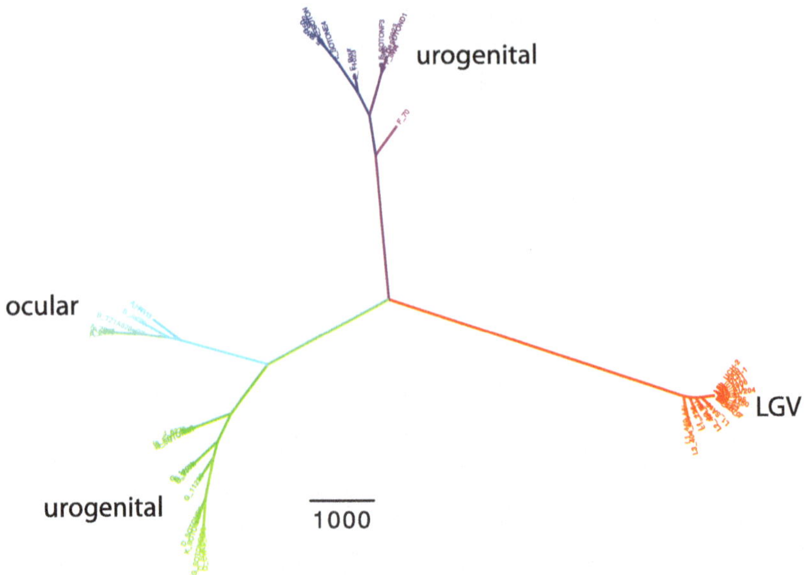

Fig. 3 Species Phylogeny of 56 whole genomes with the tropisms of the four major lineages labelled. Scale bar represents 1000 SNPs; colours indicate genotypes. The species comprises two biovars, LGV and trachoma (urogenital and ocular). Figure adapted from Harris et al. (2012)

consists of isolates collected from ocular samples. This structure is consistent with deep divisions in the phylogeny associated with the site of infection, yet the phylogenetic structure appears more complex than previously thought, why?

6 Recombination

Homologous recombination is a fundamental and powerful mechanism for creating and maintaining diversity within populations. It is a mechanism by which the impact of deleterious mutations can be rescued by purging out less favourable variation. Recombination also allows the spread of advantageous variation, as well as offering the potential to generate novel sequence within genes and genomes. Recombination has been a controversial subject in the chlamydial field over the last 10 years. Simplistically perhaps, it was thought that recombination was not a feature, or at least a significant driver, in the evolution of the Chlamydiae owing to their development in a confined and protected inclusion. Hence, the discovery from the first genome sequence that *C. trachomatis* had "considerable recombination capabilities" (Stephens et al. 1998) was unexpected and presaged the discoveries of extensive recombination between members of the species. However, with hindsight there was some evidence for recombination in the literature. As early as 1994, the *ompA* genes from novel LGV serotypes were seen to be recombinant chimeras from

L1 and L2 isolates (Hayes et al. 1994). Phylogenetic evidence that *ompA* may have been involved in recombinations was observed when the *ompA* phylogenetic signal differed from those of other genes or loci in the same genome (Brunelle and Sensabaugh 2006; Gomes et al. 2004; Millman et al. 2001) These observations extended beyond *ompA*, as loci related to tropism or virulence such as the nine genes encoding the polymorphic membrane proteins, *pmp*, showed "clear evidence for a high rate of whole-gene recombination" (Gomes et al. 2004). Specifically, the sequence of a 15 kb region encompassing *pmpE-I* found in a urogenital Da isolate was more closely related to the sequence of the orthologous genes from the ocular genotypes showing levels of variation that did not support convergent evolution, but rather recombination. Similarly, reports detailed isolates from urogenital serotypes E and F strains had exchanged *pmpB, C, D, H* and *I* genes (Gomes et al. 2006). Thus, evidence for recombination was present throughout the literature and had been gaining much acceptance across the research community. However, initially, these loci were considered to be restricted to specific regions of the genome termed "hot spots" of recombination, implying a differing propensity for recombination across the genome. It later became clear that although these regions did possess higher SNP densities, the idea of hot spots was in effect an artefact of how we recognise recombination.

6.1 Direct Experimental Evidence of Recombination

Elegant experiments in 2007 determined the potential and ease with which *C. trachomatis* recombines. Host cells were infected with two different strains, each being resistant to a different antibiotic. Post-infection, a dual antibiotic selection produced multiply-resistant recombinants (Demars et al. 2007). Furthermore, these recombinants were present amongst EBs during the early stages of development. The DNA present from autolysis of some *C. trachomatis* cells within the inclusion was postulated to be the substrate for recombination (Demars et al. 2007). In these experiments, the length of recombination regions, or blocks, was shown to range between 330 and 800 kb, with the minimum detected at 123 kb (DeMars and Weinfurter 2008). From whole-genome analysis of 12 recombinant strains generated in vitro under antibiotic selection, 190 recombination events were detected showing the extent of recombination occurring over a relatively short period of time and in a simple experimental system (Jeffrey et al. 2013). All recombination events were examples of homologous recombination, with one exception being a deletion of a sequentially duplicated rRNA sequence. No evidence supported the requirement for specific motifs involved in the recombination process.

Having established the principle in the laboratory, detecting recombination in vivo required the occurrence of co-infection of the host with distinct *C. trachomatis* strains. One study estimated that 2–13% of clinical chlamydia infections are co-infections of at least two distinct serovars (Demars et al. 2007). Assuming a 5% co-infection rate, this would result in hundreds of thousands of recombination possibilities worldwide per year. Therefore with a frequency of successful recombination events in vitro estimated between 1 in 10,000 and 1 in 1000 (Demars et al. 2007), there is ample opportunity for recombination to be an important mechanism in diversification and evolution of this pathogen.

6.2 Understanding C. Trachomatis *Population Structure*

Chlamydial population genomics studies using whole genomes have consistently shown the presence of apparent recombination regions throughout the genome, with the clearest examples involving the region surrounding *ompA* (Harris et al. 2012; Joseph et al. 2011, 2012; Putman et al. 2013). The first study of populations analysed 12 complete genomes and found widespread recombination across the genome, contrasting with earlier gene-based studies that found recombination "hot spots" (Joseph et al. 2011, 2012). The authors found eight genes to be involved in recombination with a high degree of confidence: *ompA*, three *pmp* genes (*pmpE*, *pmpF*, *pmpH*), a type III secretion protein (*yscC*), the gene encoding elongation factor Ts (*tsf*) and two hypothetical protein genes (*CT049*, *CT144*). However, many more genes showed some evidence of recombination (Joseph et al. 2011). All of these genes, as well as others, showed evidence of positive selection using a maximum likelihood estimate of dN/dS over each branch. They also found that the linkage disequilibrium (LD) decay is similar to that of other, free-living bacterial pathogens (Joseph et al. 2011).

Subsequent analysis investigated 32 genomes and continued to find evidence for extensive and pervasive recombination (Joseph et al. 2012). Contrary to the in vitro experiments, the average length of recombination regions was 357 bp, which is more consistent with those found in other bacteria (Joseph et al. 2012). These two observations of recombination fragment length are not necessarily contradictory as it may suggest that continual recombination under more complex selective forces than those used in vitro tends to produce shorter fragments encompassing the selectively advantageous loci. Alluding to the increased focus on vaccine development, the authors anticipate difficulties in finding genomically stable regions in the genome upon which to target a cross-protective vaccine (Joseph et al. 2012).

Until recently, the most comprehensive analysis encompassed 52 genomes (Harris et al. 2012). The results were generally consistent with previous studies; however, the increased sample size allowed stronger conclusions to be drawn. Namely, it was concluded that the high rates of recombination involving *ompA* had confounded our understanding of the phylogeny and epidemiology of this species because the same *ompA* genotype can exist on unrelated branches of the *C. trachomatis* phylogenetic tree. This may also explain why clinically *C. trachomatis* genovars appear epidemiologically static or invariant, as any genomic flux is masked by the *ompA* genotype, and associations with disease or patient demographic cannot be determined. It also explains in this instance why, all the existing gene-based *C. trachomatis* typing schemes can give conflicting results with the underlying whole-genome phylogeny. For example, while multi-locus sequence typing (MLST) schemes perform better, than *ompA* typing, they still fail to uncover the true phylogeny when compared to WGS.

These data showed that the recombination landscape was highly dynamic, with six regions of increased recombination detected. However, rather than these being "hot spots" as previously proposed, these regions are thought to be the product of "higher rates of fixation of recombinations in genomic regions that are under diversifying selection pressure", a finding in accordance with recent work from several groups (Harris et al. 2012; Jeffrey et al. 2010). Using a novel phylogenetic method for interpreting the recombination flux, the authors were able to show a propensity for exchange between strains with the same tropism, concordant with reports of mixed infections; however, other examples of exchange do exist especially between ocular and urogenital isolates.

The growing whole-genome data has also been used to show something altogether more subtle: there are detectable differences (not at the whole-gene level) that elude to distinct evolutionary trajectories between the different *C. trachomatis* lineages. For example, on the assumption that most of the variant alleles that were detected represent single recombination or mutational events, then it is possible to estimate the relative contribution of recombination versus mutation on the genomic evolution by simply dividing one by the other (r/m)(Joseph et al. 2012). Using this approach the r/m value for *C. trachomatis* was estimated to be 1.1. However, although this to many may be a subtle point, this rate varied between 0.31 and 1.95 across the four phylogenetic lineages (Joseph et al. 2012). These results indicated for the first time that the different lineages are acting differently in terms of their evolutionary dynamic and trajectory. It shows that recombination profiles may be lineage-specific and that we can start to define lineage-specific rather than serovar-specific differences and perhaps move towards a more detailed understanding of how *C. trachomatis* was/is evolving.

These findings have been further explored in the most recent study (Hadfield et al. 2017) which looked at over 563 full genomes from geographically diverse isolates emanating from Europe, North America, South America, Africa, Asia and Australia. They included all known genotypes, from ocular to LGV, and isolates collected between 1957 and 2012. The DNA samples for sequencing were also obtained by direct MDA of the DNA sample, IMS-MDA or SureSelect target enrichment, as well as from live culture, providing the opportunity to detect any biases in the ability to grow and sequence *C. trachomatis*.

Firstly, this data showed the robustness of the species phylogeny with the four deep branching monophyletic lineages that generally associate with tropism (Fig. 4). Moreover, it showed that the plasmid was almost entirely vertically inherited. Both of these results are important as it suggests that we are sampling from most of the genetic diversity extant within this species, at least from human clinical samples. Also, the location of genomes from cultured and culture-free extraction methods distributed throughout the tree suggested that sampling methods had not introduced significant bias into our view of the population structure.

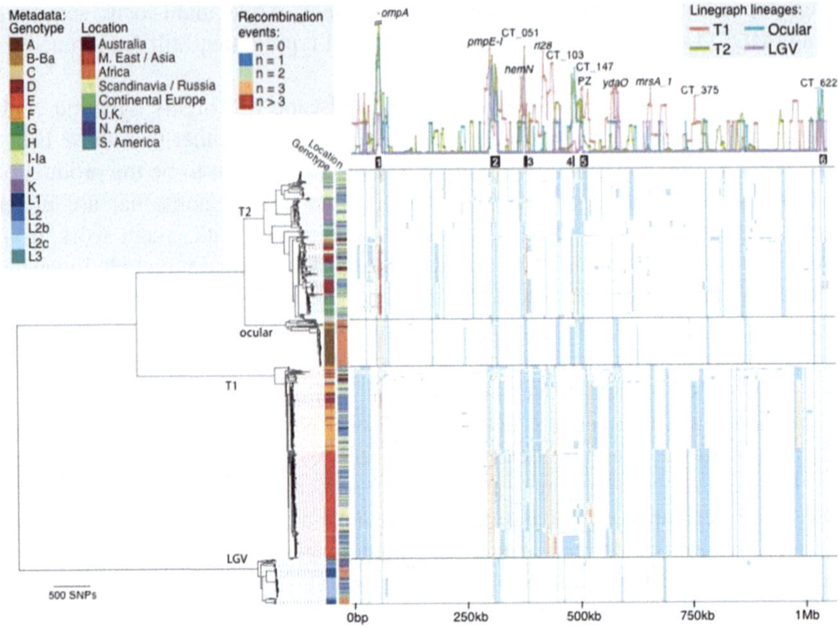

Fig. 4 Global phylogeny and recombination landscape of 563 *C. trachomatis* genomes. The phylogeny (*left*), with associated genotype and geographical data, is displayed alongside the linearised chromosome (*right*). Lineage labels are as per previous publications. Line graph (*right, upper*) shows the number of recombination events affecting individual genes and is coloured according to lineage. *Black squares* below this graph show previously identified "hot spots" of recombination (Harris et al. 2012). Coloured blocks (*right, lower*) indicate inferred recombination events each affecting selected taxa and genomic location, with colour indicating the number of inferred events. Gene annotations correspond to strain D/UW3; PZ: plasticity zone. Taken from Hadfield et al. (2017)

The great range of data generated from this study allowed the authors to dig deeper into the initial observations that had shown differential patterns of evolution between the different *C. trachomatis* lineages: T1 was believed, in comparison with T2, to contain fewer vertically inherited SNPs manifesting in shorter branch lengths of the terminal branches within the tree, once recombination had been removed (Fig. 5). The authors report that the r/m values vary by ~10-fold between lineages across the tree (r/m = 0.37 ocular to 3.11 T1; Hadfield et al. 2017). Importantly, and in consistence with the differing shape of the tree, the two urogenital lineages showed markedly different amounts of recombination (r/m 1.23–3.11) reinforcing the different impact recombination has had on their respective phylogenies.

From the same analysis, over 1100 recombination blocks (an average of 7.5 kb per recombination) were identified, which covered on average 23% of the genome (Hadfield et al. 2017). These included the six previously described "hot spots" or recombination blocks (Gomes et al. 2006; Harris et al. 2012) namely the *ompA* gene, genes *pmpE-I* and the plasticity zone amongst others (see Fig. 4). However,

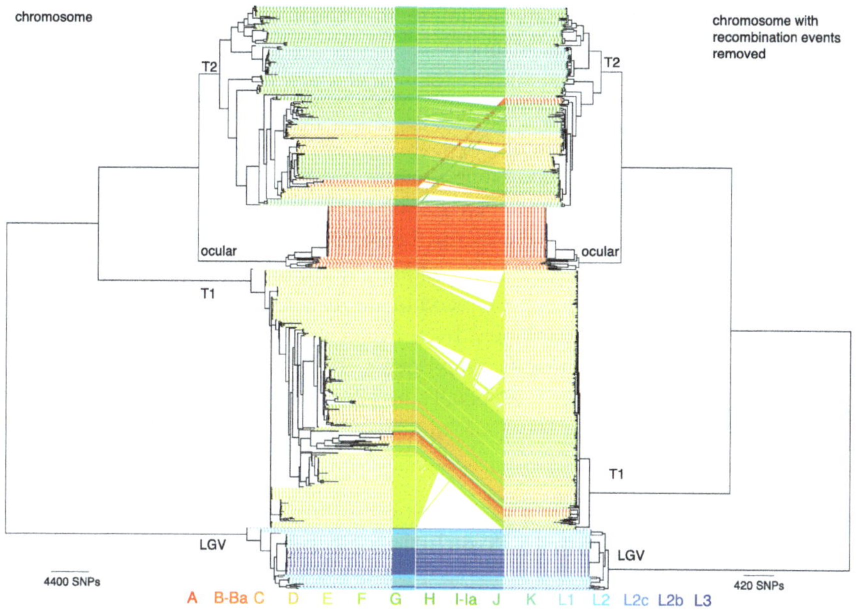

Fig. 5 Impact of recombination on the species phylogeny. A tanglegram showing the differences in tree topology between the whole genome (*left*) and the whole genome with recombinations removed (*right*). Nodes on the recombination removed tree have been rotated in order to minimise the number of differences in the ordering of tips. While T1 and T2 are clearly incongruent, the Kendall-Colijn metric shows that all lineages have different topologies as well as differences in branch lengths

while these showed elevated levels of recombination in all lineages, the majority of recombination was specific to a lineage or a clade within a lineage, showing that the "recombination landscape is more dynamic than would be expected from a small number of hot spots" and in line with the current view on the extent of recombination this bacterium is undergoing.

6.3 Lineage-Specific Patterns of Recombination

While the regions mentioned above show heightened rates of recombination across the species, which is why they stand out so prominently, Hadfield et al. (2017) show that the majority of recombination is lineage- or clade-specific, as shown by comparing the trees before and after recombination was removed (Fig. 5). These last results suggested that recombination has played a major role in driving expansion of the T1 lineage, especially when compared to T2. This is further highlighted by the fact that T1 has accumulated less background mutations, distinct from those brought in by recombination, suggesting that T1 is a more recent lineage than T2. This conclusion holds assuming that the mutation rate operates in a "clock-like", i.e. a predictable, manner.

Exploring data further, the authors highlighted many examples of genes present in all lineages that are differentially affected by recombination. These included a number of genes of unknown function as well as *incA* and *incB*, encoding for well-characterised inclusion membrane proteins. Although present in all members of the species, these genes show patterns of recombination specific to the LGV clade. Likewise, some regions known to be highly recombinogenic in some lineages are stable in other lineages. The authors chose to focus on the genotype E lineage that shows no evidence of recombination across *ompA* gene. This phenomenon is thought to be explained by a recent monophyletic expansion where recombination has not disrupted the *ompA* gene, either because of time or selection, contrasting with other lineages, especially in T2, where recombination resulted in frequent genotype switching (Harris et al. 2012).

7 Global and Temporal Population Structure of *C. trachomatis*

This extended data set also revealed significant geographical signatures in the phylogeny showing that the urogenital lineages with fewer than 210 (T1) or 280 (T2) SNP differences between genomes were more than 50% likely to originate from the same country, where recombinations are most probably masked out by sequence similarity. This compares to genotype level, where to find isolates with the same probability of sharing a common genotype you would have to draw from those with a much larger genetic distance, namely 1850 SNPs and 1470 SNPs for lineages T1 and T2, respectively. A similar analysis was not possible for the classically ocular lineage in T2 because of restricted sampling. However, this has helped refine our view on the disconnect between genotype and lineage brought about through recombination and has showed that while genotype is not a reliable phylogenetic marker, at the highest level there is a strong association between genotype and the T1, T2 or LGV lineages, as you would expect. The problem for us is largely that we are interested in the exceptions to the rule regarding genotype and tropism/pathotype where *ompA* genotype has masked interesting biological facts, as illustrated in this elegant study of *C. trachomatis* infection in the Aboriginal population of the Northern Territories of Australia (Andersson et al. 2013) (see below). The findings of this study further underline the fact that recombination must be taken into account when trying to understand the fine-scaled evolution of this species.

Understanding the relative contribution of recombination to variation helped to estimate a mutation rate (Hadfield et al. 2017). Although it can be difficult to accurately estimate mutation rate, usually because of biases in sampling, it can arguably be one of the most important pieces of information to come from genomic data. It frames the time over which the observed evolutionary changes are occurring, which allows for epidemiological information to be correlated with these changes. Hadfield et al., estimated that the mutation rate for the LGV lineage, where they had a broader temporal sampling with isolates sequenced from egg yolk dating back to the 1960s, was 0.2 SNPs per genome per year. This is consistent with estimates for other intracellular bacteria such as the aphid endosymbiont *Buchnera aphidicola* (Linz et al. 2014). This rate predicted that the most recent common ancestor (MRCA) of LGV existed just over a 1000 years ago and the MRCA of the L2b isolates being dated back to around 100 years old. These findings are consistent with epidemiological reports showing that these isolates had been around for much longer than generally thought and certainly before the reporting of the recent proctitis epidemic in men who have sex with men (Schachter and Moncada 2005). Although an accurate mutation rate could not be determined for the other *C. trachomatis* lineages, it is noteworthy that the rate observed for LGV differs from the ~175 SNPs/year estimated for *C. psittaci* (Read et al. 2013) by almost three orders of magnitude. It is difficult to resolve the two rates because this would indicate that the *C. psittaci* mutation rate lies amongst the RNA viruses (Linz et al. 2014).

8 The Plasmid

It would be impossible to ignore the contribution of the *C. trachomatis* plasmid when discussing the recent advances in our understanding of the genome. The 7.5 kb plasmid is predicted to encode eight genes and has a copy number of around 2–6 (Seth-Smith et al. 2009). Its role in virulence has been shown for both urogenital isolates in the mouse model and ocular isolates in the non-human primate model for trachoma (Kari et al. 2011). This is also evidenced by the fact that while some clinical strains are plasmid free, they are extremely rare in nature; in fact, little is known about their clinical significance. In terms of its gene content, the plasmid encodes genes that are now known to play a role in regulating expression of chromosomal genes and are considered critical for in vivo, but not in vitro, growth; in fact, studies showed that the plasmid is sometimes lost during culture passage (Carlson et al. 2008; Jeffrey et al. 2010; Rockey 2011; Song et al. 2013). Of the eight genes encoded on the plasmid, CDS1, –2, –6 and –8 are essential for plasmid maintenance, while CDS4 is a transcriptional regulator of CDS3 and a number of chromosomal genes (Carlson et al. 2008). The presence of glycogen in the inclusion is an easily observed phenotype, and plasmid-free isolates are known to display a glycogen-negative phenotype. CDS4 knockouts are, in this sense, phenotypically similar to plasmid-free strains, an observation supported by the role of CDS4 in mediating regulation of glycogen synthase (*glgA*) (Carlson et al. 2008; Song et al. 2013).

All genomic evidence to date shows that the plasmid is highly conserved at the sequence level and has been vertically inherited with the phylogeny of the plasmid matching that of the chromosome. However, there are exceptions to this rule with evidence of homologous recombination between internal regions of different plasmids as well as exchange of whole plasmids. Yet these events are also relatively rare, compared to chromosomal recombination events (Farencena et al. 1997; Peterson et al. 1990; Wang et al. 2013). As an example, only two recombination events were detected in the plasmid from the whole-genome sequence of 43 isolates (Harris et al. 2012; Seth-Smith et al. 2009). These included the complete replacement of a plasmid in a serotype Ia isolate with one from another *C. trachomatis* lineage and a single recombination event encompassing a region between pCDS3 and pCDS5 that was exchanged between ocular strains in the T2 clade and a plasmid from urogenital isolate from the T1 clade. Other variation reported in the *C. trachomatis* plasmid included the deletion in the Swedish new variant strain pE/SW2, which leads to the isolates being undetectable to molecular diagnostic tests (see below).

9 The Swedish New Variant

Due to the plasmid's copy number and its conservation across isolates, it was routinely used as the target of choice for PCR-based diagnostics. Yet in 2006, a new variant of *C. trachomatis* (nvCT) was identified in Sweden with a 377 bp deletion in CDS1 and a 44 bp duplication located at the start of CDS3 gene (Fig. 6) (Unemo and Clarke 2011; Unemo et al. 2010). This deletion disrupted a diagnostic primer binding site for the nucleic acid amplification test (NAAT), resulting in false-negative diagnosis and rapid expansion of this nvCT in Sweden, despite no apparent biological advantage (Unemo et al. 2010). As infection with strains carrying the wild-type (WT) plasmid produced a positive diagnosis, antibiotic treatment removed these strains from the population allowing this new variant to expand, undetected, within the population. This is perhaps one of the clearest examples of human-driven Darwinian selection conferred by diagnostic escape. The result was a rapid expansion of the nvCT within this population and abroad. This provided evidence that populations of *C. trachomatis* given the correct selective pressure are highly dynamic and can expand dramatically. Should *C. trachomatis* become resistant to treatment and it has not so far, then the spread of the nvCT shows how rapidly these isolates would rise to dominance. Luckily widespread resistance has not been observed so far, a topic that will be further discussed below.

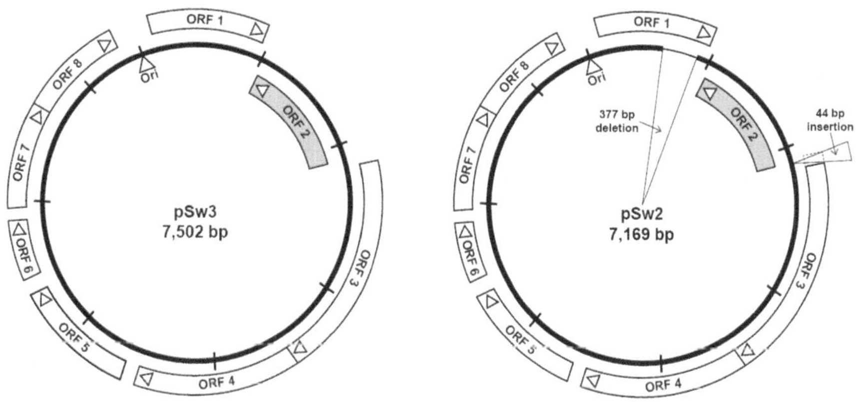

Fig. 6 Genetic architecture of a representative wild-type *C. trachomatis* virulence plasmid encoding eight genes (*right*; pSw3) compared with that of the Swedish new variant plasmid (*left*) which escaped PCR detection (*inner*). Figure taken from Thomson and Clarke (2010)

10 Antimicrobial Resistance in *C. trachomatis*

The literature on antimicrobial resistance (AMR) in *C. trachomatis* is quite broad including multiple reports on the ability to isolate in vitro strains with mutations conferring significant AMR to clinically relevant antimicrobial compounds (reviewed in Sandoz and Rockey 2010), to reports of sporadic clinical resistance through treatment failure (Hogan et al. 2004; O'Neill et al. 2013; Sandoz and Rockey 2010). However, outside of these experimental settings and sporadic reports, stable AMR has not been shown conclusively in a clinical setting (Sandoz and Rockey 2010). Although isolates included in the study by Hadfield et al. (2017) were not collected to study clinical resistance, they were nevertheless representative of isolates circulating in the human population. From analysing these data, the authors found no evidence for the presence of characteristic mutations associated with azithromycin resistance in the chlamydial reads, either fixed (in all reads) or as SNPs in low abundance.

However, these data did highlight important considerations when using mapping-based approaches to identify point mutations in highly conserved regions of a genome, like those associated with macrolide resistance in the 23S rRNA gene. Regions within the 23S rRNA gene are highly conserved across bacteria. Hence, unlike almost all other areas of the genome, DNA from these regions can be "pulled down" by direct sequencing approaches and if so will map convincingly to the chlamydial 23S rRNA gene. By differential mapping of reads to multiple 23S rRNA operons and restricting the analysis to only paired reads, the authors showed that any read with SNPs associated with resistance mapped, in their correct pairs, more strongly to other bacterial species sequences, suggesting that the reads were from contaminants in the original sample (Hadfield et al. 2017). The most common contaminant read belonged to *Lactobacillus* species. As a result, all reads containing resistance SNPs no longer mapped to the *C. trachomatis* 23S rRNA gene; hence, there was no evidence of chlamydial resistance mutations in the samples sequenced.

The main interest in this finding does not lie within the probability of such resistant mutation occurring but rather in the fact that these mutations have not become fixed in the circulating populations, unlike in most other bacterial species, suggesting that there may be a strong fitness cost to their maintenance that precludes antibiotic resistance developing. This is certainly a positive note on which to end this section.

11 *Chlamydia trachomatis* in the Field

Applying genome-based technologies to field samples has also revealed some surprises. In fact, much of our previous understanding of the genomic diversity of this bacterium was limited by having to culture the isolate, based on serotype/genotype or derived from a limited number of samples. One such surprise, amongst several others associated with exchange of the *ompA* gene, was presented by Andersson et al. who describe a recent "mother-child" study carried out on isolates collected in Aboriginal communities in the Northern Territories of Australia between 1985 and 1993 (Andersson et al. 2013). The prevalence of trachoma in this community ranged between 12 and 28% in 0- to 14-year olds (Dixon 1992). Serological data for isolates taken from ocular sites or from the nasopharynx in the original study was consistent with the expected associations between serovar and anatomical site of isolation (serotypes B, Ba, B/Ba & C). In fact, these isolates sequenced more than twenty years later showed the sequence data to be consistent with that derived from the original study. However, the remaining >99% of the genomes of these isolates suggested very different findings. Once recombination blocks had been excluded, the Australian isolates were seen to comprise three separate lineages, all of which fell outside the single classical ocular lineage associated with trachoma, instead falling amongst the urogenital isolates in T1 and T2. The five isolates within T2 were all of genotype B and most closely related to urogenital genotypes D and K. The isolates in T1 comprised C and Ba genotypes, each forming its own monophyletic sublineage. It is noteworthy that these isolates corresponded to the age group with the highest prevalence for trachoma infection, the Northern Territories of Australia being reported as a trachoma endemic region. Perhaps more importantly, *C. trachomatis* Ba and C serovars were only observed in the ocular site, not in the genital tract, whereas the B genotypes from this study were found in both sites. It is also important to note that the disease grading in these children fell below what would be classified as trachoma in hyper-endemic trachoma regions such as Africa. However, this has been the subject of extensive discussion; using the original grading scheme in this region, then 53% of disease cases and 59% of PCR positivity are seen in people graded lower than the WHO grade for trachoma (Michel et al. 2011; West et al. 1991)

Looking across the genomes of Australian Ba and C isolates, the genes encoding the polymorphic membrane proteins (*pmpEFGH*), which are associated with virulence, showed higher conservation with orthologues in isolates belonging to the classical ocular lineage compared to those present in the closest urogenital relatives. However there was still significant divergence between orthologues as well as evidence of a different mosaic structures for these genes in the Ba and C clades. This observation was also supported by a genome-wide association study of the ocular phenotype which showed that the only loci with a significant association were *ompA* and *pmpEFGH*. The remaining portions of the genome showed a stronger association with urogenital lineages. These observations naturally challenge how we think about the emergence of the ocular tropism. The emergence of these isolates has almost certainly been influenced by the differing ecologies, burdens of disease but also most likely by host factors as well. The authors state that "environmental conditions favouring long-term ocular infection lead to the parallel evolution of multiple *ompA* and *pmpEFGH* variants, which aid adaptation to that niche". If these "ocular" alleles were present in what we now know to be an extensive recombining gene pool, then they could be shared and "when environmental/social conditions favour the emergence of trachoma, the strains that have acquired these "ocular" alleles will be at a selective advantage and rapidly emerge as "trachoma" strains between strains through horizontal gene transfer". However novel these observations may be, they have broad implications and should be considered in context. One thing is clear: genomically we have much still to discover from this enigmatic bacterium.

References

Al-Rifai KM (1988) Trachoma through history. Int Ophthalmol 12(1):9–14

Amann R, Springer N, Schonhuber W, Ludwig W, Schmid EN, Muller KD, Michel R (1997) Obligate intracellular bacterial parasites of acanthamoebae related to Chlamydia spp. Appl Environ Microbiol 63(1):115–121

Andersson P, Klein M, Lilliebridge RA, Giffard PM (2013) Sequences of multiple bacterial genomes and a *Chlamydia trachomatis* genotype from direct sequencing of DNA derived from a vaginal swab diagnostic specimen. Clin Microbiol Infect 19(9):E405–E408. doi:10.1111/1469-0691.12237

Bavoil PM, Wyrick PB (2006) Chlamydia genomics and pathogenesis. Horizon Scientific Press

Blanco L, Bernad A, Lazaro JM, Martin G, Garmendia C, Salas M (1989) Highly efficient DNA synthesis by the phage phi 29 DNA polymerase. Symmetrical mode of DNA replication. J Biol Chem 264(15):8935–8940

Brunelle BW, Sensabaugh GF (2006) The ompA gene in *Chlamydia trachomatis* differs in phylogeny and rate of evolution from other regions of the genome. Infect Immun 74(1):578–585. doi:10.1128/IAI.74.1.578-585.2006

Caldwell HD, Wood H, Crane D, Bailey R, Jones RB, Mabey D, McClarty G (2003) Polymorphisms in *Chlamydia trachomatis* tryptophan synthase genes differentiate between genital and ocular isolates. J Clin Invest 111(11):1757–1769. doi:10.1172/JCI17993

Carlson JH, Porcella SF, McClarty G, Caldwell HD (2005) Comparative genomic analysis of *Chlamydia trachomatis* oculotropic and genitotropic strains. Infect Immun 73(10):6407–6418. doi:10.1128/IAI.73.10.6407-6418.2005

Carlson JH, Whitmire WM, Crane DD, Wicke L, Virtaneva K, Sturdevant DE, Caldwell HD (2008) The *Chlamydia trachomatis* plasmid is a transcriptional regulator of chromosomal genes and a virulence factor. Infect Immun 76(6):2273–2283. doi:10.1128/IAI.00102-08

Chilamakuri CS, Lorenz S, Madoui MA, Vodak D, Sun J, Hovig E, Meza-Zepeda LA (2014) Performance comparison of four exome capture systems for deep sequencing. BMC Genom 15:449. doi:10.1186/1471-2164-15-449

Christiansen MT, Brown AC, Kundu S, Tutill HJ, Williams R, Brown JR, Breuer J (2014) Whole-genome enrichment and sequencing of *Chlamydia trachomatis* directly from clinical samples. BMC Infect Dis 14:591. doi:10.1186/s12879-014-0591-3

Dean FB, Nelson JR, Giesler TL, Lasken RS (2001) Rapid amplification of plasmid and phage DNA using Phi 29 DNA polymerase and multiply-primed rolling circle amplification. Genome Res 11(6):1095–1099. doi:10.1101/gr.180501

DeMars R, Weinfurter J (2008) Interstrain gene transfer in *Chlamydia trachomatis* in vitro: mechanism and significance. J Bacteriol 190(5):1605–1614. doi:10.1128/JB.01592-07

Demars R, Weinfurter J, Guex E, Lin J, Potucek Y (2007) Lateral gene transfer in vitro in the intracellular pathogen *Chlamydia trachomatis*. J Bacteriol 189(3):991–1003. doi:10.1128/JB.00845-06

Dixon B (1992) Northern Territory Aboriginal Eye Health Committee Inc. Biennial Report July 1990–June 1992 Centre for Disease Control, Department of Health, Northern Territory. http://nthealth.intersearch.com.au/cgi-bin/koha/opac-detail.pl?biblionumber=8482

Domman D, Collingro A, Lagkouvardos I, Gehre L, Weinmaier T, Rattei T, Horn M (2014) Massive expansion of Ubiquitination-related gene families within the Chlamydiae. Mol Biol Evol 31(11):2890–2904. doi:10.1093/molbev/msu227

Farencena A, Comanducci M, Donati M, Ratti G, Cevenini R (1997) Characterization of a new isolate of *Chlamydia trachomatis* which lacks the common plasmid and has properties of biovar trachoma. Infect Immun 65(7):2965–2969

Fehlner-Gardiner C, Roshick C, Carlson JH, Hughes S, Belland RJ, Caldwell HD, McClarty G (2002) Molecular basis defining human *Chlamydia trachomatis* tissue tropism. A possible role for tryptophan synthase. J Biol Chem 277(30):26893–26903. doi:10.1074/jbc.M203937200

Garcia-Garcia G, Baux D, Faugere V, Moclyn M, Koenig M, Claustres M, Roux AF (2016) Assessment of the latest NGS enrichment capture methods in clinical context. Sci Rep 6:20948. doi:10.1038/srep20948

Gomes JP, Bruno WJ, Borrego MJ, Dean D (2004) Recombination in the genome of *Chlamydia trachomatis* involving the polymorphic membrane protein C gene relative to ompA and evidence for horizontal gene transfer. J Bacteriol 186(13):4295–4306. doi:10.1128/JB.186.13.4295-4306.2004

Gomes JP, Nunes A, Bruno WJ, Borrego MJ, Florindo C, Dean D (2006) Polymorphisms in the nine polymorphic membrane proteins of *Chlamydia trachomatis* across all serovars: evidence for serovar Da recombination and correlation with tissue tropism. J Bacteriol 188(1):275–286. doi:10.1128/JB.188.1.275-286.2006

Hadfield J, Harris SR, Seth-Smith HMB, Parmar S, Andersson P, Giffard PM, Thomson NR (2017) Comprehensive global genome dynamics of *Chlamydia trachomatis* show ancient diversification followed by contemporary mixing and recent lineage expansion. Genome Res. doi:10.1101/gr.212647.116

Harris SR, Clarke IN, Seth-Smith HM, Solomon AW, Cutcliffe LT, Marsh P,… Thomson NR (2012) Whole-genome analysis of diverse *Chlamydia trachomatis* strains identifies phylogenetic relationships masked by current clinical typing. Nat Genet 44(4):413–419, S411. doi:10.1038/ng.2214

Hayes LJ, Yearsley P, Treharne JD, Ballard RA, Fehler GH, Ward ME (1994) Evidence for naturally occurring recombination in the gene encoding the major outer membrane protein of

lymphogranuloma venereum isolates of *Chlamydia trachomatis*. Infect Immun 62(12): 5659–5663
Hogan RJ, Mathews SA, Mukhopadhyay S, Summersgill JT, Timms P (2004) Chlamydial persistence: beyond the biphasic paradigm. Infect Immun 72(4):1843–1855
Horn M (2008) Chlamydiae as symbionts in eukaryotes. Annu Rev Microbiol 62:113–131. doi:10.1146/annurev.micro.62.081307.162818. Review PMID:18473699
Horn M, Collingro A, Schmitz-Esser S, Beier CL, Purkhold U, Fartmann B, Wagner M (2004) Illuminating the evolutionary history of chlamydiae. Science 304(5671):728–730. doi:10.1126/science.1096330
Horz HP, Scheer S, Vianna ME, Conrads G (2010) New methods for selective isolation of bacterial DNA from human clinical specimens. Anaerobe 16(1):47–53. doi:10.1016/j.anaerobe.2009.04.009
Hosono S, Faruqi AF, Dean FB, Du Y, Sun Z, Wu X, Lasken RS (2003) Unbiased whole-genome amplification directly from clinical samples. Genome Res 13(5):954–964. doi:10.1101/gr.816903
Hybiske K, Stephens RS (2007) Mechanisms of host cell exit by the intracellular bacterium Chlamydia. Proc Natl Acad Sci U S A 104(27):11430–11435. doi:10.1073/pnas.0703218104
Jeffrey BM, Suchland RJ, Quinn KL, Davidson JR, Stamm WE, Rockey DD (2010) Genome sequencing of recent clinical *Chlamydia trachomatis* strains identifies loci associated with tissue tropism and regions of apparent recombination. Infect Immun 78(6):2544–2553. doi:10.1128/IAI.01324-09
Jeffrey BM, Suchland RJ, Eriksen SG, Sandoz KM, Rockey DD (2013) Genomic and phenotypic characterization of in vitro-generated *Chlamydia trachomatis* recombinants. BMC Microbiol 13:142. doi:10.1186/1471-2180-13-142
Joseph SJ, Didelot X, Gandhi K, Dean D, Read TD (2011) Interplay of recombination and selection in the genomes of *Chlamydia trachomatis*. Biol Direct 6:28. doi:10.1186/1745-6150-6-28
Joseph SJ, Didelot X, Rothschild J, de Vries HJ, Morre SA, Read TD, Dean D (2012) Population genomics of *Chlamydia trachomatis*: insights on drift, selection, recombination, and population structure. Mol Biol Evol 29(12):3933–3946. doi:10.1093/molbev/mss198
Joseph SJ, Li B, Ghonasgi T, Haase CP, Qin ZS, Dean D, Read TD (2014) Direct amplification, sequencing and profiling of *Chlamydia trachomatis* strains in single and mixed infection clinical samples. PLoS ONE 9(6):e99290. doi:10.1371/journal.pone.0099290
Kari L, Whitmire WM, Olivares-Zavaleta N, Goheen MM, Taylor LD, Carlson JH, Caldwell HD (2011) A live-attenuated chlamydial vaccine protects against trachoma in nonhuman primates. J Exp Med 208(11):2217–2223. doi:10.1084/jem.20111266
Lagkouvardos I, Weinmaier T, Lauro FM, Cavicchioli R, Rattei T, Horn M (2014) Integrating metagenomic and amplicon databases to resolve the phylogenetic and ecological diversity of the Chlamydiae. ISME J 8(1):115–125. doi:10.1038/ismej.2013.142
Lasken RS (2012) Genomic sequencing of uncultured microorganisms from single cells. Nature Rev Microbiol 10:631–640
Liechti GW, Kuru E, Hall E, Kalinda A, Brun YV, VanNieuwenhze M, Maurelli AT (2014) A new metabolic cell-wall labelling method reveals peptidoglycan in *Chlamydia trachomatis*. Nature 506(7489):507–510. doi:10.1038/nature12892
Linz B, Windsor HM, McGraw JJ, Hansen LM, Gajewski JP, Tomsho LP, Marshall BJ (2014) A mutation burst during the acute phase of Helicobacter pylori infection in humans and rhesus macaques. Nat Commun 5:4165. doi:10.1038/ncomms5165
Longbottom D, Coulter LJ (2003) Animal chlamydioses and zoonotic implications. J Comp Pathol 128(4):217–244
Michel CE, Roper KG, Divena MA, Lee HH, Taylor HR (2011) Correlation of clinical trachoma and infection in aboriginal communities. PLoS Negl Trop Dis 5(3):e986. doi:10.1371/journal.pntd.0000986
Millman KL, Tavare S, Dean D (2001) Recombination in the ompA gene but not the omcB gene of Chlamydia contributes to serovar-specific differences in tissue tropism, immune

surveillance, and persistence of the organism. J Bacteriol 183(20):5997–6008. doi:10.1128/JB.183.20.5997-6008.2001

Newman L, Rowley J, Vander Hoorn S, Wijesooriya NS, Unemo M, Low N, Temmerman M (2015) Global estimates of the prevalence and incidence of four curable sexually transmitted infections in 2012 based on systematic review and global reporting. PLoS One 10(12): e0143304. doi:10.1371/journal.pone.0143304

O'Neill CE, Seth-Smith HM, Van Der Pol B, Harris SR, Thomson NR, Cutcliffe LT, Clarke IN (2013) *Chlamydia trachomatis* clinical isolates identified as tetracycline resistant do not exhibit resistance in vitro: whole-genome sequencing reveals a mutation in porB but no evidence for tetracycline resistance genes. Microbiology 159(Pt 4):748–756. doi:10.1099/mic.0.065391-0

Peterson EM, Markoff BA, Schachter J, de la Maza LM (1990) The 7.5-kb plasmid present in *Chlamydia trachomatis* is not essential for the growth of this microorganism. Plasmid 23 (2):144–148

Putman TE, Suchland RJ, Ivanovitch JD, Rockey DD (2013) Culture-independent sequence analysis of *Chlamydia trachomatis* in urogenital specimens identifies regions of recombination and in-patient sequence mutations. Microbiology 159(Pt 10):2109–2117. doi:10.1099/mic.0.070029-0

Read TD, Joseph SJ, Didelot X, Liang B, Patel L, Dean D (2013) Comparative analysis of Chlamydia psittaci genomes reveals the recent emergence of a pathogenic lineage with a broad host range. MBio 4(2):604–612. doi:10.1128/mBio.00604-12

Read TD, Myers GS, Brunham RC, Nelson WC, Paulsen IT, Heidelberg J, Fraser CM (2003) Genome sequence of *Chlamydophila caviae* (Chlamydia psittaci GPIC): examining the role of niche-specific genes in the evolution of the Chlamydiaceae. Nucleic Acids Res 31(8): 2134–2147

Rockey DD (2011) Unraveling the basic biology and clinical significance of the chlamydial plasmid. J Exp Med 208(11):2159–2162. doi:10.1084/jem.20112088

Sandoz KM, Rockey DD (2010) Antibiotic resistance in Chlamydiae. Future Microbiol 5(9): 1427–1442. doi:10.2217/fmb.10.96

Schachter J, Caldwell HD (1980) Chlamydiae. Annu Rev Microbiol 34:285–309. doi:10.1146/annurev.mi.34.100180.001441

Schachter J, Moncada J (2005) Lymphogranuloma venereum: how to turn an endemic disease into an outbreak of a new disease? Start looking. Sex Transm Dis 32(6):331–332

Seth-Smith HM, Harris SR, Persson K, Marsh P, Barron A, Bignell A, Clarke IN (2009) Co-evolution of genomes and plasmids within *Chlamydia trachomatis* and the emergence in Sweden of a new variant strain. BMC Genom 10:239. doi:10.1186/1471-2164-10-239

Seth-Smith HM, Harris SR, Scott P, Parmar S, Marsh P, Unemo M, Thomson NR (2013a) Generating whole bacterial genome sequences of low-abundance species from complex samples with IMS-MDA. Nat Protoc 8(12):2404–2412. doi:10.1038/nprot.2013.147

Seth-Smith HM, Harris SR, Skilton RJ, Radebe FM, Golparian D, Shipitsyna E, Thomson NR (2013b) Whole-genome sequences of *Chlamydia trachomatis* directly from clinical samples without culture. Genome Res 23(5):855–866. doi:10.1101/gr.150037.112

Song L, Carlson JH, Whitmire WM, Kari L, Virtaneva K, Sturdevant DE, Caldwell HD (2013) *Chlamydia trachomatis* plasmid-encoded Pgp4 is a transcriptional regulator of virulence-associated genes. Infect Immun 81(3):636–644. doi:10.1128/IAI.01305-12

Stephens RS, Kalman S, Lammel C, Fan J, Marathe R, Aravind L, Davis RW (1998) Genome sequence of an obligate intracellular pathogen of humans: *Chlamydia trachomatis*. Science 282 (5389):754–759

Taylor LD, Nelson DE, Dorward DW, Whitmire WM, Caldwell HD (2010) Biological characterization of *Chlamydia trachomatis* plasticity zone MACPF domain family protein CT153. Infect Immun 78(6):2691–2699. doi:10.1128/IAI.01455-09

Taylor-Brown A, Vaughan L, Greub G, Timms P, Polkinghorne A (2015) Twenty years of research into Chlamydia-like organisms: a revolution in our understanding of the biology and pathogenicity of members of the phylum Chlamydiae. Pathog Dis 73(1):1–15. doi:10.1093/femspd/ftu009

Thomson NR, Clarke IN (2010) *Chlamydia trachomatis*: small genome, big challenges. Future Microbiol 5(4):555–561. doi:10.2217/fmb.10.31

Thomson NR, Holden MT, Carder C, Lennard N, Lockey SJ, Marsh P, Clarke IN (2008) *Chlamydia trachomatis*: genome sequence analysis of lymphogranuloma venereum isolates. Genome Res 18(1):161–171. doi:10.1101/gr.7020108

Unemo M, Clarke IN (2011) The Swedish new variant of *Chlamydia trachomatis*. Curr Opin Infect Dis 24(1):62–69. doi:10.1097/QCO.0b013e32834204d5

Unemo M, Seth-Smith HM, Cutcliffe LT, Skilton RJ, Barlow D, Goulding D, Clarke IN (2010) The Swedish new variant of *Chlamydia trachomatis*: genome sequence, morphology, cell tropism and phenotypic characterization. Microbiology 156(Pt 5):1394–1404. doi:10.1099/mic.0.036830-0

Wang Y, Cutcliffe LT, Skilton RJ, Persson K, Bjartling C, Clarke IN (2013) Transformation of a plasmid-free, genital tract isolate of *Chlamydia trachomatis* with a plasmid vector carrying a deletion in CDS6 revealed that this gene regulates inclusion phenotype. Pathog Dis 67(2):100–103. doi:10.1111/2049-632X.12024

Ward ME (1983) Chlamydial classification, development and structure. Br Med Bull 39(2): 109–115

West SK, Rapoza P, Munoz B, Katala S, Taylor HR (1991) Epidemiology of ocular chlamydial infection in a trachoma-hyperendemic area. J Infect Dis 163(4):752–756

WHO-report (2014) WHO Alliance for the Global Elimination of Blinding Trachoma by the year 2020. Progress report on elimination of trachoma, 2013. *Wkly Epidemiol Rec, 89*(39), 421–428

Yilmaz S, Singh AK (2012) Single cell genome sequencing. Curr Op Biotechnol 23:437–443

Advances and Obstacles in the Genetic Dissection of Chlamydial Virulence

Julie A. Brothwell, Matthew K. Muramatsu, Guangming Zhong and David E. Nelson

Abstract Obligate intracellular pathogens in the family *Chlamydiaceae* infect taxonomically diverse eukaryotes ranging from amoebae to mammals. However, many fundamental aspects of chlamydial cell biology and pathogenesis remain poorly understood. Genetic dissection of chlamydial biology has historically been hampered by a lack of genetic tools. Exploitation of the ability of chlamydia to recombine genomic material by lateral gene transfer (LGT) ushered in a new era in chlamydia research. With methods to map mutations in place, genetic screens were able to assign functions and phenotypes to specific chlamydial genes. Development of an approach for stable transformation of chlamydia also provided a mechanism for gene delivery and platforms for disrupting chromosomal genes. Here, we explore how these and other tools have been used to test hypotheses concerning the functions of known chlamydial virulence factors and discover the functions of completely uncharacterized genes. Refinement and extension of the existing genetic tools to additional *Chlamydia* spp. will substantially advance understanding of the biology and pathogenesis of this important group of pathogens.

Julie A. Brothwell and Matthew K. Muramatsu—Equal contributions

---

J. A. Brothwell · M. K. Muramatsu · D. E. Nelson (✉)
Department of Microbiology and Immunology, Indiana University School of Medicine, Indianapolis, IN, USA
e-mail: nelsonde@indiana.edu

G. Zhong
Department of Microbiology, Immunology and Molecular Genetics, University of Texas Health Science Center at San Antonio, San Antonio, TX, USA

Current Topics in Microbiology and Immunology (2018) 412:133–158
DOI 10.1007/82_2017_76

Published Online: 01 November 2017

Contents

1 Introduction

Bacteria in the phylum *Chlamydiae* share a characteristic biphasic intracellular developmental cycle and reside within a parasitophorous vacuole (termed the inclusion) (Moulder 1985). This obligate intracellular lifestyle and protected intracellular niche limit opportunities for chlamydia to exchange genetic material with other microorganisms and pose barriers to their genetic manipulation in the laboratory. There are few examples of genetic exchange between chlamydiae and other organisms, and *Chlamydia* spp. generally have few mobile genetic elements and other horizontally acquired genes compared to free-living bacteria (Stephens et al. 1998; Kalman et al. 1999; Read et al. 2000; Horn et al. 2004; Collingro et al. 2011).

Genome sequencing and comparative genomics have played especially important roles in the investigation of chlamydial biology because methods for targeted genetic manipulation only became available recently. The first sequenced *C. trachomatis* genomes were highly similar, suggesting that static genomes might be another obstacle that would hinder genetic manipulation. However, subsequent comparisons of hundreds of genomes and the recapitulation of chlamydial recombination and transformation in vitro confirmed that some *Chlamydia* spp. readily exchange DNA, but usually only with close relatives (DeMars et al. 2007; Wang et al. 2011; Hadfield et al. 2017). Another barrier to genetic manipulation of members of *Chlamydia* spp. is that more than half of their pan-genome is comprised of a core set of orthologous genes that are present in all *Chlamydiae* (Collingro et al. 2011). Many of these core genes are predicted to mediate essential and conserved features of chlamydial development, such as maintenance of the chlamydial inclusion and the transitions between the extracellular infectious elementary body (EB) and intracellular replicative reticulate body (RB) forms, and may not be dispensable even in vitro.

Chlamydiae are estimated to have diverged from other eubacteria 2 billion years ago, and vertebrate pathogens in the family *Chlamydia* species diverged from environmental Chlamydia-like organisms (CLOs) 700 million years ago (Weisburg et al. 1986; Everett et al. 1999; Horn et al. 2004). Partial or full genome sequences from eight CLO families (*Parachlamydieaceae*, *Waddliaceae*, *Simkaniaceae*, *Rhabdochlamydiaceae*, *Criblamydiaceae* *Chlavichlamydiaceae*, and *Parilichlamydiaceae*) have been described, and there is evidence that as many as 200 more exist (Lagkouvardos et al. 2014; Taylor-Brown et al. 2015). CLO genomes contain numerous rearrangements and share little synteny with one another, which may reflect the broad taxonomic range of the hosts that these organisms parasitize (Collingro et al. 2011). Some members of *Criblamydiaceae*, *Chlavichlamydiaceae*, and *Parilichlamydiaceae* spp. are important fish pathogens (Draghi et al. 2004; Karlsen et al. 2008; Stride et al. 2013). Other CLOs can enter and proliferate in cultured human cells (Greub et al. 2003; Collingro et al. 2005; Casson et al. 2006). *S. nevegensis*, *P. acanthaomoebae*, *W. condrophila* and *Rabdochlamydia* spp. have been associated with disease in humans and livestock (Taylor-Brown et al. 2015). *Parachlamydia* can also elicit respiratory disease in experimental mouse and cattle challenge models, which is consistent with the hypothesis that they are mammalian pathogens (Casson et al. 2008; Lohr et al. 2015). The predicted expanded metabolic and recombination capacities of some CLOs, compared to *Chlamydia* spp., suggest that they might be excellent candidates for the development of both genetic tools and axenic culture, although no attempts to genetically modify CLOs have been described (Collingro et al. 2011; Omsland et al. 2014).

Unlike CLO genomes, *Chlamydiaceae* genomes share substantial synteny with one another (Read et al. 2000; Read et al. 2003; Collingro et al. 2011; Nunes and Gomes 2014). Eleven *Chlamydia* spp. (*C. trachomatis, C. muridarum, C. pneumoniae, C. psittaci, C. pecorum, C. abortus, C. felis, C. suis, C. cavie, C. gallinacea, C. avium*) are recognized, and reference genomes are available for representatives of all of these except *C. avium* (Stephens et al. 1998; Kalman et al. 1999; Read et al. 2000; Read et al. 2003; Thomson et al. 2005; Azuma et al. 2006; Mojica et al. 2011; Schofl et al. 2011; Donati et al. 2014; Sachse et al. 2014; Holzer et al. 2016). Extant members of the genus *Chlamydia* separate into two well-supported clades based on their 16S rRNA gene sequences (Stephens et al. 2009; Sachse and Laroucau 2015). One clade contains the mouse pathogen *C. muridarum*, the pig pathogen *C. suis,* and various human pathogens in the species *C. trachomatis*, and the other clade contains the remaining species.

Little genetic distance can separate *Chlamydia* spp. and strains that infect different hosts and cause distinct diseases. For example, 99% of *C. muridarum* genes have high similarity orthologues in *C. trachomatis* serovar D (Read et al. 2000). Genomes of *C. trachomatis* strains that cause blinding trachoma (serovars A-C, trachoma), mucosa-restricted sexually transmitted infections (serovars D-K, chlamydia), and the invasive sexually transmitted disease lymphogranuloma venereum (Lymphogranuloma venereum (LGV) serovars L1-L3) share more than 99% nucleotide sequence identity (Stephens et al. 1998; Carlson et al. 2005; Thomson et al. 2008). This phenotypic diversity in the context of little genetic distance led to the proposal that host and tissue tropism of *Chlamydia* spp. is determined by a small group of niche-specific genes (Read et al. 2003). These genes are attractive targets for manipulation because their variable presence in different isolates that can be cultivated in the same conditions suggests that they are dispensable (Kari et al. 2011). In this review, we describe recent advances in the development of tools for genetic manipulation of pathogenic *Chlamydia*, the uses and limitations of these tools, and how these might be improved for dissecting mechanisms of chlamydial cell biology and pathogenesis.

2 Chlamydial Genomes Are Malleable

Statements that chlamydiae are genetically "intractable" were fixtures in the literature until recently, but evidence that this was not so emerged earlier. For example, a study in 1983 showed that temperature-sensitive (TS) *C. abortus* mutants could be isolated from infected cell cultures treated with the alkylating mutagen *N*-methyl-*N* '-nitro-*N*-nitrosoguanidine (NTG) (Rodolakis 1983). One of these TS mutants was a potent attenuated vaccine strain that afforded strong protection against the virulent parent organism in sheep (Rodolakis and Souriau 1983, 1986). Sequencing of this mutant 30 years later confirmed that it contained multiple mutations consistent with the effects of NTG (Burall et al. 2009).

Antibiotic resistance studies provided additional evidence that chlamydial genomes are malleable. Treharne observed that *C. trachomatis* became rifampin resistant when passed in increasing concentrations of this antibiotic (Treharne et al. 1989). Another study identified a fluoroquinolone-resistant chlamydial *gyrA* allele by sequencing candidate resistance alleles in drug-resistant mutants isolated by serial passage (Dessus-Babus et al. 1998). Endogenous chlamydial resistance alleles for other antibiotics were identified using similar strategies (Dreses-Werringloer et al. 2003; McCoy et al. 2003; Misiurina et al. 2004; Binet and Maurelli 2007; Demars et al. 2007). The ease with which *Chlamydia* spp. developed resistance to antibiotics in vitro initially seemed inconsistent with the paucity of antibiotic-resistant *C. trachomatis* clinical isolates. Subsequent studies showed that laboratory selected endogenous resistance alleles have fitness costs in the absence of antibiotic explained this paradox (Binet and Maurelli 2005, 2009; Binet et al. 2010). Chlamydial metabolism has also been investigated using mutants derived by passage in toxic precursors. For example, hydroxyurea, thioguanine, trimethoprim, and sulfisoxazole-resistant *C. trachomatis* mutants provided insights into the mechanisms of chlamydial nucleotide metabolism (Tipples and McClarty 1991; Qin and McClarty 1992; Wylie et al. 1996).

Other groups have harnessed spontaneous mutants to study chlamydial pathogenesis. To test if detrimental mutations accumulate in cell culture, a *C. trachomatis* reference isolate was passaged in a murine genital tract (GT) model, and the genomes of the resulting progeny were compared to the reference isolate (Sturdevant et al. 2010). Decreased virulence of the starting reference strain compared to progeny shed late from the murine GT mapped to a frameshift mutation in *ct135*. Analogous mutations accumulated in a *C. muridarum ct135* orthologue (*tc0412)*, and cell culture propagation selects against intact *ct135* (Ramsey et al. 2009; Borges et al. 2013). Another study compared the virulence of a *C. muridarum* parent isolate and its cell culture-adapted progeny in mice. Two alleles, *tc0237* and *tc0668*, that mediate *C. muridarum* attachment and pathogenicity were identified (Chen et al. 2015a; Conrad et al. 2015).

Studies of rare, naturally plasmid-negative *Chlamydia* isolates and later of parent and chemically cured strain pairs demonstrated that some key chlamydial virulence determinants are dispensable in vitro (Peterson et al. 1990; Farencena et al. 1997; Stothard et al. 1998; O'Connell and Nicks 2006). Most natural *Chlamydia* isolates, except *C. pneumoniae*, contain a highly conserved ~7.5 kb plasmid that encodes 8 open reading frames (ORFs) and at least two small noncoding RNAs (sRNAs) (Palmer and Falkow 1986; Thomas et al. 1997; Pickett et al. 2005; Albrecht et al. 2010; Zhong 2017). The ubiquity of plasmids in *C. trachomatis* reference and clinical isolates suggested that these plasmids play key roles in chlamydial biology and pathogenesis. Plasmid-free *C. trachomatis* (pCT^-) isolates grow with near-normal kinetics in vitro, but do not accumulate glycogen and have reduced infectivity (Matsumoto et al. 1998; Russell et al. 2011). However, plasmid-free *C. muridarum* (pCM^-) is highly attenuated, unable to elicit pathology, and unable to compete with wild type *C. muridarum* in the murine GT (O'Connell et al. 2007; Russell et al. 2011). Studies of pCM^- and wild-type strain pairs have now shown that the plasmid plays a central role in *C. muridarum* GT virulence, dissemination from the murine upper GT to the gastrointestinal (GI) tract, and colonization of the murine GI tract (Carlson et al. 2008; Lei et al. 2014; Chen et al. 2015b; Shao et al. 2017; Zhong 2017). Collectively, these studies defined plasmid-associated phenotypes and laid the groundwork for contemporary studies of plasmid ORFs using transformation and plasmid genetic engineering (discussed below).

3 Moving Genes Between and into Chlamydial Genomes with Recombination and Lateral Gene Transfer

Major outer membrane protein (MOMP) gene (*ompA*) sequencing began to replace *C. trachomatis* serotyping in the early 1990s. The resulting sequences revealed that many un-typeable clinical *C. trachomatis* isolates contained chimeric *ompA* alleles (Dean et al. 1992; Fitch et al. 1993; Lampe et al. 1993; Brunham et al. 1994; Hayes et al. 1994). Hayes understood the significance of these chimeras and proposed, "efforts to manipulate the chlamydial genome in vitro by recombination should be intensified" (Hayes et al. 1994). Sequencing of the polymorphic membrane protein (*pmp*) genes later revealed identical *pmpC* sequences associated with different *ompA* genotypes in *C. trachomatis* clinical isolates, showing that recombination between *Chlamydia* isolates could extend beyond *ompA* (Gomes et al. 2004).

Recapitulation of lateral gene transfer (LGT) in vitro confirmed that chlamydiae can exchange chromosomal DNA and led to the development LGT-based mutation mapping (discussed below) (Demars et al. 2007; DeMars and Weinfurter 2008). Demars and colleagues first demonstrated that doubly antibiotic-resistant isolates arose from co-infections with various combinations of antibiotic-resistant *C. trachomatis* L1 parents 1000- to 10,000-fold more frequently than did spontaneous double mutants from single infections with either parent alone (Demars et al. 2007). Recombination between endogenous ofloxacin resistant *C. trachomatis* serovar L1 and rifampicin resistant *C. trachomatis* serovar D parents showed that LGT could be used to exchange DNA between dissimilar parents and that large genomic regions (123–790 kb) could be exchanged (DeMars and Weinfurter 2008). Exchange of a *C. suis* tetracycline resistance island between *C. suis*, *C. muridarum*, and *C. trachomatis* in another study showed that LGT between different chlamydial species and heterologous regions of chlamydial genomes was possible (Suchland et al. 2009). LGT does not appear to require that the donor and recipient reside in the same vacuole for *C. trachomatis* because wild-type and non-fusogenic *incA*$^{-}$ parents produced LGT recombinants at similar frequencies (Jeffrey et al. 2013). If LGT can occur between other non-fusogenic *Chlamydia* spp. is unknown. So far, analyses of genomes from dozens of LGT recombinants has not yet identified any clear recombination hotspots associated with this process (Jeffrey et al. 2010, 2013; Brothwell et al. 2016; Muramatsu et al. 2016). The mechanisms of LGT also remain mysterious, but many *Chlamydia* spp. encode low identity orthologues of the *B. subtilis* competence genes *comEC* and *mec*, so it is plausible that DNA exchange between competent RBs mediates LGT (Stephens et al. 1998; Demars et al. 2007; DeMars and Weinfurter 2008).

Two LGT-based mutation-mapping approaches have been described, positive selection LGT (LGT) and counterselection LGT (csLGT). In LGT, host cells are co-infected with a parent that has a phenotype of interest and is resistant to an antibiotic (e.g., spectinomycin, rifampicin, trimethoprim) and a second parent that does not have the phenotype but is resistant to a second antibiotic (Nguyen and Valdivia 2012). Comparison of the genomes of the resulting doubly antibiotic-resistant progeny that have either maintained or lost the phenotype of interest can identify which allele is responsible for the phenotype (Nguyen and Valdivia 2013). Importantly, reciprocal LGT of these progenies with a third antibiotic-resistant parent can permit resistance allele recycling and serial mapping attempts (Nguyen and Valdivia 2012). In csLGT, healthy recombinant progeny is generated from parents that both have conditional or nonconditional growth defects (Brothwell et al. 2016; Muramatsu et al. 2016). For example, an LGT cross of two TS parent strains performed at the non-permissive temperature will yield temperature-resistant progeny (Brothwell et al. 2016). Similar to LGT, comparing parent and recombinant progeny genomes can then identify the alleles linked to the phenotypes of the parents. The advantages of csLGT include avoidance of the fitness costs associated with some endogenous antibiotic resistance alleles and generation of progeny-parent pairs that differ only in the detrimental allele. Unlike LGT, enrichment of recombinants by csLGT is dependent upon the strength of the counter-selectable phenotypes of the parents.

Binet and Maurelli showed that homologous dsDNA sequences can also be directly introduced into *C. psittaci* using electroporation and recombined into the chlamydial chromosome (Binet and Maurelli 2009a, b). This clever study took advantage of the single copy rRNA operon in *C. psittaci* and distinct SNPs in the 16S rRNA gene that confer resistance to kasugamycin and spectinomycin. The engineered resistance alleles contained a silent mutation that destroyed a restriction site to monitor allelic exchange verses spontaneous antibiotic resistance and flanking homologous sequences that targeted the allele to the chromosome. This promising approach has not been replicated in other *Chlamydia* spp. or used to manipulate other genes.

4 Transformation of Chlamydia with Plasmid Shuttle Vectors

The potential of the chlamydial plasmid for genetic engineering was appreciated upon its discovery, but was not realized until almost 35 years later when *C. trachomatis* L2 was stably transformed with a vector constructed from its corresponding plasmid (pL2) (Wang et al. 2011). Electroporation of *C. trachomatis* EBs with a vector constructed from pCT and an *E. coli* plasmid (pBGS9) in which the pBGS9 chloramphenicol acetyltransferase (*cat*) gene was controlled by a *Chlamydia* promoter provided the first evidence that transformation was possible (Tam et al. 1994). Chloramphenicol resistant organisms and RBs containing the vector detected in the transformed cultures could survive up to four passages in chloramphenicol but were eventually lost. In hindsight, the shuttle vector may have been unstable because the *E. coli* plasmid elements disrupted a pCT maintenance gene (Song et al. 2013). Nonetheless, careful descriptions of positive and negative results in this study provided a roadmap for future attempts.

An approach developed by the Clarke group is the basis for most contemporary transformation protocols (Wang et al. 2011). Their initial vector consisted of a portion of pBR325 encoding β-lactamase (*bla*) and pBR *oriC* ligated into the pL2 plasmid (pBR325::L2). The shuttle vector and EBs were incubated in $CaCl_2$-Tris buffer, and McCoy cells infected with this mixture yielded stable penicillin-resistant transformants. Transformation of the glycogen-deficient pCT^- *C. trachomatis* isolate 25667R with pBR325::L2 restored glycogen accumulation. This confirmed that plasmid loss–not background mutations—caused the glycogen deficiency of pCT^- strains and was the first example of genetic complementation in *Chlamydia*. Finally, a similar vector containing a green fluorescent protein (GFP) gene under a *Neisseria* promoter was introduced into the backbone of the new Swedish variant plasmid (pSW2), which contains a deletion in CDS1 and a duplication in CDS3 (Seth-Smith et al. 2009). The transformants stably expressed GFP. This demonstrated that pCT-derived vectors can express foreign transgenes and that some regions of chlamydial plasmids are dispensable for their in vitro maintenance.

5 Applications of the Plasmid as a Shuttle Vector

The ability to deliver and express transgenes facilitated the development of many new approaches for investigating chlamydial biology. For example, Agaisse and Derré developed vectors that express GFP, mCherry, and cyan fluorescent protein genes under the control of chlamydial promoters (Agaisse and Derre 2013). This permitted real-time visualization of developing inclusions and their interactions with host cell organelles. Introduction of a tetracycline promoter and operator sequences upstream of a multiple cloning site in pASK permitted anhydrotetracycline-regulated expression of transgenes in *C. trachomatis* (Wickstrum et al. 2013). Further tuning of a tetracycline-regulated vector permitted comprehensive interrogation of the secretion and localization of known and putative inclusion membrane proteins (Incs) (Bauler and Hackstadt 2014; Weber et al. 2015). New chlamydial expression and shuttle vectors and are evolving rapidly, and we refer readers to a more extensive review of this topic (Bastidas and Valdivia 2016).

Despite remarkable progress and recent demonstration of transformation in additional *Chlamydia* spp., chlamydial transformation still has many limitations (Ding et al. 2013, Song et al. 2014). Inability to transform specific constructs, achieve expression of specific products from vectors and/or complement chromosomal defects is common (Nelson DE, unpublished) (Weber et al. 2015, 2017). We and others have observed subtle—and sometimes not so subtle—growth defects in transformants (Nelson and Zhong, unpublished; Wang et al. 2011). Possible explanations for these vector effects could include inappropriate timing of gene expression during the developmental cycle and/or improper levels of gene expression from multi-copy vectors (Wickstrum et al. 2013). Recently identified roles of the plasmid in the regulation of chlamydial virulence, chromosomal gene expression, and lytic exit suggest multiple reasons why manipulation of the chlamydial plasmid could elicit unanticipated phenotypes (discussed below). Considering these limitations, it is essential that vector controls be included in complementation experiments when feasible. Alternately, complementation results can sometimes be validated using phenotypic complementation and/or ectopic expression of the chlamydial gene in host cells (Clifton et al. 2004; Nelson et al. 2007).

6 Reverse Genetic Dissection of Chlamydia Plasmids

Development of transformation permitted reverse genetic dissection of the functions of chlamydial plasmids. The inability to transform non-LGV strains with pBR325::L2 or pGFP::SW2 suggested that plasmid or chromosomal determinants dictated plasmid tropism. *C. trachomatis* serovar *A* and *C. muridarum* could only be stably transformed with shuttle vectors constructed from their corresponding plasmids, indicating that plasmid sequences mediate stable transformation (Song et al. 2014). Forcing recombination between *C. muridarum* and LGV plasmids in another study revealed that CDS2 is a key determinant of plasmid tropism (Wang et al. 2014). Inactivation of specific plasmids ORFs revealed that Pgp1, 2 and 6 proteins and *pgp8*, but not Pgp8, are also essential for plasmid maintenance and identified additional *cis*-acting plasmid regulatory regions (Gong et al. 2013; Song et al. 2013; Liu et al. 2014; Zhong 2017). Pgp4 is dispensable for plasmid maintenance, but regulates multiple chromosomal genes including *glgA* (Carlson et al. 2008; Song et al. 2013). Loss of *pgp4* is also sufficient to elicit glycogen deficiency (Song et al. 2013). Pgp4 also plays an essential and type III secretion-dependent role in the lytic exit of *C. trachomatis* (Yang et al. 2015). Collectively, these studies revealed that chlamydial plasmids play central roles in multiple aspects of chlamydial metabolism and pathogenesis.

7 Genetic Manipulation of Chlamydial Chromosomes

Four approaches for genetic analysis of chlamydial chromosomal gene functions have been reported (Table 1): Targeting Induced Local Lesions in Genomes (TILLING), TILLING by sequencing, TargeTron®, and Fluorescence-Reported Allelic Exchange Mutagenesis (FRAEM) (Kari et al. 2011; Johnson and Fisher 2013; Kokes et al. 2015; Mueller et al. 2016). Chemical mutagens are used to generate libraries of random mutants in the TILLING approaches, whereas TargeTron and FRAEM permit targeted mutagenesis (Fig. 1).

Two methods to identify naturally occurring or mutagen-induced mutations in a gene of interest have been described: TILLING and TILLING by sequencing. TILLING was adapted from plant genetics for application in *Chlamydia* in 2011 (McCallum et al. 2000; Kari et al. 2011). Mutants that contained less than one mutation per genome on average were generated by ethyl methanesulfonate (EMS) mutagenesis and were expanded in pools in HeLa cells. The tryptophan synthase operon (*trpBA*) was PCR amplified from genomic DNA from each of these pools. Cleavage of the PCR products with a mismatch-specific endonuclease (CEL-I) then identified pools that contained both wild-type and mutant *trpBA* amplicons. Multiple *trpBA* mutants were identified, including an isogenic *trpB* null (*trpB*) mutant. Unlike the library parent, growth of the isogenic *trpB*$^-$ mutant was not rescued from tryptophan starvation by indole, which is consistent with the predicted function of TrpB (Fehlner-Gardiner et al. 2002; Caldwell et al. 2003; Carlson et al. 2005). A similar approach was used to isolate a near-isogenic *C. trachomatis pmpD*$^-$ mutant (Kari et al. 2014). Although the *pmpD*$^-$ mutant behaved similarly to its parent in the murine GT, it was highly attenuated in a macaque trachoma model, again demonstrating that key chlamydial virulence factors can be dispensable in vitro.

Other TILLING studies have used higher mutagen doses and different *Chlamydia* species. TILLING of a highly mutagenized *C. trachomatis* serovar D library identified three *chxR*$^-$ mutants and five ChxR regulated genes (Yang et al. 2017). The *chxR*$^-$ mutants were attenuated in mice, suggesting that ChxR is a

Table 1 Genetic analysis of chlamydial chromosomal gene functions

Method	Strain	Gene(s)	Advantage	Caveat	References
Serial passage with increasing selection Non-mutagenized organisms were serially passaged in increasing concentrations of a selection agent	*C. trachomatis* L2	Various	Mutants with one or a few mutations per genome	Mutants may not arise; isolation of mutants highly dependent on selection conditions	Tipples and McClarty (1991)
In vitro serial passage Organisms were passaged 10 X in between embryonating hen's eggs and 17 X in HeLa 229 cells. Virulence selection in mice	*C. trachomatis* D/UW-3/CX	*ct135*	Isolate phenotypic mutants with one or a few mutations per genome	Mutants may not arise; isolation of mutants highly dependent on selection conditions	Sturdevant et al. (2010)
In vitro serial passage and selection *C. muridarum* was passaged for 28 generation in vitro using unassisted and assisted attachment infection models	*C. muridarum*	*tc0237*, *tc0412*, *tc0668*	Isolate phenotypic mutants with one or a few mutations per genome	Mutants may not arise; isolation of mutants highly dependent on selection conditions	Chen et al. (2015a, b)
Chemical mutagenesis NTG mutagenesis and screening for temperature-sensitive mutants	*C. psittaci* AB7	TS genes	Identify multiple phenotypically related mutants; mutate essential genes	Multiple mutations requiring mapping to determine the causative TS allele(s)	Rodolakis (1983)
Chemical mutagenesis & antibiotic LGT EMS mutagenesis and screening for diverse plaque morphologies Antibiotic recombination to map causative alleles	*C. trachomatis* L2	Glycogen genes	Identify multiple phenotypically related mutants; map causative alleles	Labor intensive library creation, screening, and mapping; compare multiple recombinants to identify causative allele; antibiotic recombinants may have growth defects	Nguyen and Valdivia (2012)

(continued)

Table 1 (continued)

Method	Strain	Gene(s)	Advantage	Caveat	References
Chemical mutagenesis & WGS EMS or ENU mutagenesis and screening for mutants that failed to promote F-actin assembly	*C. trachomatis* L2	*inaC*	Identify multiple phenotypically related mutants; rapidly map causative alleles	WGS of a large mutant library may be cost prohibitive; mutants may not share the same mutation related to phenotype of interest	Kokes et al. (2015)
Chemical mutagenesis & csLGT EMS mutagenesis of a GFP-expressing parent and screening for mutants. Counter selection recombination to map causative alleles	*C. trachomatis* L2	TS & IFN-γ persistance genes	Identify multiple phenotypically related mutants; map multiple causative alleles at the same time and isolate isogenic recombinants	Labor intensive library creation, screening, and mapping; selection of recombinants limited by strength of phenotype	Brothwell et al. (2016), Muramatsu et al. (2016)
Allelic exchange Homologous recombination of linear and circular suicide plasmids	*C. psittaci* 6BC	*16S rRNA*	Modify genes with specific mutations	Electroporation equipment; suicide vector may be maintained episomally after a number of passages	Binet and Maurelli (2009a, b)
TILLING for null mutant EMS mutagenesis and screening for null mutants within a subset of mutants found to have mismatched sequence in a region of interest	*C. trachomatis* D/UW-3/CX	*trpB*	Knock out any nonessential gene; mutate essential genes	Labor-intensive library creation, screening, and mapping; potential for multiple chromosomal mutations that need to be mapped and complemented	Kari et al. (2011)
TargeTron—gene disruption Homologous Recombination of a group II Intron on a suicide plasmid	*C. trachomatis* L2	*incA*	Disrupt any nonessential gene	Proprietary algorithm to determine appropriate targeting sites; potential lack of insertion sites in 5′ sequence of the gene of interest; transformation efficiency	Johnson and Fisher (2013)

(continued)

Table 1 (continued)

Method	Strain	Gene(s)	Advantage	Caveat	References
FRAEM—gene knockout Homologous recombination of an insertional cassette using a conditional suicide plasmid	*C. trachomatis* L2	*trpA*; *ctl063-065*	Knock out any nonessential gene(s); transient suicide plasmid with fluorescent reporter	Polar effects; transformation efficiency	Mueller et al. (2016)

Abbreviations used: *NTG N*-methyl-*N′*-nitro-*N*-nitrosoguanidine; *EMS* ethyl methanesulfonate; *ENU N*-ethylnitrosourea; *WGS* whole genome sequencing; *TILLING* targeting induced local lesions in genomes; *FRAEM* fluorescence reported allelic exchange mutagenesis; *LGT* lateral gene transfer; *cs* counterselction; *TS* temperature sensitive

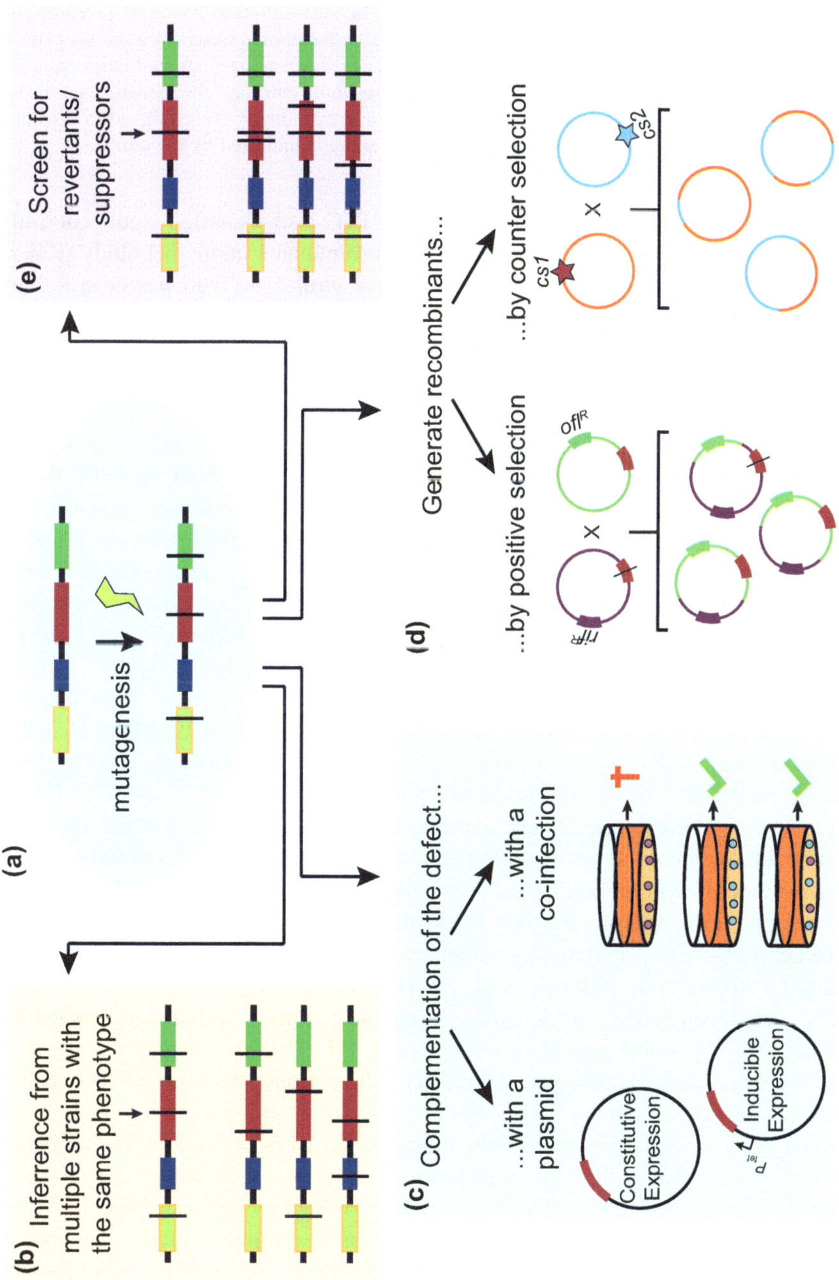
(a)
mutagenesis
(b) Inferrence from multiple strains with the same phenotype
(c) Complementation of the defect...
...with a plasmid
Constitutive Expression
Inducible Expression
P_{tet}
...with a co-infection
(d) Generate recombinants...
...by positive selection
ri^R
ofl^R
...by counter selection
cs1
cs2
(e) Screen for revertants/ suppressors

◂**Fig. 1** Mutation mapping in chlamydia. **a** Chemical mutagenesis strategies can result in multiple mutations (denoted by black lines). Multiple approaches can resolve which mutation(s) (shown in red) are linked to a phenotype. **b** Additional mutants with the same phenotype that have different mutant alleles of the same gene can be isolated. **c** A plasmid that expresses the wild-type allele of the gene can be used to complement the phenotype. Alternately, co-infection with wild-type chlamydia and/or ectopic expression of the gene in host cells can be used to complement phenotypes associated with secreted effectors, inclusion membrane transporters, or enzymes that detoxify the inclusion. **d** LGT can generate recombinants using endogenous antibiotic resistance or counter-selectable alleles. **e** Continued passage of a mutant in detrimental screening conditions can also generate revertants and intragenic suppressors that can identify genes linked to detrimental phenotypes (Nelson, unpublished). The original mutation is indicated by the arrow

conserved chlamydial virulence factor. TILLING also identified a collection of *C. muridarum* plasticity zone (PZ) ORF nonsense mutants in another study (Rajaram et al. 2015). These PZ mutants were similarly virulent to their parent in a murine GT model, but some were profoundly attenuated in a mouse GI tract model (Nelson, unpublished).

Kokes et al. coupled chemical mutagenesis with genome sequencing to produce a mutant library for simultaneous forward (discussed below) and reverse genetic analyses using a strategy that we refer to as "TILLING by sequencing" (Kokes et al. 2015). A rifampicin resistant *C. trachomatis* L2 isolate was mutagenized with either EMS or *N*-ethylnitrosourea (ENU) and the resulting mutants were plaque-cloned. Sequencing of the mutants in pools identified over 8,000 different mutations, including nonsense mutations in 84 *C. trachomatis* ORFs. Detection of nonsense mutations in genes that play roles in carbon metabolism, DNA damage repair, and virulence revealed that a variety of cellular processes are dispensable for chlamydial survival in vitro. Use of a rifampicin-resistant parent in this study also facilitated downstream LGT mapping efforts used to link phenotypes to specific mutations.

Major limitations of TILLING by sequencing compared to TILLING include the higher costs of library construction, genome sequencing, analysis, and the general requirement for more sophisticated technology. However, since TILLING by sequencing libraries are clonal, multiple isolates with distinct mutant alleles of a gene of interest can be identified by inspection of the corresponding genome sequences (Kokes et al. 2015). These libraries are also amenable to phenotypic screening. For example, Snavely et al. identified chlamydial protease-like activity factor (CPAF) null mutants by screening for isolates that failed to stain with the anti-CPAF antibody (Snavely et al. 2014). Theoretically, any *Chlamydia* spp. that can be propagated in vitro, mutagenized, and clonally isolated is amenable to TILLING. The most important limitation of TILLING is mapping phenotypes to genotypes. These approaches invariably suffer from the trade-off between the overall size of the mutant library and difficulty of mapping mutations of interest in the library isolates. Fewer heavily mutagenized isolates need to be screened to identify a mutant with a given phenotype of interest, but linking phenotypes to genotypes become more difficult as numbers of background mutations increase.

The Fisher group successfully adapted an insertional mutagenesis approach (TargeTron®, Sigma Inc.) to target type II introns to specific locations on the chlamydial chromosome (Johnson and Fisher 2013). A type II intron carrying a *bla* cassette and *incA* targeting sequences was transformed into *C. trachomatis* L2 using a suicide vector. Integrants *(incA::bla)* were selected with ampicillin and confirmed by PCR and Southern blot. Similar to naturally occurring *incA* mutant strains, inclusions of the *incA::bla* mutant were non-fusogenic (Suchland et al. 2000; Johnson and Fisher 2013). Subsequently, a spectinomycin resistant intron was developed to create an *incA::aad*A *rsbV1::bla* double mutant (Lowden et al. 2015). TargeTron has now been used to disrupt multiple genes including the chaperones *groEL2* and *groEL3*, *cpoS*, *ct813/inaC*, and various *inc* genes in *C. trachomatis* L2 (Illingworth et al. 2017; Sixt et al. 2017; Weber et al. 2017, Wesolowski et al. 2017). The applicability of the TargeTron approach is limited by the presence of optimal intron targeting sequences within the gene of interest (Hooppaw and Fisher 2016; Key and Fisher 2017). Although insertional mutagenesis approaches can disrupt specific genes, they can also induce polar effects and are less suitable than chemical mutagenesis for generation of partial loss of function alleles.

FRAEM insertional mutagenesis utilizes DNA homology to target genomic regions of interest and introduce a selection cassette and dual reporter genes to facilitate identification of recombinants (Mueller et al. 2016). The FRAEM vector is a conditional suicide vector that places the plasmid maintenance gene (*pgp6*) under control of tetracycline-regulated operator sequence. This permits expansion of shuttle vector transformants within the population to increase the possibility of recombination between homologous sequences on the chromosome and vector, while still maintaining the ability to cure the FRAEM vector. The selection cassette contains *bla* for penicillin selection of recombinants, and GFP to monitor transformation and integration of the selection cassette into the chromosome. Finally, visual screening of single and double crossover (allelic exchange) events is facilitated by a mCherry gene located outside of the selection cassette and flanking chromosomal homology regions. *C. trachomatis* L2 *trpA* was deleted and replaced with the shuttle-vector selection cassette in a proof of principle experiment. The limitations of FRAEM include its relative complexity, the risk of deletion of unknown *cis*-acting chromosomal sequences, and polar effects (Mueller et al. 2017). Nonetheless, FRAEM is clearly a powerful tool for targeted manipulation of chlamydial genomes.

8 Forward Genetic Analysis of Chlamydial Genomes

Forward genetic screens have identified genes that mediate multiple aspects of chlamydial development, virulence, and immune evasion. These screens have relied on chemically mutagenized libraries because the TargeTron and FRAEM approaches are low-throughput (Table 1). In addition to the relative ease of mutagenesis, chemically mutagenized libraries contain a mixture of isolates with total and partial loss of function alleles, which permits interrogation of essential gene functions.

Nguyen and Valdivia compared the plaque morphologies of a collection of EMS mutagenized isolates derived from a rifampicin resistant *C. trachomatis* L2 parent (Nguyen and Valdivia 2012). The mutations causing altered plaque phenotypes were mapped using LGT and phenotypic linkage analysis. Three mutants that produced granular plaques had distinct missense mutations in *glgB*, a glycogen-branching enzyme. One of these missense mutations segregated with the granular plaque phenotypes when the mutant was crossed by LGT with spectinomycin and trimethoprim resistant *C. trachomatis* parents. Missense mutations in the type II secretion gene, *gspE*, were also linked to granular and small plaque phenotypes.

The same library of mutagenized *C. trachomatis* L2 isolates was screened for mutants that failed to promote F-actin assembly at the inclusion (Kokes et al. 2015). LGT with a spectinomycin parent linked this phenotype to a nonsense mutation in an uncharacterized *inc* gene, *inaC/ctl0184*. InaC expression from a plasmid complemented the *inaC* mutant, confirming the results of the LGT mapping. Another screen identified mutants that elicited increased lactose dehydrogenase (LDH) release from HeLa cells, which is an indicator of host cell death (Sixt et al. 2017). A nonsense mutation in the Inc gene *ctl0481* (renamed cpoS for chlamydia promoter of survival) was linked to the early cell death phenotype.

Two screens from the Nelson laboratory utilized an EMS-mutagenized library derived from a wild-type *C. trachomatis* L2 isolate transformed with pGFP::SW2 to avoid fitness costs associated with chromosomal antibiotic resistance alleles (Brothwell et al. 2016; Muramatsu et al. 2016). The use of pGFP::SW2 (L2-GFP) facilitated visual screens of mutant phenotypes and GFP expression served as a reporter of chlamydial metabolic activity. TS mutants that produced a reduced ratio of inclusions at 32°C versus 37°C (cold sensitive, CS) or 40°C versus. 37°C (heat sensitive, HS), compared to the library parent, were identified in the first screen (Brothwell et al. 2016). Thirty-one unique mutants with CS, TS or CS/TS phenotypes were identified and the mutations in 14 of these were mapped by csLGT. TS alleles of genes that play roles in protein synthesis, DNA replication, fatty acid biosynthesis, and carbohydrate metabolism in other bacteria as well as conserved chlamydial genes of unknown function were identified. A second screen identified six mutants that were sensitive to interferon (IFN)-γ-mediated persistence (Sip) (Muramatsu et al. 2016). Three *sip* alleles were mapped using csLGT. One Sip mutant contained a missense mutation in *trpB*, which is consistent with the known role of *trpB* in *C. trachomatis* during indole-rescue from IFN-γ-mediated tryptophan starvation (Fehlner-Gardiner et al. 2002; Kari et al. 2011). The other two mutants had missense mutations in a predicted oxidative stress protein gene *cysJ* and a predicted small neutral amino acid transporter. These mutants suggested that the chlamydial response to IFN-γ involves more than tryptophan metabolism.

Successful genetic screens in chlamydiae hinge upon both library diversity and the ability to map specific mutations to the phenotype of interest. Multiple approaches can link phenotypes to genotypes (Fig. 1). As with TILLING, fewer isolates need to be screened to achieve saturation when a higher concentration of mutagen is employed, but parsing out the relevant mutation becomes more difficult downstream. Additionally, high mutation burdens increase the occurrence of both directly and synthetically lethal mutations. Despite the initial challenges of library construction, forward genetic screens are powerful tools for identifying the functions of chlamydial genes, which can then be validated using the reverse genetics approaches discussed above.

9 Overview and Future Perspectives

When the field of molecular microbial pathogenesis began to expand in the 1980s Stanley Falkow proposed a guide that was later deemed Koch's postulate of molecular pathogenesis (Falkow 1988). Paraphrasing these postulates: (1) the phenotype under investigation should be associated with a pathogen; (2) specific inactivation of the gene associated with the virulence phenotype should reduce pathogenicity; and (3) reversion or replacement of the mutant gene should restore pathogenicity. Falkow also stressed that genetic approaches for testing these postulates were not rigid, and that a lack of relevant in vivo models was a serious obstacle for identifying virulence factors of many genetically tractable pathogens. The latter points may be especially pertinent to the current state of chlamydial genetics where our perspective is that the excitement about the latest tools has sometimes led to incomplete consideration of their limitations as well as the best model systems in which the mutation associated phenotypes would be apparent.

There is no single or perfect approach for genetic manipulation of chlamydiae for all applications and choosing the best method for a given study requires consideration of the strengths and weaknesses of the existing tools. For example, forward genetic screens that employ TILLING approaches benefit from the ability of mutagens to introduce desirable point mutations that are less likely to cause *cis-* and *trans*-acting effects, but are limited by downstream mutation mapping. A report describing two *C. trachomatis* Himar transposon mutants suggests that transposon mutant libraries that could help circumvent this limitation may soon be available (Fischer et al. 2017). TargeTron and FRAEM can alter specific genes, but these approaches introduce disruptions and/or deletions that could disrupt *cis-* and *trans*-acting sequences. These limitations have been circumvented in other bacteria using CRISPR/Cas9 gene editing since inactivation of specific targets is achieved without altering the larger genomic context, and adaptation of this approach for chlamydiae could be valuable (Luo et al. 2016; Zhang et al. 2017). Looking more long-term, adaptation of methods pioneered in *E. coli* for markerless allelic exchange and single copy gene expression from neutral loci seem like promising approaches for inactivating chlamydial genes while avoiding *cis*-and *trans*-acting effects and for expressing chlamydial proteins at physiological levels (Datsenko and Wanner 2000). Multiple tools in the chlamydial genetic toolbox remain limited by transformation efficiency, and further optimization of transformation techniques including electroporation and dendrimer-based approaches could be fruitful (Tam et al. 1994; Binet and Maurelli 2009a, b; Mishra et al. 2012; Gerard et al. 2013; Kannan et al. 2013). Probably the most significant impediment in the genetic dissection of chlamydial pathogenesis remains that these organisms need to be propagated in host cells. Genetic manipulation of other "obligate" intracellular organisms has clearly benefited from the development of anexic growth media, and promising findings that might be on the horizon for chlamydiae too (Omsland et al. 2009, 2012; Haider et al. 2010).

Finally, the overwhelming focus on the development of tools for a single model strain, *C. trachomatis* L2 434/Bu, has limited our ability to use genetic approaches to dissect crucial aspects of chlamydial pathogenesis. Despite the lack of a good in vivo model for *C. trachomatis* L2, the advent of genetic approaches has greatly enhanced our understanding of chlamydial biology. The challenge is now to extend these approaches to other *Chlamydia* spp.—especially those for which relevant animal models exist. LGV biology differs from the more common and medically important trachoma biovar strains in many ways. Trachoma biovar strains primarily infect columnar epithelial cells that protect the conjunctiva, urethra, GI, lung, cervix, and upper female reproductive tract. In contrast, LGV biovar strains infect via epithelial micro-abrasions where they enter into and proliferate in lymphatic cells. Innate immunity also rapidly clears *C. trachomatis* strains in mice (Morrison and Caldwell 2002). In contrast, *C. muridarum* can cause long-lasting infections in mice that are cleared by adaptive immunity (Barron et al. 1981; Morrison and Caldwell 2002). Existing murine *C. muridarum* pulmonary and GI infection models also mimic aspects of these infections with *C. trachomatis* STI strains in humans and the latter model was crucial to the discovery of the virulence role of chlamydial plasmids (Morrison and Caldwell 2002; Ramsey et al. 2009; Yeruva et al. 2013; Rank and Yeruva 2014). Virulence factors initially identified in the mouse GT were more important for *C. muridarum* GI colonization, showing that the tissue choice can also profoundly impact relevance of specific chlamydial virulence factors in the same animals (Shao et al. 2017). Beyond *C. muridarum*, *C. caviae* Guinea pig models can investigate urethral infections and sexual transmission (Rank et al. 2003; Wang et al. 2010). Primate models of trachoma and cervicitis exist that use the same isolates that cause these diseases in humans (Wolner-Hanssen et al. 1991; Kari et al. 2008). Understanding the animal and tissue-specific context in which chlamydial virulence genes are required during infection will shed light on both chlamydial biology and the limits of a given infection model. Looking forward, adapting the existing genetic tools to additional species and strains could enhance the utility of genetic approaches for dissecting mechanisms of chlamydial pathogenesis.

Acknowledgements DE Nelson was supported by grants AI099278 and AI116706, and G Zhong was supported by grants AI121989, AI105712, AI047997, from the United States National Institutes of Health, Division of Allery and Infectious Diseases. We would like Drs. Harlan Caldwell and Derek Fisher for discussion and insights regarding aspects of this manuscript. Finally, any oversights of relevant studies were not intentional and the authors would like to apologize for any instance of this in advance.

References

Agaisse H, Derre I (2013) A *C. trachomatis* cloning vector and the generation of *C. trachomatis* strains expressing fluorescent proteins under the control of a *C. trachomatis* promoter. PLoS ONE 8(2):e57090

Albrecht M, Sharma CM, Reinhardt R, Vogel J, Rudel T (2010) Deep sequencing-based discovery of the *Chlamydia trachomatis* transcriptome. Nucleic Acids Res 38(3):868–877

Azuma Y, Hirakawa H, Yamashita A, Cai Y, Rahman MA, Suzuki H, Mitaku S, Toh H, Goto S, Murakami T, Sugi K, Hayashi H, Fukushi H, Hattori M, Kuhara S, Shirai M (2006) Genome sequence of the cat pathogen, Chlamydophila felis. DNA Res 13(1):15–23

Barron AL, White HJ, Rank RG, Soloff BL, Moses EB (1981) A new animal model for the study of *Chlamydia trachomatis* genital infections: infection of mice with the agent of mouse pneumonitis. J Infect Dis 143(1):63–66

Bastidas RJ, Valdivia RH (2016) Emancipating Chlamydia: advances in the genetic manipulation of a recalcitrant intracellular pathogen. Microbiol Mol Biol Rev 80(2):411–427

Bauler LD, Hackstadt T (2014) Expression and targeting of secreted proteins from *Chlamydia trachomatis*. J Bacteriol 196(7):1325–1334

Binet R, Maurelli AT (2005) Fitness cost due to mutations in the 16S rRNA associated with spectinomycin resistance in *Chlamydia psittaci* 6BC. Antimicrob Agents Chemother 49 (11):4455–4464

Binet R, Maurelli AT (2007) Frequency of development and associated physiological cost of azithromycin resistance in *Chlamydia psittaci* 6BC and *C. trachomatis* L2. Antimicrob Agents Chemother 51(12):4267–4275

Binet R, Maurelli AT (2009a) The chlamydial functional homolog of KsgA confers kasugamycin sensitivity to *Chlamydia trachomatis* and impacts bacterial fitness. Bmc Microbiology 9

Binet R, Maurelli AT (2009b) Transformation and isolation of allelic exchange mutants of *Chlamydia psittaci* using recombinant DNA introduced by electroporation. Proc Natl Acad Sci USA 106(1):292–297

Binet R, Bowlin AK, Maurelli AT, Rank RG (2010) Impact of azithromycin resistance mutations on the virulence and fitness of Chlamydia caviae in guinea pigs. Antimicrob Agents Chemother 54(3):1094–1101

Borges V, Ferreira R, Nunes A, Sousa-Uva M, Abreu M, Borrego MJ, Gomes JP (2013) Effect of long-term laboratory propagation on *Chlamydia trachomatis* genome dynamics. Infect Genet Evol 17:23–32

Brothwell JA, Muramatsu MK, Toh E, Rockey DD, Putman TE, Barta ML, Hefty PS, Suchland RJ, Nelson DE (2016) Interrogating genes that mediate *Chlamydia trachomatis* survival in cell culture using conditional mutants and recombination. J Bacteriol 198 (15):2131–2139

Brunham R, Yang C, Maclean I, Kimani J, Maitha G, Plummer F (1994) *Chlamydia trachomatis* from individuals in a sexually transmitted disease core group exhibit frequent sequence variation in the major outer membrane protein (omp1) gene. J Clin Invest 94(1):458–463

Burall LS, Rodolakis A, Rekiki A, Myers GS, Bavoil PM (2009) Genomic analysis of an attenuated Chlamydia abortus live vaccine strain reveals defects in central metabolism and surface proteins. Infect Immun 77(9):4161–4167

Caldwell HD, Wood H, Crane D, Bailey R, Jones RB, Mabey D, Maclean I, Mohammed Z, Peeling R, Roshick C, Schachter J, Solomon AW, Stamm WE, Suchland RJ, Taylor L, West SK, Quinn TC, Belland RJ, McClarty G (2003) Polymorphisms in *Chlamydia trachomatis* tryptophan synthase genes differentiate between genital and ocular isolates. J Clin Invest 111(11):1757–1769

Carlson JH, Porcella SF, McClarty G, Caldwell HD (2005) Comparative genomic analysis of *Chlamydia trachomatis* oculotropic and genitotropic strains. Infect Immun 73(10):6407–6418

Carlson JH, Whitmire WM, Crane DD, Wicke L, Virtaneva K, Sturdevant DE, Kupko JJ 3rd, Porcella SF, Martinez-Orengo N, Heinzen RA, Kari L, Caldwell HD (2008) The *Chlamydia trachomatis* plasmid is a transcriptional regulator of chromosomal genes and a virulence factor. Infect Immun 76(6):2273–2283

Casson N, Medico N, Bille J, Greub G (2006) Parachlamydia acanthamoebae enters and multiplies within pneumocytes and lung fibroblasts. Microbes Infect 8(5):1294–1300

Casson N, Entenza JM, Borel N, Pospischil A, Greub G (2008) Murine model of pneumonia caused by Parachlamydia acanthamoebae. Microb Pathog 45(2):92–97

Chen C, Zhou Z, Conrad T, Yang Z, Dai J, Li Z, Wu Y, Zhong G (2015a) In vitro passage selects for Chlamydia muridarum with enhanced infectivity in cultured cells but attenuated pathogenicity in mouse upper genital tract. Infect Immun 83(5):1881–1892

Chen J, Yang Z, Sun X, Tang L, Ding Y, Xue M, Zhou Z, Baseman J, Zhong G (2015b) Intrauterine infection with plasmid-free Chlamydia muridarum reveals a critical role of the plasmid in chlamydial ascension and establishes a model for evaluating plasmid-independent pathogenicity. Infect Immun 83(6):2583–2592

Clifton DR, Fields KA, Grieshaber SS, Dooley CA, Fischer ER, Mead DJ, Carabeo RA, Hackstadt T (2004) A chlamydial type III translocated protein is tyrosine-phosphorylated at the site of entry and associated with recruitment of actin. Proc Natl Acad Sci USA 101(27):10166–10171

Collingro A, Poppert S, Heinz E, Schmitz-Esser S, Essig A, Schweikert M, Wagner M, Horn M (2005) Recovery of an environmental Chlamydia strain from activated sludge by co-cultivation with Acanthamoeba sp. Microbiology 151(Pt 1):301–309

Collingro A, Tischler P, Weinmaier T, Penz T, Heinz E, Brunham RC, Read TD, Bavoil PM, Sachse K, Kahane S, Friedman MG, Rattei T, Myers GS, Horn M (2011) Unity in variety–the pan-genome of the Chlamydiae. Mol Biol Evol 28(12):3253–3270

Conrad TA, Gong S, Yang Z, Matulich P, Keck J, Beltrami N, Chen C, Zhou Z, Dai J, Zhong G (2015) The chromosome-encoded hypothetical protein TC0668 Is an upper genital tract pathogenicity factor of Chlamydia muridarum. Infect Immun 84(2):467–479

Datsenko KA, Wanner BL (2000) One-step inactivation of chromosomal genes in Escherichia coli K-12 using PCR products. Proc Natl Acad Sci USA 97(12):6640–6645

Dean D, Schachter J, Dawson CR, Stephens RS (1992) Comparison of the major outer membrane protein variant sequence regions of B/Ba isolates: a molecular epidemiologic approach to *Chlamydia trachomatis* infections. J Infect Dis 166(2):383–392

DeMars R, Weinfurter J (2008) Interstrain gene transfer in *Chlamydia trachomatis* in vitro: mechanism and significance. J Bacteriol 190(5):1605–1614

DeMars R, Weinfurter J, Guex E, Lin J, Potucek Y (2007) Lateral gene transfer in vitro in the intracellular pathogen *Chlamydia trachomatis*. J Bacteriol 189(3):991–1003

Dessus-Babus S, Bebear CM, Charron A, Bebear C, de Barbeyrac B (1998) Sequencing of gyrase and topoisomerase IV quinolone-resistance-determining regions of *Chlamydia trachomatis* and characterization of quinolone-resistant mutants obtained In vitro. Antimicrob Agents Chemother 42(10):2474–2481

Ding H, Gong S, Tian Y, Yang Z, Brunham R, Zhong G (2013) Transformation of sexually transmitted infection-causing serovars of *Chlamydia trachomatis* using Blasticidin for selection. PLoS ONE 8(11):e80534

Donati M, Huot-Creasy H, Humphrys M, Di Paolo M, Di Francesco A, Myers GS (2014) Genome Sequence of Chlamydia suis MD56, isolated from the conjunctiva of a weaned piglet. Genome Announc 2(3):e00425

Draghi A 2nd, Popov VL, Kahl MM, Stanton JB, Brown CC, Tsongalis GJ, West AB, Frasca S Jr (2004) Characterization of "Candidatus piscichlamydia salmonis" (order Chlamydiales), a chlamydia-like bacterium associated with epitheliocystis in farmed Atlantic salmon (Salmo salar). J Clin Microbiol 42(11):5286–5297

Dreses-Werringloer U, Padubrin I, Kohler L, Hudson AP (2003) Detection of nucleotide variability in rpoB in both rifampin-sensitive and rifampin-resistant strains of *Chlamydia trachomatis*. Antimicrob Agents Chemother 47(7):2316–2318

Everett KD, Bush RM, Andersen AA (1999) Emended description of the order Chlamydiales, proposal of Parachlamydiaceae fam. nov. and Simkaniaceae fam. nov., each containing one monotypic genus, revised taxonomy of the family Chlamydiaceae, including a new genus and five new species, and standards for the identification of organisms. Int J Syst Bacteriol 49(Pt 2):415–440

Falkow S (1988) Molecular Koch's postulates applied to microbial pathogenicity. Rev Infect Dis 10(Suppl 2):S274–276

Farencena A, Comanducci M, Donati M, Ratti G, Cevenini R (1997) Characterization of a new isolate of *Chlamydia trachomatis* which lacks the common plasmid and has properties of biovar trachoma. Infect Immun 65(7):2965–2969

Fehlner-Gardiner C, Roshick C, Carlson JH, Hughes S, Belland RJ, Caldwell HD, McClarty G (2002) Molecular basis defining human *Chlamydia trachomatis* tissue tropism. A possible role for tryptophan synthase. J Biol Chem 277(30):26893–26903

Fischer A, Harrison KS, Ramirez Y, Auer D, Chowdhury BK, Prusty BK, Sauer F, Dimond Z, Kisker C, Scott Hefty P, Rudel T (2017) *Chlamydia trachomatis*-containing vacuole serves as deubiquitination platform to stabilize Mcl-1 and to interfere with host defense. Elife 6

Fitch WM, Peterson EM, de la Maza LM (1993) Phylogenetic analysis of the outer-membrane-protein genes of Chlamydiae, and its implication for vaccine development. Mol Biol Evol 10(4):892–913

Gerard HC, Mishra MK, Mao G, Wang S, Hali M, Whittum-Hudson JA, Kannan RM, Hudson AP (2013) Dendrimer-enabled DNA delivery and transformation of *Chlamydia pneumoniae*. Nanomedicine 9(7):996–1008

Gomes JP, Bruno WJ, Borrego MJ, Dean D (2004) Recombination in the genome of *Chlamydia trachomatis* involving the polymorphic membrane protein C gene relative to ompA and evidence for horizontal gene transfer. J Bacteriol 186(13):4295–4306

Gong S, Yang Z, Lei L, Shen L, Zhong G (2013) Characterization of *Chlamydia trachomatis* plasmid-encoded open reading frames. J Bacteriol 195(17):3819–3826

Greub G, Berger P, Papazian L, Raoult D (2003) Parachlamydiaceae as rare agents of pneumonia. Emerg Infect Dis 9(6):755–756

Hadfield J, Harris SR, Seth-Smith HMB, Parmar S, Andersson P, Giffard PM, Schachter J, Moncada J, Ellison L, Vaulet MLG, Fermepin MR, Radebe F, Mendoza S, Ouburg S, Morre SA, Sachse K, Puolakkainen M, Korhonen SJ, Sonnex C, Wiggins R, Jalal H, Brunelli T, Casprini P, Pitt R, Ison C, Savicheva A, Shipitsyna E, Hadad R, Kari L, Burton MJ, Mabey D, Solomon AW, Lewis D, Marsh P, Unemo M, Clarke IN, Parkhill J, Thomson NR (2017) Comprehensive global genome dynamics of *Chlamydia trachomatis* show ancient diversification followed by contemporary mixing and recent lineage expansion. Genome Res 27(7):1220–1229

Haider S, Wagner M, Schmid MC, Sixt BS, Christian JG, Hacker G, Pichler P, Mechtler K, Muller A, Baranyi C, Toenshoff ER, Montanaro J, Horn M (2010) Raman microspectroscopy reveals long-term extracellular activity of Chlamydiae. Mol Microbiol 77(3):687–700

Hayes LJ, Yearsley P, Treharne JD, Ballard RA, Fehler GH, Ward ME (1994) Evidence for naturally occurring recombination in the gene encoding the major outer membrane protein of lymphogranuloma venereum isolates of *Chlamydia trachomatis*. Infect Immun 62(12):5659–5663

Holzer M, Laroucau K, Creasy HH, Ott S, Vorimore F, Bavoil PM, Marz M, Sachse K (2016) Whole-genome sequence of Chlamydia gallinacea type strain 08-1274/3. Genome Announc 4 (4):e00708

Hooppaw AJ, Fisher DJ (2016) A coming of age story: Chlamydia in the Post-Genetic Era. Infect Immun 84(3):612–621

Horn M, Collingro A, Schmitz-Esser S, Beier CL, Purkhold U, Fartmann B, Brandt P, Nyakatura GJ, Droege M, Frishman D, Rattei T, Mewes HW, Wagner M (2004) Illuminating the evolutionary history of chlamydiae. Science 304(5671):728–730

Illingworth M, Hooppaw AJ, Ruan L, Fisher DJ, Chen L (2017) Biochemical and genetic analysis of the Chlamydia GroEL Chaperonins. J Bacteriol 199(12):e00844

Jeffrey BM, Suchland RJ, Quinn KL, Davidson JR, Stamm WE, Rockey DD (2010) Genome sequencing of recent clinical *Chlamydia trachomatis* strains identifies loci associated with tissue tropism and regions of apparent recombination. Infect Immun 78(6):2544–2553

Jeffrey BM, Suchland RJ, Eriksen SG, Sandoz KM, Rockey DD (2013) Genomic and phenotypic characterization of in vitro-generated *Chlamydia trachomatis* recombinants. BMC Microbiol 13:142

Johnson CM, Fisher DJ (2013) Site-specific, insertional inactivation of incA in *Chlamydia trachomatis* using a group II intron. PLoS ONE 8(12):e83989

Kalman S, Mitchell W, Marathe R, Lammel C, Fan J, Hyman RW, Olinger L, Grimwood J, Davis RW, Stephens RS (1999) Comparative genomes of *Chlamydia pneumoniae* and *C. trachomatis*. Nat Genet 21(4):385–389

Kannan RM, Gerard HC, Mishra MK, Mao G, Wang S, Hali M, Whittum-Hudson JA, Hudson AP (2013) Dendrimer-enabled transformation of *Chlamydia trachomatis*. Microb Pathog 65:29–35

Kari L, Whitmire WM, Carlson JH, Crane DD, Reveneau N, Nelson DE, Mabey DC, Bailey RL, Holland MJ, McClarty G, Caldwell HD (2008) Pathogenic diversity among *Chlamydia trachomatis* ocular strains in nonhuman primates is affected by subtle genomic variations. J Infect Dis 197(3):449–456

Kari L, Goheen MM, Randall LB, Taylor LD, Carlson JH, Whitmire WM, Virok D, Rajaram K, Endresz V, McClarty G, Nelson DE, Caldwell HD (2011) Generation of targeted *Chlamydia trachomatis* null mutants. Proc Natl Acad Sci USA 108(17):7189–7193

Kari L, Southern TR, Downey CJ, Watkins HS, Randall LB, Taylor LD, Sturdevant GL, Whitmire WM, Caldwell HD (2014) *Chlamydia trachomatis* polymorphic membrane protein D is a virulence factor involved in early host-cell interactions. Infect Immun 82(7):2756–2762

Karlsen M, Nylund A, Watanabe K, Helvik JV, Nylund S, Plarre H (2008) Characterization of 'Candidatus Clavochlamydia salmonicola': an intracellular bacterium infecting salmonid fish. Environ Microbiol 10(1):208–218

Key CE, Fisher DJ (2017) Use of group II intron technology for targeted mutagenesis in *Chlamydia trachomatis*. Methods Mol Biol 1498:163–177

Kokes M, Dunn JD, Granek JA, Nguyen BD, Barker JR, Valdivia RH, Bastidas RJ (2015) Integrating chemical mutagenesis and whole-genome sequencing as a platform for forward and reverse genetic analysis of Chlamydia. Cell Host Microbe 17(5):716–725

Lagkouvardos I, Jehl MA, Rattei T, Horn M (2014) Signature protein of the PVC superphylum. Appl Environ Microbiol 80(2):440–445

Lampe MF, Suchland RJ, Stamm WE (1993) Nucleotide sequence of the variable domains within the major outer membrane protein gene from serovariants of *Chlamydia trachomatis*. Infect Immun 61(1):213–219

Lei L, Chen J, Hou S, Ding Y, Yang Z, Zeng H, Baseman J, Zhong G (2014) Reduced live organism recovery and lack of hydrosalpinx in mice infected with plasmid-free Chlamydia muridarum. Infect Immun 82(3):983–992

Liu Y, Chen C, Gong S, Hou S, Qi M, Liu Q, Baseman J, Zhong G (2014) Transformation of Chlamydia muridarum reveals a role for Pgp5 in suppression of plasmid-dependent gene expression. J Bacteriol 196(5):989–998

Lohr M, Prohl A, Ostermann C, Liebler-Tenorio E, Schroedl W, Aeby S, Greub G, Reinhold P (2015) A bovine model of a respiratory Parachlamydia acanthamoebae infection. Pathog Dis 73(1):1–14

Lowden NM, Yeruva L, Johnson CM, Bowlin AK, Fisher DJ (2015) Use of aminoglycoside 3' adenyltransferase as a selection marker for *Chlamydia trachomatis* intron-mutagenesis and in vivo intron stability. BMC Res Notes 8:570

Luo ML, Leenay RT, Beisel CL (2016) Current and future prospects for CRISPR-based tools in bacteria. Biotechnol Bioeng 113(5):930–943

Matsumoto A, Izutsu H, Miyashita N, Ohuchi M (1998) Plaque formation by and plaque cloning of *Chlamydia trachomatis* biovar trachoma. J Clin Microbiol 36(10):3013–3019

McCallum CM, Comai L, Greene EA, Henikoff S (2000) Targeted screening for induced mutations. Nat Biotechnol 18(4):455–457

McCoy AJ, Sandlin RC, Maurelli AT (2003) In vitro and in vivo functional activity of Chlamydia MurA, a UDP-*N*-acetylglucosamine enolpyruvyl transferase involved in peptidoglycan synthesis and fosfomycin resistance. J Bacteriol 185(4):1218–1228

Mishra MK, Gerard HC, Whittum-Hudson JA, Hudson AP, Kannan RM (2012) Dendrimer-enabled modulation of gene expression in *Chlamydia trachomatis*. Mol Pharm 9 (3):413–421

Misiurina O, Shipitsina EV, Finashutina Iu P, Lazarev VN, Akopian TA, Savicheva AM, Govorun VM (2004) Analysis of point mutations in the ygeD, gyrA and parC genes in fluoroquinolones resistant clinical isolates of *Chlamydia trachomatis*. Mol Gen Mikrobiol Virusol 3:3–7

Mojica S, Huot Creasy H, Daugherty S, Read TD, Kim T, Kaltenboeck B, Bavoil P, Myers GS (2011) Genome sequence of the obligate intracellular animal pathogen Chlamydia pecorum E58. J Bacteriol 193(14):3690

Morrison RP, Caldwell HD (2002) Immunity to murine chlamydial genital infection. Infect Immun 70(6):2741–2751

Moulder JW (1985) Comparative biology of intracellular parasitism. Microbiol Rev 49(3):298–337

Mueller KE, Wolf K, Fields KA (2016) Gene deletion by fluorescence-reported allelic exchange mutagenesis in *Chlamydia trachomatis*. MBio 7(1):e01817–01815

Mueller KE, Wolf K, Fields KA (2017) *Chlamydia trachomatis* Transformation and Allelic Exchange Mutagenesis. Curr Protoc Microbiol 45: 11A 13 11–11A 13 15

Muramatsu MK, Brothwell JA, Stein BD, Putman TE, Rockey DD, Nelson DE (2016) Beyond tryptophan synthase: identification of genes that contribute to *Chlamydia trachomatis* survival during IFN-gamma induced persistence and reactivation. Infect Immun

Nelson DE, Taylor LD, Shannon JG, Whitmire WM, Crane DD, McClarty G, Su H, Kari L, Caldwell HD (2007) Phenotypic rescue of *Chlamydia trachomatis* growth in IFN-gamma treated mouse cells by irradiated Chlamydia muridarum. Cell Microbiol 9(9):2289–2298

Nguyen BD, Valdivia RH (2012) Virulence determinants in the obligate intracellular pathogen *Chlamydia trachomatis* revealed by forward genetic approaches. Proc Natl Acad Sci USA 109 (4):1263–1268

Nguyen BD, Valdivia RH (2013) Forward genetic approaches in *Chlamydia trachomatis*. J Vis Exp 80:e50636

Nunes A, Gomes JP (2014) Evolution, phylogeny, and molecular epidemiology of Chlamydia. Infect Genet Evol 23:49–64

O'Connell CM, Nicks KM (2006) A plasmid-cured Chlamydia muridarum strain displays altered plaque morphology and reduced infectivity in cell culture. Microbiology 152(Pt 6):1601–1607

O'Connell CM, Ingalls RR, Andrews CW Jr, Scurlock AM, Darville T (2007) Plasmid-deficient Chlamydia muridarum fail to induce immune pathology and protect against oviduct disease. J Immunol 179(6):4027–4034

Omsland A, Cockrell DC, Howe D, Fischer ER, Virtaneva K, Sturdevant DE, Porcella SF, Heinzen RA (2009) Host cell-free growth of the Q fever bacterium Coxiella burnetii. Proc Natl Acad Sci USA 106(11):4430–4434

Omsland A, Sager J, Nair V, Sturdevant DE, Hackstadt T (2012) Developmental stage-specific metabolic and transcriptional activity of *Chlamydia trachomatis* in an axenic medium. Proc Natl Acad Sci USA 109(48):19781–19785

Omsland A, Sixt BS, Horn M, Hackstadt T (2014) Chlamydial metabolism revisited: interspecies metabolic variability and developmental stage-specific physiologic activities. FEMS Microbiol Rev 38(4):779–801

Palmer L, Falkow S (1986) A common plasmid of *Chlamydia trachomatis*. Plasmid 16(1):52–62

Peterson EM, Markoff BA, Schachter J, de la Maza LM (1990) The 7.5-kb plasmid present in *Chlamydia trachomatis* is not essential for the growth of this microorganism. Plasmid 23 (2):144–148

Pickett MA, Everson JS, Pead PJ, Clarke IN (2005) The plasmids of *Chlamydia trachomatis* and Chlamydophila pneumoniae (N16): accurate determination of copy number and the paradoxical effect of plasmid-curing agents. Microbiology-Sgm 151:893–903

Qin B, McClarty G (1992) Effect of 6-thioguanine on *Chlamydia trachomatis* growth in wild-type and hypoxanthine-guanine phosphoribosyltransferase-deficient cells. J Bacteriol 174(9):2865–2873

Rajaram K, Giebel AM, Toh E, Hu S, Newman JH, Morrison SG, Kari L, Morrison RP, Nelson DE (2015) Mutational analysis of the Chlamydia muridarum plasticity zone. Infect Immun 83(7):2870–2881

Ramsey KH, Sigar IM, Schripsema JH, Denman CJ, Bowlin AK, Myers GA, Rank RG (2009) Strain and virulence diversity in the mouse pathogen Chlamydia muridarum. Infect Immun 77 (8):3284–3293

Rank RG, Yeruva L (2014) Hidden in plain sight: chlamydial gastrointestinal infection and its relevance to persistence in human genital infection. Infect Immun 82(4):1362–1371

Rank RG, Bowlin AK, Reed RL, Darville T (2003) Characterization of chlamydial genital infection resulting from sexual transmission from male to female guinea pigs and determination of infectious dose. Infect Immun 71(11):6148–6154

Read TD, Brunham RC, Shen C, Gill SR, Heidelberg JF, White O, Hickey EK, Peterson J, Utterback T, Berry K, Bass S, Linher K, Weidman J, Khouri H, Craven B, Bowman C, Dodson R, Gwinn M, Nelson W, DeBoy R, Kolonay J, McClarty G, Salzberg SL, Eisen J, Fraser CM (2000) Genome sequences of *Chlamydia trachomatis* MoPn and *Chlamydia pneumoniae* AR39. Nucleic Acids Res 28(6):1397–1406

Read TD, Myers GS, Brunham RC, Nelson WC, Paulsen IT, Heidelberg J, Holtzapple E, Khouri H, Federova NB, Carty HA, Umayam LA, Haft DH, Peterson J, Beanan MJ, White O, Salzberg SL, Hsia RC, McClarty G, Rank RG, Bavoil PM, Fraser CM (2003) Genome sequence of *Chlamydophila caviae* (*Chlamydia psittaci* GPIC): examining the role of niche-specific genes in the evolution of the Chlamydiaceae. Nucleic Acids Res 31(8):2134–2147

Rodolakis A (1983) In vitro and in vivo properties of chemically induced temperature-sensitive mutants of *Chlamydia psittaci* var. ovis: screening in a murine model. Infect Immun 42 (2):525–530

Rodolakis A, Souriau A (1983) Response of ewes to temperature-sensitive mutants of *Chlamydia psittaci* (var ovis) obtained by NTG mutagenesis. Ann Rech Vet 14(2):155–161

Rodolakis A, Souriau A (1986) Response of goats to vaccination with temperature-sensitive mutants of *Chlamydia psittaci* obtained by nitrosoguanidine mutagenesis. Am J Vet Res 47 (12):2627–2631

Russell M, Darville T, Chandra-Kuntal K, Smith B, Andrews CW Jr, O'Connell CM (2011) Infectivity acts as in vivo selection for maintenance of the chlamydial cryptic plasmid. Infect Immun 79(1):98–107

Sachse K, Laroucau K (2015) Two more species of Chlamydia-does it make a difference? Pathog Dis 73(1):1–3

Sachse K, Laroucau K, Riege K, Wehner S, Dilcher M, Creasy HH, Weidmann M, Myers G, Vorimore F, Vicari N, Magnino S, Liebler-Tenorio E, Ruettger A, Bavoil PM, Hufert FT, Rossello-Mora R, Marz M (2014) Evidence for the existence of two new members of the family Chlamydiaceae and proposal of Chlamydia avium sp. nov. and Chlamydia gallinacea sp. nov. Syst Appl Microbiol 37(2):79–88

Schofl G, Voigt A, Litsche K, Sachse K, Saluz HP (2011) Complete genome sequences of four mammalian isolates of Chlamydophila psittaci. J Bacteriol 193(16):4258

Seth-Smith HM, Harris SR, Persson K, Marsh P, Barron A, Bignell A, Bjartling C, Clark L, Cutcliffe LT, Lambden PR, Lennard N, Lockey SJ, Quail MA, Salim O, Skilton RJ, Wang Y, Holland MJ, Parkhill J, Thomson NR, Clarke IN (2009) Co-evolution of genomes and plasmids within *Chlamydia trachomatis* and the emergence in Sweden of a new variant strain. BMC Genom 10:239

Shao L, Melero J, Zhang N, Arulanandam B, Baseman J, Liu Q, Zhong G (2017) The cryptic plasmid is more important for Chlamydia muridarum to colonize the mouse gastrointestinal tract than to infect the genital tract. PLoS ONE 12(5):e0177691

Sixt BS, Bastidas RJ, Finethy R, Baxter RM, Carpenter VK, Kroemer G, Coers J, Valdivia RH (2017) The *Chlamydia trachomatis* inclusion membrane protein CpoS counteracts STING-mediated cellular surveillance and suicide programs. Cell Host Microbe 21(1):113–121

Snavely EA, Kokes M, Dunn JD, Saka HA, Nguyen BD, Bastidas RJ, McCafferty DG, Valdivia RH (2014) Reassessing the role of the secreted protease CPAF in *Chlamydia trachomatis* infection through genetic approaches. Pathog Dis 71(3):336–351

Song L, Carlson JH, Whitmire WM, Kari L, Virtaneva K, Sturdevant DE, Watkins H, Zhou B, Sturdevant GL, Porcella SF, McClarty G, Caldwell HD (2013) *Chlamydia trachomatis* plasmid-encoded Pgp4 is a transcriptional regulator of virulence-associated genes. Infect Immun 81(3):636–644

Song L, Carlson JH, Zhou B, Virtaneva K, Whitmire WM, Sturdevant GL, Porcella SF, McClarty G, Caldwell HD (2014) Plasmid-mediated transformation tropism of chlamydial biovars. Pathog Dis 70(2):189–193

Stephens RS, Kalman S, Lammel C, Fan J, Marathe R, Aravind L, Mitchell W, Olinger L, Tatusov RL, Zhao Q, Koonin EV, Davis RW (1998) Genome sequence of an obligate intracellular pathogen of humans: *Chlamydia trachomatis*. Science 282(5389):754–759

Stephens RS, Myers G, Eppinger M, Bavoil PM (2009) Divergence without difference: phylogenetics and taxonomy of Chlamydia resolved. FEMS Immunol Med Microbiol 55 (2):115–119

Stothard DR, Williams JA, Van Der Pol B, Jones RB (1998) Identification of a *Chlamydia trachomatis* serovar E urogenital isolate which lacks the cryptic plasmid. Infect Immun 66 (12):6010–6013

Stride MC, Polkinghorne A, Miller TL, Groff JM, Lapatra SE, Nowak BF (2013) Molecular characterization of "Candidatus Parilichlamydia carangidicola," a novel Chlamydia-like epitheliocystis agent in yellowtail kingfish, Seriola lalandi (Valenciennes), and the proposal of a new family, "Candidatus Parilichlamydiaceae" fam. nov. (order Chlamydiales). Appl Environ Microbiol 79(5):1590–1597

Sturdevant GL, Kari L, Gardner DJ, Olivares-Zavaleta N, Randall LB, Whitmire WM, Carlson JH, Goheen MM, Selleck EM, Martens C, Caldwell HD (2010) Frameshift mutations in a single novel virulence factor alter the in vivo pathogenicity of *Chlamydia trachomatis* for the female murine genital tract. Infect Immun 78(9):3660–3668

Suchland RJ, Rockey DD, Bannantine JP, Stamm WE (2000) Isolates of *Chlamydia trachomatis* that occupy nonfusogenic inclusions lack IncA, a protein localized to the inclusion membrane. Infect Immun 68(1):360–367

Suchland RJ, Sandoz KM, Jeffrey BM, Stamm WE, Rockey DD (2009) Horizontal transfer of tetracycline resistance among Chlamydia spp. in vitro. Antimicrob Agents Chemother 53 (11):4604–4611

Tam JE, Davis CH, Wyrick PB (1994) Expression of recombinant DNA introduced into *Chlamydia trachomatis* by electroporation. Can J Microbiol 40(7):583–591

Taylor-Brown A, Vaughan L, Greub G, Timms P, Polkinghorne A (2015) Twenty years of research into Chlamydia-like organisms: a revolution in our understanding of the biology and pathogenicity of members of the phylum Chlamydiae. Pathog Dis 73(1):1–15

Thomas NS, Lusher M, Storey CC, Clarke IN (1997) Plasmid diversity in Chlamydia. Microbiology 143(Pt 6):1847–1854

Thomson NR, Yeats C, Bell K, Holden MT, Bentley SD, Livingstone M, Cerdeno-Tarraga AM, Harris B, Doggett J, Ormond D, Mungall K, Clarke K, Feltwell T, Hance Z, Sanders M, Quail MA, Price C, Barrell BG, Parkhill J, Longbottom D (2005) The Chlamydophila abortus genome sequence reveals an array of variable proteins that contribute to interspecies variation. Genome Res 15(5):629–640

Thomson NR, Holden MT, Carder C, Lennard N, Lockey SJ, Marsh P, Skipp P, O'Connor CD, Goodhead I, Norbertzcak H, Harris B, Ormond D, Rance R, Quail MA, Parkhill J,

Stephens RS, Clarke IN (2008) *Chlamydia trachomatis*: genome sequence analysis of lymphogranuloma venereum isolates. Genome Res 18(1):161–171
Tipples G, McClarty G (1991) Isolation and initial characterization of a series of *Chlamydia trachomatis* isolates selected for hydroxyurea resistance by a stepwise procedure. J Bacteriol 173(16):4932–4940
Treharne JD, Yearsley PJ, Ballard RC (1989) In vitro studies of *Chlamydia trachomatis* susceptibility and resistance to rifampin and rifabutin. Antimicrob Agents Chemother 33 (8):1393–1394
Wang Y, Nagarajan U, Hennings L, Bowlin AK, Rank RG (2010) Local host response to chlamydial urethral infection in male guinea pigs. Infect Immun 78(4):1670–1681
Wang Y, Kahane S, Cutcliffe LT, Skilton RJ, Lambden PR, Clarke IN (2011) Development of a transformation system for *Chlamydia trachomatis*: restoration of glycogen biosynthesis by acquisition of a plasmid shuttle vector. PLoS Pathog 7(9):e1002258
Wang YB, Cutcliffe LT, Skilton RJ, Ramsey KH, Thomson NR, Clarke IN (2014) The genetic basis of plasmid tropism between *Chlamydia trachomatis* and Chlamydia muridarum. Pathogens and Disease 72(1):19–23
Weber MM, Bauler LD, Lam J, Hackstadt T (2015) Expression and localization of predicted inclusion membrane proteins in *Chlamydia trachomatis*. Infect Immun 83(12):4710–4718
Weber MM, Lam JL, Dooley CA, Noriea NF, Hansen BT, Hoyt FH, Carmody AB, Sturdevant GL, Hackstadt T (2017) Absence of specific *Chlamydia trachomatis* inclusion membrane proteins triggers premature inclusion membrane lysis and host cell death. Cell Rep 19(7):1406–1417
Weisburg WG, Hatch TP, Woese CR (1986) Eubacterial origin of chlamydiae. J Bacteriol 167 (2):570–574
Wesolowski J, Weber MM, Nawrotek A, Dooley CA, Calderon M, St Croix CM, Hackstadt T, Cherfils J, Paumet F (2017) Chlamydia hijacks ARF GTPases to coordinate microtubule posttranslational modifications and golgi complex positioning. MBio 8(3):e02280
Wickstrum J, Sammons LR, Restivo KN, Hefty PS (2013) Conditional gene expression in *Chlamydia trachomatis* using the tet system. PLoS ONE 8(10):e76743
Wolner-Hanssen P, Patton DL, Holmes KK (1991) Protective immunity in pig-tailed macaques after cervical infection with *Chlamydia trachomatis*. Sex Transm Dis 18(1):21–25
Wylie JL, Wang LL, Tipples G, McClarty G (1996) A single point mutation in CTP synthetase of *Chlamydia trachomatis* confers resistance to cyclopentenyl cytosine. J Biol Chem 271 (26):15393–15400
Yang C, Starr T, Song L, Carlson JH, Sturdevant GL, Beare PA, Whitmire WM, Caldwell HD (2015) Chlamydial lytic exit from host cells is plasmid regulated. MBio 6(6):e01648–01615
Yang C, Kari L, Sturdevant GL, Song L, Patton MJ, Couch CE, Ilgenfritz JM, Southern TR, Whitmire WM, Briones M, Bonner C, Grant C, Hu P, McClarty G, Caldwell HD (2017) *Chlamydia trachomatis* ChxR is a transcriptional regulator of virulence factors that function in in vivo host-pathogen interactions. Pathog Dis 75(3):ftx035
Yeruva L, Spencer N, Bowlin AK, Wang Y, Rank RG (2013) Chlamydial infection of the gastrointestinal tract: a reservoir for persistent infection. Pathog Dis 68(3):88–95
Zhang H, Cheng QX, Liu AM, Zhao GP, Wang J (2017) A novel and efficient method for bacteria genome editing employing both CRISPR/Cas9 and an antibiotic resistance cassette. Front Microbiol 8:812
Zhong G (2017) Chlamydial plasmid-dependent pathogenicity. Trends Microbiol 25(2):141–152

Chlamydia trachomatis as the Cause of Infectious Infertility: Acute, Repetitive or Persistent Long-Term Infection?

Larissa Schuchardt and Jan Rupp

Abstract *Chlamydia trachomatis* is the most frequently detected agent of sexually transmitted infections worldwide. Infection of the lower female genital tract (FGT) can cause cervicitis and if ascending to the upper FGT may result in serious sequelae such as pelvic inflammatory disease (PID), salpingitis and tubal factor infertility (TFI). The factors leading to this complication are still not completely understood. We elaborate four different models for host–pathogen interactions in *C. trachomatis* infections that may promote disease development: (1) acute infection, (2) repeated infections, (3) chronic/persistent infections and (4) non-inflammatory colonization. Whereas experimental data exist for all of these models in vitro, ex vivo and in vivo, we were interested in seeing what clinical evidence we have supporting one or the other model. We particularly focused on data that favour the one or the other model for TFI development in *C. trachomatis* infection and speculate on future studies that could integrate in vitro findings for a better characterization of the situation in vivo.

Abbreviations

BV	Bacterial vaginosis
DFO	Deferoxamine
EB	Elementary body
EP	Ectopic pregnancy
FGT	Female genital tract
HSP60	Heat-shock protein 60
IFN-γ	Interferon-γ
OmpA	Outer membrane protein A
PID	Pelvic inflammatory disease
RB	Reticulate body
TFI	Tubal factor infertility

L. Schuchardt · J. Rupp (✉)
Department of Infectious Diseases and Microbiology, University of Lübeck, Ratzeburger Allee 160, 23538 Lübeck, Germany
e-mail: Jan.Rupp@uksh.de

Current Topics in Microbiology and Immunology (2018) 412:159–182
DOI 10.1007/82_2016_15

Published Online: 02 July 2016

Contents

1 Introduction

Infection with *Chlamydia trachomatis* is the most common bacteria sexually transmitted infection in the world. *Chlamydia* is an obligate intracellular bacterial pathogen with a unique biphasic developmental cycle. Its infectious elementary bodies (EBs) are able to attach to and penetrate into the cell, where they form inclusions that escape the mechanism of phagocytosis. They differentiate into the metabolically more active but non-infectious reticulate bodies (RBs) that are able to divide by binary fission. After retransformation, infectious EBs are released from the cell and initiate another developmental cycle, approximately 48–72 h post-infection (Wyrick 2000). In addition to those two developmental life stages, a third stage has been shown to play an important role, the "aberrant" RB. It has also been referred to as "persistent", since it seems to be metabolically less active and, more importantly, proves difficult to be eliminated by antibiotic treatment or the host's immune system. Numerous in vitro models showing the induction of aberrant RBs have been established and investigated in the past, but its relevance for the situation in vivo and infections in humans is still controversially discussed.

In humans, chlamydial infection of the female genital tract has been shown to cause cervicitis and, if ascending, may lead to pelvic inflammatory disease (PID) and serious complications such as infectious infertility or ectopic pregnancies. Infectious infertility is also being referred to as tubal factor infertility (TFI), since the main pathomechanism is the occlusion of the fallopian tubes through scarring. It is of great importance to understand the exact nature of these processes and the mechanisms that are involved. Acute and/or chronic infections may be the pivotal driver of these processes just as chlamydial "persistence" could play a major role. An extensive number of cell culture models have been used in order to elucidate the complicated relationship between micro-environmental factors that influence the infection and the resulting course of disease. Cell cultures allow us to modify certain conditions, but are limited when it comes to long-term consequences and can merely be an approach to the in vivo infection in humans. Also, a great number of studies has been carried out in humans and animals, with *Chlamydia muridarum* infections in mice and *Chlamydia suis* infections in pigs having currently the most translational impact for the situation in humans (see also De Clercq et al. 2013). Animal models are suitable to only a limited extent but still necessary, since longitudinal studies in humans are difficult to perform. In this review, we want to elaborate trials that have been conducted in humans but also recent studies from cell culture and animals that we considered relevant in the context of *C. trachomatis* infection and TFI development.

Different disease models and how they might be linked to TFI development We will discuss four potential scenarios on how *C. trachomatis* infections could result in severe inflammatory diseases of the urogenital tract in females: (1) the single acute infection, (2) multiple unrelated (repeated) infections, (3) the long-time, chronic or persistent infection and (4) colonization of the gastrointestinal tract with its possibility of frequent autoreinfection. Often these scenarios may overlap and make a clear discrimination impossible. Chronic infections may arise from a single infection, but also after a longer episode of multiple infections. Multiple infections, in its sense mostly repetitive infections after clearance or treatment of a previous acute infection, could also unmask as intermitting acute episodes when chronic infection alternates between persistent and non-persistent forms (in this case labelled "recurrent infection"). The topic is even more complicated by the fact that clear definitions for the terms "chronic" or "persistent" in *C. trachomatis* infections in humans have not been characterized and defined very well. Thus, we will present evidence for the impact of single and multiple infections on TFI development and elaborate the chronic infection model from studies on chlamydial persistence in vitro. Furthermore, we will briefly address the possible role of gastrointestinal colonization.

2 Acute Infections with *C. trachomatis*

A woman's risk for at least a single infection with *C. trachomatis* is estimated to be 42.9 % by the age of 44 (Kavanagh et al. 2013). For the differentiation between single and repeated infections, women should be tested at least for the presence of serum antibodies against *C. trachomatis* before entering a study. The fact that not all studies exclude women with earlier infections, either self-reported or tested, may obscure the results obtained in different study designs. Therefore, findings especially from studies dealing with single vs. repeated infections have to be interpreted carefully. This should also be kept in mind for other aspects that are discussed in this part: prevalence and incidence of chlamydial infections as well as risk factors and possible mechanisms for developing tubal impairment.

2.1 Prevalence, Incidence, Screening and Treatment of Acute Chlamydial Infection

According to recently published data, global estimates show that approximately 357 million new infections with the 4 most prevalent sexually transmitted pathogens *Chlamydia trachomatis*, *Neisseria gonorrhoea*, *Treponema pallidum* and *Trichomonas vaginalis* occur every year. Of these, at least 100 million are estimated to be infections with *C. trachomatis* (Newman et al. 2015) with more than 1.4 million reported cases in the USA alone. The prevalence of chlamydial infections was found to be 1.7 % in 14–39-year-old women, but 4.7 % in sexually active 14–24-year-old women (Torrone et al. 2014). Therefore, annual screening in females <25 years is strongly recommended (Geisler 2015). Chlamydial prevalence might even be higher in groups of females who are more difficult to engage in screening programmes such as younger females and females living in disadvantaged areas (Macleod et al. 2005). Acute infection with *C. trachomatis* can be accompanied by symptoms of urethritis, cervicitis or PID, but is asymptomatic in 50–70 % of all infections (Carey and Beagley 2010). This notably high number of undetected cases makes the definition of a risk population necessary. Recommended treatment regimens include azithromycin or doxycycline, but there is a lack of studies directly comparing antibiotic efficacies in particular patient groups (Geisler et al. 2015).

2.2 What Are the Risk Factors?

Who is at risk to get infected with *Chlamydia*? Most studies agree that younger females who have more than one sexual partner are more at risk than women over the age of 25 and without a frequent partner change. Walker et al. (2012) conducted a study in Australia with women aged 16–25 and considered the 16–20 age group the most vulnerable. Scott Lamontagne et al. (2007) could narrow it down even further to 16–17-year-olds in a group of 16–24-year-old women in the UK. They also reported non-white ethnicity and a self-reported history of chlamydial infections to be risk factors. Additionally, low education seems to be another risk factor (Walker et al. 2012). In a group of 16–27-year-old women, risk for incident *Chlamydia* infection correlated with having a new sexual partner, smoking, bacterial vaginosis (BV) and coinfection with high-risk types of the human papillomavirus (Aghaizu et al. 2014). The same applied for concurrent *N. gonorrhoea* infections (Batteiger et al. 2010). These findings may be biased due to the fact that most of the studies recruited women in STD or family planning clinics, which may be not representative for the whole population.

2.3 Paradigms for the Development of Infectious Infertility

Several paradigms exist on the pathogenesis of *C. trachomatis* infections of the urogenital tract and disease progression to infectious infertility. Stephens earlier introduced a broad hypothesis concerning the development of fibrosis in the FGT and made the distinction between an "immunological" and a "cellular" genesis of the disease (Stephens 2003). The immunological paradigm was described as delayed-type hypersensitivity and the induction of autoimmunity. The concept of autoimmunity comprised the recognition of a chlamydial antigen (e.g. HSP60) that can also be found in human cells and is therefore attacked by TH1 cells and/or specific antibodies. Recent studies nowadays favour the concept of immunological host responses that includes not only T cells, but also polymorphonuclear neutrophil granulocytes (PMNs) and NK cells (Frazer et al. 2011; Marks et al. 2010). It overlaps with the cellular paradigm that includes pro-inflammatory cytokines such as IL-8, IL-6 or TNF-alpha and growth factors such as EGF or VEGF as major drivers in promoting, tissue remodelling and fibrosis that may finally lead to tubal scarring and occlusion with the clinical consequences of tubal factor infertility or ectopic pregnancies.

In a recent review, Menon et al. (2015) also addressed the question whether the described mechanisms might apply for some women and not for others. They distinguished chlamydial (e.g. serovars), immunological (e.g. innate response, antibody levels) factors in reproductive tissues and additional host factors (e.g. microbiome, hormonal status) and proposed that each of these factors might be associated with an increased risk of pathology development. However, studies often did not include all of these factors together so that further analyses for direct correlations are warranted in predicting the risk for individual females.

3 Multiple Infections

When speaking about multiple infections, we have to discriminate between repeated and recurrent infections. By the term "repeated infection", we refer to women who have two or more *Chlamydia* infections that are completely unrelated to each other or reinfection by having sex with an untreated partner. Detection of the pathogen after a longer episode of negative tests and without apparent risk of reinfection may be referred to as persistent infections and/or treatment failure ("recurrent infection"). Not all studies distinguish as clearly or have conducted tests in between two infection episodes to prove intercurrent chlamydial negativity. Possibly, one could think these repeated cases could be avoided more easily as the tested women usually had medical counselling during their first infection episode and thus are more attentive towards the disease. Therefore, questions that are being addressed in this paragraph are the frequency of occurrence of repeated infections, risk factors and whether several infection episodes have more severe consequences than a single incidental one.

3.1 Is Reinfection a Common Problem?

In a review from 2009, Hosenfeld et al. stated the overall median proportion of reinfections to be 13.9 % with maximum rates of 19.0–20.0 % at 8 or 10 months after the previous episode (Hosenfeld et al. 2009). Similar studies mention rates between 12.9 and 19.4 % (Xu et al. 2011), 20.3 % (Walker et al. 2012) or even 25.5 % (Aghaizu et al. 2014). These studies have to be interpreted carefully as they do not provide further characterization of the reinfection episode. In contrast, Batteiger et al. (2010) performed OmpA genotyping and discriminated between definite reinfections (negative tests in between or different OmpA genotype), probable reinfections (unprotected sex) and treatment failure. Within the group with more than 2 episodes, they classified more than 84 % of the *C. trachomatis* infections as definite or probably reinfections and not due to antimicrobial treatment failure. However, comparisons between different studies are often difficult to perform because of differences in the study design, the follow-up periods, applied examination methods and the investigated population.

3.2 Are Women More Susceptible to C. trachomatis *upon Reinfection?*

Considering these high rates of repeated infections, it seems only plausible that women who were once subjected to chlamydial infection are predestined for a second infection episode. Interestingly, additional infection episodes do not seem to proceed like the first one. In their study in Australian women, Walker et al. (2012) found the bacterial load to be significantly lower in the second infection episode when compared to the first one. These results are consistent with a characterization of protective immunity in murine models (Morrison and Caldwell 2002), showing immunity in over 60 % of the mice after resolved chlamydial infection and decreased EB shedding in recurring infections. These findings could be translated to the human in vivo situation, where the risk for reinfection was calculated to be 4 times higher in women who had an infection that did not spontaneously resolve and had to be treated compared to women with an infection resolving on its own (Geisler et al. 2013). However, it is interesting to note that this did not happen in all women (in this study in 22 % of the cases), and there is also not much known about the involved immune pathways. Independently, they could name risk factors for reinfection such as being aged <25 years. Also frequent change of partners and incomplete partner treatment are stated as risk factors (Scott Lamontagne et al. 2007), surprisingly just like the combination of treated partners and reliable use of condoms. In general, risk factors for single and repeated infections seem to be similar.

3.3 *What Is the Risk for TFI After Chlamydial Infection and Is It Increased by Multiple Infections?*

Several studies have tried to determine the risk for developing tubal factor infertility in *Chlamydia*-positive women, regardless of number or length of infection. In women tested culture-positive in screening programmes, van Valkengoed et al. (2004) calculated the risk for developing PID to be 0.43 % and for TFI to be 0.02 %. Land et al. estimated a risk between 0.1 and 6 % for developing TFI. If serum antibody testing was included, a risk of up to 4.6 % was calculated (van Valkengoed et al. 2004; Land et al. 2010). Also more recent studies presume risks in the same range, 0.9–1.4 % for TFI after past or current chlamydial infection tested by culture or urine sampling. Additionally, these numbers are relatively consistent over all age groups between 16 and 44 years (Kavanagh et al. 2013). Previous studies suggested higher numbers (10 % according to Marrazzo et al. 1997, 20% according to Paavonen et al. 1998). However, these studies should be interpreted carefully as they vary in study design and diagnostic methods or omit risk assessment for a *Chlamydia*-negative control group and coinfections with pathogens such as *N. gonorrhoea* (Wallace et al. 2008). The Uppsala cohort study, one of the most extensive studies so far, correlates chlamydia (culture) test status with infertility (Low et al. 2006). Their results confirm risk numbers from aforementioned studies, but they show a stronger correlation between the risk for sequelae and lower education level than between the risk for sequelae and chlamydia test status.

Still, none of these studies give attention to reinfection compared to single infections. A retrospective cohort study that was conducted with 11,000 women from Wisconsin/USA could show an augmented risk for chlamydial sequelae after ≥2 infection episodes confirmed by either culture or serology. According to this study, the increase in the risk for ectopic pregnancy (EP) was 2.1 and 4.5 for women with 2 and ≥3 infections, respectively. For hospitalization due to PID, the risk increased to 4.0 and 6.5 for women with 2 and ≥3 infections, respectively (Hillis et al. 1997). A similar study design was performed, and similar results were obtained by Bakken et al. (2007) who stated the risk for EP to be twice as high after ≥2 chlamydial infections. The main problem when trying to elucidate these questions further is that any study design would be considered unethical, since treatment for chlamydial infection is strongly recommended and developing sequelae after long-term infection should be avoided. Murine models can exemplify reinfections to only a certain limit, since mice develop partial or complete immunity after a first infection has ceased. Nevertheless, factors such as organism load, duration of the following infections and altered immune response should generally be considered surrogates, in animals and humans likewise. Interestingly, a recent study showed that repeated, abbreviated infection with either wild-type or attenuated plasmid strains of *C. muridarum* could not prevent reinfection of the mice but interrupted the development of pathology (Riley et al. 2012). The study found a significant decrease in inflammatory leucocyte infiltration and an augmented T cell response during the second infection. Studies exploring this particular question in humans could not reproduce the results. However, a correlation between an increased number of infection episodes and an increased risk for TFI seems to be supported by the currently available studies.

4 Chronic Infections

In addition to the well-studied biphasic life cycle of *Chlamydia,* the concept of a "persistent" state has been established. Chlamydiae that are subjected to persistence-inducing stimuli in vitro appear to be viable but, as can be deduced from reinfection experiments, have lost their infectivity. Furthermore, they show an altered morphology in terms of smaller inclusions with enlarged, aberrant reticulate bodies (aRBs). Both infectivity and morphological appearance can mostly be restored after removal of the inducing stimulus (Wyrick 2010). However, the "persistent infection" in women is still in need of a clear definition. It is commonly associated with prolonged *Chlamydia* positivity, with incompletely cleared and thus recurrent infections or with chronic inflammation. But a direct correlation to the in vitro appearance of aberrant *Chlamydiae* cannot be drawn. Thus, the term "persistence" should be used carefully as it describes not very well-defined entities in vitro and in vivo (Bavoil 2014).

4.1 The Induction of Aberrant RBs In Vitro

As reviewed earlier by Beatty et al. (1994), Hogan et al. (2004) and Wyrick (2010), aberrant RBs are induced by a variety of different stimuli. The following list is not exhaustive, and many questions concerning further inductors or the involved intracellular pathways are still to be investigated. We will focus on those that might be of physiological relevance, either because the respective factors naturally occur in the FGT in physiological concentrations or because we considered them to be of clinical significance.

4.1.1 Iron Depletion

Iron is known to be an essential factor in growth and survival of *C. trachomatis*. In infected cells, transferrin receptor (TfR)-enriched vesicles could be found close to *Chlamydia* vacuoles (Al-Younes et al. 1999), indicating interaction between *Chlamydia* and the host cells' iron metabolism (Vardhan et al. 2009). Already prior to that, Raulston reported that the infectivity of *C. trachomatis* serovar E was greatly reduced in HEC-1B cells treated with the iron chelator deferoxamine (DFO) (Raulston et al. 2007). While chlamydial inclusions appeared smaller, enlarged RBs could be found inside. Similar experiments have been conducted since then by Al-Younes et al. (2001), Dill et al. (2009) and Thompson and Carabeo (2011), who introduced another iron-deficiency model using the membrane-permeable iron chelator 2,2-bipyridyl. Using this model, they could not only show reduced infectivity and the aberrant morphology, but moreover prolonged expression of the early chlamydial gene *euo* and repression of the late gene *omcB*. These effects that are typically found in aberrant Chlamydiae usually showed a regress after the addition of iron, with chlamydial inclusions again producing viable and infectious EBs.

4.1.2 IFN-γ

Interferon gamma is considered to be one of the most important immunological mediators causing chlamydial growth restriction in epithelial cells. Byrne et al. (1986) could show that IFN-γ induces the cellular enzyme indoleamine-2, 3-dioxygenase (IDO) and thus creates intracellular degradation of the amino acid tryptophan. Thereby, development of *C. trachomatis* is inhibited, as they rely on exogenous tryptophan sources. This happens in a concentration-dependent manner reaching from termination of the infection to the formation of morphological aberrant RBs (Shemer and Sarov 1985). IFN-γ might also act via other mechanisms (Ramsey et al. 2001), but since the addition of indole causes IFN-γ-mediated aRBs of genital serovars (Caldwell et al. 2003) to return to the normal chlamydial developmental cycle, IDO upregulation is considered one of the most important (Beatty et al. 1994).

4.1.3 Antibiotics

Kramer and Gordon (1971) and Johnson and Hobson (1977) both described that penicillin changed chlamydial morphology to large, aberrant RBs with the formation of membranes inside and outside of the RBs. After changing to penicillin-free media, maturation to normal RBs and then to EBs followed (Matsumoto and Manire 1970). Tanami and Yamada (1973) described an unequal cellular division with the formation of miniature RBs in *C. psittaci*, which Phillips et al. (1984) could also detect in *C. muridarum*-infected mouse oviducts in vivo. Only recently, Klöckner et al. (2014) introduced AmiA as a penicillin-sensitive enzyme, which its activity might be crucial for coordinated chlamydial cell division and which moreover could be involved in peptidoglycan degradation. Thus, it could cause the formation of enlarged aRBs and also interfere with the host's immune response.

But not only Penicillin, also other antibacterial substances such as Chlortetracycline (Kramer and Gordon 1971), Erythromycin (Clark et al. 1982), Ciprofloxacin and Ofloxacin (Dreses-Werringloer et al. 2000) induced morphological and functional abnormalities. This was shown for *C. trachomatis* in physiologically relevant concentrations of the aforementioned substances (Kintner et al. 2014) as well as for subinhibitory conditions of many first-line antibiotics for the treatment of chlamydial infections (Gieffers et al. 2004).

4.1.4 Coinfection with Herpes Simplex Virus

Coinfection with HSV1/HSV2 abrogates the production of infectious chlamydial EBs and leads to swollen, aberrant RBs (Deka et al. 2006, 2007). As Vanover et al. (2010) could show later, no productive viral replication was necessary, just interaction of viral particles such as glycoprotein D (gD) with the host cell surface. As supplementation of nutrients or suppression of IDO or the IFN-γ-mediated pathways could not rescue chlamydial infectivity (Vanover et al. 2008), Prusty et al. revealed that chlamydial aRBs were possibly induced via elevated ROS levels. They could show that HSV1-coinfection-induced loss of infectivity could be reverted when ROS scavenging DTT was added to the culture (Prusty et al. 2012). In HSV-coinfection, nectin-1 was established as the necessary coreceptor involved, which suggests that the HSV-gD/nectin-1 interaction triggers an intracellular calcium release. This in turn elevates ROS production. Through this pathway, both the decline of EBs and the altered RB morphology could be explained (Hall et al. 2014).

4.2 *What Would Be the Clinical Relevance, if We Could Translate the In Vitro Findings to the In Vivo Situation?*

If a long-term relationship with the host is established, it may lead to chronic inflammation that can easily cause damage to the reproductive tract. If we hypothesize that aberrant RBs observed in vitro may exhibit similar characteristics within the FGT in vivo, several questions concerning clinical appearance of the infection, diagnosis and treatment have to be considered. When we take into account that iron levels in the FGT fluctuate according to the menstrual cycle (Kelver et al. 1996), the probability of persistent infection increases, depending on the hormonal status at the time the infection takes place. Since this cannot easily be determined in women, we have to revert to animal models to learn more about a possible connection. The same applies to HSV coinfection, as an already existing HSV infection could influence the infection towards persistence. Here, only longitudinal studies following women from puberty on over decades might show a correlation between HSV–*C. trachomatis* coinfections and long-term consequences such as infectious infertility.

Azithromycin as a standard treatment for genital *C. trachomatis* infection showed reduced bactericidal effects when used on penicillin-induced aberrant RBs (Wyrick and Knight 2004). This could be of great clinical importance, as—with regard to our hypothesis—other stimuli could cause a treatment-resistant state and thus decrease the effectiveness of azithromycin. A decrease in natural immunity with its main mediator IFN-γ, however, is possible in patients with bacterial vaginosis (BV). Lewis et al. (2014) found that indole was present in vaginal secretions of women with BV. Thus, reduced efficacy of IFN-γ could subsequently result in a reduced clearance of the pathogen and may drive the formation of aRBs. In combination with studies showing an increased likelihood for women with BV to contract a *C. trachomatis* infection (Yoshimura et al. 2009), this could be of great epidemiological importance.

4.3 What Evidence Do We Have for Finding Persistence In Vivo?

There is evidence that persistent *Chlamydiae* exist in the FGT. In general, when using the term "persistence", we do not refer to chlamydial morphology but to a long-term relationship with the infected host. Clinical evidence for persistence comes from culture-negative women with tubal biopsy specimens testing positive in immunocytochemistry, in situ hybridization or serum antibodies (Patton et al. 1994). Also *Chlamydia*-positive tests in women up to 3 months after azithromycin treatment despite the women denying re-exposition by sexual contact (Golden et al. 2005) could be due to treatment failure or behavioural misreports, just like prolonged PCR positivity in the first weeks after clearing of the infection (Geisler 2015). Still, the possibility of chlamydial persistence should be taken into account. In persisting infections, reactivation would be possible, matching in vitro experiments after drug removal (Kintner et al. 2014). The hypothesis of persisting infections is supported by data from Dean et al. (2000) showing that recurrent infections in women over years were often isolates of the same omp1 genotype, which makes independent, casual reinfections seem unlikely. In addition, they revealed that culture-negative samples in between culture-positive episodes became positive when tested with nucleic acid amplification techniques.

Clinically, the concept of persistent *Chlamydia* infection is easily conceivable. But evidence has yet to be supplied that in vitro experiments showing aRBs truly reflect in vivo conditions. The detection of abnormal RB morphology in human samples after azithromycin treatment failure (Bragina et al. 2001) or in a patient with mucopurulent cervicitis (Lewis et al. 2014) provides further evidence here. The latter study in particular could correlate aRBs in in vivo cytobrush samples with a low IFU number and high IFN-γ levels in vaginal fluids of the same patient, which parallels the aforementioned in vitro studies. Phillips-Campbell et al. (2012) were the first to induce *C. muridarum* aRBs in a mouse model via amoxicillin treatment with strongly reduced vaginal shedding and aRBs visible in TEM. Carey et al. (2013) intranasally vaccinated *C. muridarum*-infected mice and demonstrated that the transcriptome of oviduct specimens mostly overlapped with the transcriptome of penicillin-induced persistence in McCoy cells. They concluded that cellular in vitro and mouse in vivo models match, even though they did not show further proof for persistence in the mouse model. A recent study in female baboons with hormone-based intrauterine contraception devices (IUD) showed a delayed endocervical clearance of *C. trachomatis* infection compared to baboons without IUDs (Liechty et al. 2015). Interestingly, they did not detect alterations in the vaginal microbial communities due to either IUD or *C. trachomatis* infection.

All in all, these morphologically persistent-like *Chlamydiae* that can be found in vivo could indicate a correlation with reports of clinical long-term infection. But if so, what would be the consequences? Would a protracted infection necessarily mean increased damage on the FGT tissue or do other factors such as the patient's immune response, genetic disposition or micro-environmental conditions play a bigger role than the length of the infection? Could chlamydial antigens that persist after clearing of the infection cause similar damage? Since studies in humans with prolonged, untreated infections would be considered unethical, the mouse model or pig models with *C. suis* have to be developed further. Particular attention should be paid to differences in detection, treatment and long-term outcome of persistent infections. For example, one drawback for successful treatment could be a reduced response to antibiotic treatment such as Phillips-Campbell et al. could show in amoxicillin-induced "persistence" of *C. muridarum*. In humans, large-scale studies should be conducted longitudinally with culture, PCR and cytobrush samples taken on a regular basis to not only detect chlamydial infection, but also obtain information concerning morphological aberrance and comparison with in vitro persistence models (Phillips-Campbell et al. 2014).

In vivo studies arguing for the induction of persistent-like chlamydial development by established persistence-inducing stimuli in vitro are shown in Table 1.

Table 1 Selection of references giving evidence for the existence of persistent infections in vivo

Putative persistence-inducing stimulus	Evidence towards in vivo persistence
Iron depletion	– Differences in gene haplotypes that are connected to iron metabolism, e.g. haptoglobin, are associated with varied risk for active ocular trachoma in Gambian children (Savy et al. 2010) – Patient sera samples were found to have high concentrations of antibodies against YtgA, an iron-responsive chlamydial antigen that is apparently induced in iron-limited in vitro cell cultures (Raulston 1997)
IFN-γ	– Apoptosis of epithelial cells is inhibited especially in cells containing IFN-γ-induced aberrant vacuoles in vitro (Perfettini et al. 2002). Also in vivo, IFN-γ-deficient *C. muridarum*-infected mice showed a lot more apoptotic cells compared to wild-type mice, which may contribute to the hypothesis that IFN-γ induces long-term infections by preventing apoptosis of infected cells – In a study that investigated chlamydial growth patterns in infected women, two patients stood out because of remarkably different chlamydial morphology. One patient showed normal EBs and RBs inside the inclusions, whereas the other held abnormally large RBs that displayed unequal binary fission. While both had high genome copy numbers, the first patient had a high IFU count, whereas the latter had a very low IFU count, and, most interestingly, had high levels of IFN-γ found in genital secretions when compared to patient 1. Furthermore, patient 2 showed high RNA levels of *euo*, a gene that is supposed to be involved in chlamydial persistence, whereas patient 1 had higher levels of *omcB*, a gene involved in the differentiation to infective EBs. This is the first description of a *C. trachomatis* infection in vivo that runs completely concordant with in vitro experiments when subjected to IFN-γ treatment (Lewis et al. 2014) – T cell responses and different disease patterns were correlated with IFN-γ levels and spontaneous resolution or TFI development (Picard et al. 2015)
Subinhibitory antibiotic concentrations	– Women with recurrent infections with the same serovars (according to omp1 genotyping) showed culture-negative results between two episodes, but remained positive by NAAT (Dean et al. 2000) – EM pictures were taken from clinical samples of patients who still had positive cell cultures after azithromycin treatment for chlamydial infection. Inside the inclusions, atypical RBs, some of them in the process of dividing, but no EBs, were detected (Bragina et al. 2001) – *C. muridarum*-infected mice were treated with subinhibitory doses of amoxicillin that reduced vaginal shedding by >99 % but not 16s-rRNA levels when compared to untreated mice, indicating a loss of infectivity. TEM analysis of uterine tissue

(continued)

Table 1 (continued)

Putative persistence-inducing stimulus	Evidence towards in vivo persistence
	furthermore showed large, aberrant RBs in amoxicillin-treated mice, which leads to the conclusion that this mouse model excellently represents in vitro experiments with antibiotic-induced persistence in *C. muridarum*-infected mice (Phillips-Campbell et al. 2012) – When mice in the same experimental setup were subsequently treated with azithromycin, treatment failure was increased in the amoxicillin pretreated animals, suggesting that amoxicillin-induced changes to the chlamydial growth render them less susceptible to antichlamydial treatment in vivo (Phillips-Campbell et al. 2014)
Co-infection with HSV-2	– In a *C. muridarum (Cm)*/HSV-2 co-infection model in mice viable *Chlamydiae* were able to induce a transient protection from HSV-2-induced neurologic disease. When mice were superinfected with *Cm* 3 days after infection with HSV-2, chlamydial shedding was significantly lower on day 6, but remained at higher levels compared to single *Cm* infected mice up to day 18 (Slade et al. 2016)

4.4 Is the Induction of Chlamydial Aberrant RBs a Necessary Survival Mechanism or Merely a Stress Response to Unfavourable Circumstances?

It has often been speculated whether the formation of aberrant RBs is an alternative stage in the chlamydial developmental cycle or simply a stress response to unfavourable conditions in the environment. Kahane and Friedman (1992) found that heat shock causes an aberrant morphology, which could also explain HSP (heat-shock protein) 60 upregulation found in aberrant cultures (Morrison et al. 1989). The same was applied for amino acid and glucose deprivation (Harper et al. 2000). With regard to these findings, even the occasional aRB observation in productive infections in vitro (Wolf et al. 2000; Tan et al. 2010) could be due to local nutrient depletion within the cell culture, as Hogan et al. (2004) suspected. However, transcriptome analysis revealed that there is a complete set of genes being up- or downregulated after IFN-γ treatment. These include several stress response genes, but according to Belland et al. (2003), aRBs are subjected to more extensive transcriptome alterations than a simple stress response would cause. Upon removal of the inducing stimulus, *Chlamydia* easily switches back to transcribing genes that support EB production without further after-effects, which also suggests that aberrant RBs are a desired adaptation to hostile conditions that enables the pathogen to survive and even withstand the host immune response. But as aRB morphology and growth characteristics in vitro show great differences depending on the stimulus, it is very well possible that each inductor has parts from both sides, i.e. that the transformation into aRBs is partly a general stress response and partly a stimulus-specific coping mechanism to ensure survival.

4.5 Can a Human Fallopian Tube Cell Model Further Elucidate the Connection Between In Vivo and In Vitro?

Conventional *Chlamydia* infection cell models usually work with immortalized cell lines, the most common one being the HeLa cancer cell line. Since HeLa cells are easy to handle and to infect with *C. trachomatis,* they work as an excellent model for chlamydial infection. Nevertheless, the process of immortalization and the fact that the cells grow segregated from their normal surrounding in the FGT make those cell models a less-than-ideal solution when it comes to translating the findings to the in vivo situation. Isolation and propagation of human fallopian tube cells as firstly described by Levanon et al. (2010) is one possibility to optimize the experimental set-up. In previous studies, this model has been successfully used to study biomarkers for ovarian cancer, genotoxic stress to FT epithelial cells and differences between secretory and ciliated cells in the response to DNA damage (Levanon et al. 2010). A similar model was used for elucidating the impact of ovulation on ovarian carcinogenesis, as the addition of human follicular fluids to FT cells induced precancerous lesions in FT cells (Bahar-Shany et al. 2014). But also whole organ tissue models of human fallopian tubes are suitable for the analyses of host–pathogen interactions on a cellular level, with the limitation that the dynamics of inflammatory cell influx cannot be monitored (Jerchel et al. 2012; Kessler et al. 2012).

Human fallopian tubes and/or FT cells may better reflect the situation in vivo, but several factors have to be considered. Age, hormonal status, comorbidities, history of previous STIs and differences in the vaginal/cervical microbiome are only some of the apparent interindividual changes that may directly have an impact on the experiments. On the other hand, integrating those data in the interpretation of the *C. trachomatis* infection effectivity, intracellular progeny, etc., ex vivo may further guide our efforts in identifying factors that promote or inhibit chlamydial development. Comparing *C. trachomatis* infections between HeLa and FT cells, the infectivity dose needs to be roughly 30 times higher for achieving similar infection rates in the latter, but sometimes infections are not even visible in FT cells using higher doses (data not shown). Another difference is the regulation of the MAP kinase signalling cascades. Whereas phosphorylation of the p44/42 MAPkinase is strongly induced upon infection with *C. trachomatis* in HeLa cells, no significant upregulation is observed in FT cells that already express higher basal levels of the protein.

Gathering data on further differences between HeLa and FT cells with respect to mitochondrial activation, metabolism and immune function will foster our understanding of the control of chlamydial infections in the female genital tract.

5 Chronic Colonization of the Gastrointestinal Tract

It is long known that animals that appear clinically healthy can be chlamydia positive when tissue from intestinal sites is examined. Rank and Yeruva suggested the possibility that *Chlamydiae* are commensals in the gut, just like *E. coli* and other bacteria that have established themselves in the intestinal environment but cause pathogenic reactions when transferred to other sites of the body (Rank and Yeruva 2014). Arguments supporting this would be the complete lack of inflammatory reaction even after long-term infection of >8 months (Igietseme et al. 2001) as well as the low IFU number that is required for oral infection (Yeruva et al. 2013a), making easy passage through the mouth seem quite likely. Possibly, intestinal *Chlamydiae* remain in a chronic, silent state from which opportunistic acute infections can arise.

5.1 How Does Intestinal Colonization Happen and How Often Does It Affect Humans?

As Perry et al. (1999) could show with *C. muridarum*, the bacteria most likely spread from the genital mucosa to the intestinal mucosa, probably by autoinoculation as well as via oral ingestion of faeces. Varying animal studies show similar results for *C. suis* in pigs (Pospischil et al. 2009) or *C. muridarum* in mice (Zhang et al. 2015) as well as in a number of other animals. In studies that tested for rectal involvement during chlamydial infection in humans, a substantial proportion of both women and men were found to be positive. Women in rural South Africa had a genital prevalence of 16 % and a rectal prevalence of 7.1 % while being mainly asymptomatic (Peters et al. 2014). In a study that screened >3,000 female patients at a STI clinic in Canada, rectal chlamydial prevalence was shown to be between 11.7 and 13.5 % (Gratrix et al. 2015), including 133 rectal-only cases. Trebach et al. (2015) tested >10,000 patients from STI clinics and concluded that 13.8 % of extragenital *C. trachomatis* infections would have been missed with urogenital-only testing. Van Liere et al. (2014) on the other hand reported that 94.5 % of all anorectal *Chlamydia* cases also had urogenital infections, and 74.1 % of urogenital infections also showed positive anorectal tests, which implies a high co-occurrence and displayed hardly any rectal-only cases. According to them, sexual behaviour could not be linked to anorectal test results and also *C. trachomatis* strain and anatomical location showed no correlation (Versteeg et al. 2014). In the context of possible persistence in humans, gastrointestinal colonization gains importance, since this could represent a reservoir for Chlamydiae from which genital infections can reappear and thus impede successful treatment.

5.2 What Would Be the Consequences?

There are two major questions whether gastrointestinal (GIT) colonization is relevant in humans, one more theoretical and one more practical in nature. The first one deals with the integration of the colonization concept into previous *Chlamydia* research. Does asymptomatic colonization complement or replace the concept of long-term infection of the FGT? Are the bacteria able to persist, no matter of their location in GIT or FGT? And is the aberrant morphology such as it was found in pigs (Pospischil et al. 2009) equivalent to persisting infection in the GIT as we presume it to be in the FGT?

On the other hand, is it possible that persistence in the FGT does not play a major role at all, and recurring infections can be attributed to chronic GIT infection that has spread anew to the FGT? With the help of direct sequencing of clinical isolates from different sites, one could try to obtain more insights into the in vivo relevance of GI colonization.

The second question addresses the guidelines for screening and therapy, because even if the topic of persistence is set aside, rectal *Chlamydia* positivity raises the question for the need of antibiotic treatment. Eradicating *Chlamydia* from the GIT in mice can prove difficult (Yeruva et al. 2013b) and in humans the impact of antibiotic treatment on the normal gastrointestinal flora could do more harm than it benefits. On the other hand, the possibility of frequent reinfection with the development of TFI as a potential consequence should be prevented. Rectal screening of high-risk women, as Gratrix et al. (2015) proposed, and subsequent higher-frequent urogenital screening if the rectal test is positive, could be a compromise, but cost-effectiveness analyses should be conducted. But also treatment should be reconsidered, since azithromycin shows less potency in GIT infections in mice (Yeruva et al. 2013b). Transferring these studies to humans and calculated with the help of a mathematical model, its effectiveness is reduced to 82 %, while effectiveness of doxycycline is still at 97 % (Craig et al. 2015). In the end, also the possibility of vaccination has to be re-evaluated, if the immune system is not able to effectively clear intestinal *Chlamydia* infection.

6 Conclusions

It is important to understand how *Chlamydia*–host relationships as well as micro-environmental influences shape the course of disease and determine subsequent results such as infertility (Fig. 1). If we can assign women to risk groups for

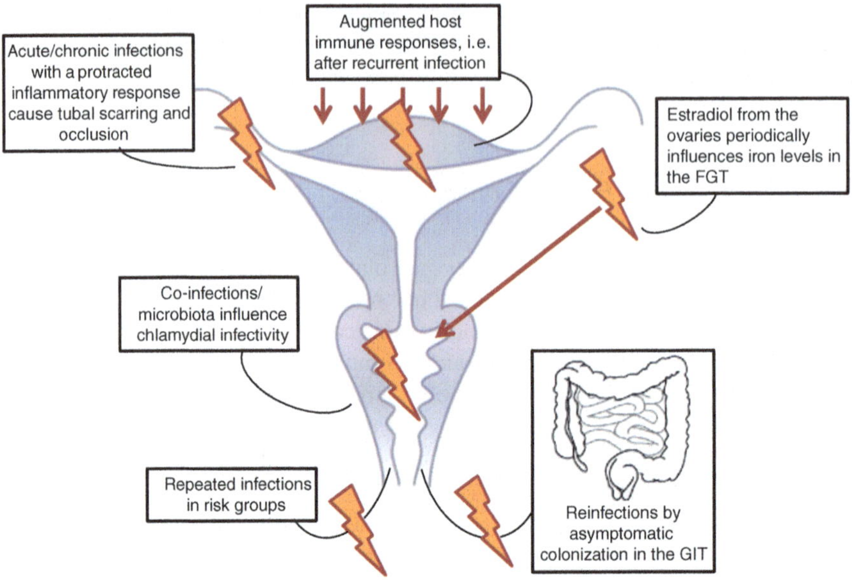

Fig. 1 Mechanisms that may contribute to *C. trachomatis* induced pathology in the female urogenital tract. The authors are grateful to Mathilde Cosse, Paris, for supplying the depiction of the female reproductive tract

reinfection for or long-term infection, or identify women with rectal-positive *Chlamydia* tests, we might be able to give proper attention to those women more individually. Particularly in the current context of personalized medicine, the choice of antibiotic treatment or the frequency of medical check-ups could be adjusted according to individual risk group. Pursuing this way further by implementing more accurate diagnostic algorithms, the progress to infertility or other pathologies could be reduced. Thanks to numerous studies, we have quite a good idea as to how faithfully the different disease models reflect reality, but proof of our prospect is still missing. Therefore, further investigation is necessary, especially in vivo studies as well as carefully verified in vitro models. An extensive longitudinal study with a large number of women would probably be useful, particularly if individuals could be followed from before their first sexual contact and possible *Chlamydia* exposure, to minimize confounding by potential asymptomatic infections that remained unnoticed. Also sensible screening frequencies should be established for each risk group and age group, as well as further research should be conducted into the development of vaccines. This review intends to facilitate understanding of the complex host–pathogen interaction from a novel perspective and aims at instigating further research into the role that this unique pathogen plays in the development of TFI.

References

Aghaizu A, Reid F, Kerry S, Hay PE, Mallinson H, Jensen JS, Kerry S, Kerry S, Oakeshott P (2014) Frequency and risk factors for incident and redetected Chlamydia trachomatis infection in sexually active, young, multi-ethnic women: a community based cohort study. Sex Transm Infect. 90(7):524–528

Al-Younes HM, Rudel T, Meyer TF (1999) Characterization and intracellular trafficking pattern of vacuoles containing Chlamydia pneumoniae in human epithelial cells. Cell Microbiol 1 (3):237–247

Al-Younes HM, Rudel T, Brinkmann V, Szczepek AJ, Meyer TF (2001) Low iron availability modulates the course of *Chlamydia pneumoniae* infection. Cell Microbiol 3(6):427–437

Bahar-Shany K, Brand H, Sapoznik S, Jacob-Hirsch J, Yung Y, Korach J, Perri T, Cohen Y, Hourvitz A, Levanon K (2014) Exposure of fallopian tube epithelium to follicular fluid mimics carcinogenic changes in precursor lesions of serous papillary carcinoma. Gynecol Oncol 132 (2):322–327

Bakken IJ, Skjeldestad FE, Nordbø SA (2007) *Chlamydia trachomatis* infections increase the risk for ectopic pregnancy: a population-based, nested case-control study. Sex Transm Dis 34 (3):166–169

Batteiger BE, Tu W, Ofner S, Van Der Pol B, Stothard DR, Orr DP, Katz BP, Fortenberry JD (2010) Repeated *Chlamydia trachomatis* genital infections in adolescent women. J Infect Dis 201(1):42–51

Bavoil PM (2014) What's in a word: the use, misuse, and abuse of the word "persistence" in Chlamydia biology. Front Cell Infect Microbiol 4:27

Beatty WL, Morrison RP, Byrne GI (1994) Persistent chlamydiae: from cell culture to a paradigm for chlamydial pathogenesis. Microbiol Rev 58(4):686–699

Belland RJ, Nelson DE, Virok D, Crane DD, Hogan D, Sturdevant D, Beatty WL, Caldwell HD (2003) Transcriptome analysis of chlamydial growth during IFN-gamma-mediated persistence and reactivation. Proc Natl Acad Sci USA. 100(26):15971–15976

Bragina EY, Gomberg MA, Dmitriev GA (2001) Electron microscopic evidence of persistent chlamydial infection following treatment. J Eur Acad Dermatol Venereol 15(5):405–409

Byrne GI, Lehmann LK, Landry GJ (1986) Induction of tryptophan catabolism is the mechanism for gamma-interferon-mediated inhibition of intracellular *Chlamydia psittaci* replication in T24 cells. Infect Immun 53(2):347–351

Caldwell HD, Wood H, Crane D et al (2003) Polymorphisms in *Chlamydia trachomatis* tryptophan synthase genes differentiate between genital and ocular isolates. J Clin Invest. 111 (11):1757–1769

Carey AJ, Beagley KW (2010) Chlamydia trachomatis, a hidden epidemic: effects on female reproduction and options for treatment. Am J Reprod Immunol 63(6):576–586

Carey AJ, Huston WM, Cunningham KA, Hafner LM, Timms P, Beagley KW (2013) Characterization of in vitro *Chlamydia muridarum* persistence and utilization in an in vivo mouse model of Chlamydia vaccine. Am J Reprod Immunol 69(5):475–485

Clark RB, Schatzki PF, Dalton HP (1982) Ultrastructural analysis of the effects of erythromycin on the morphology and developmental cycle of *Chlamydia trachomatis* HAR-13. Arch Microbiol 133(4):278–282

Craig AP, Kong FY, Yeruva L, Hocking JS, Rank RG, Wilson DP, Donovan B (2015) Is it time to switch to doxycycline from azithromycin for treating genital chlamydial infections in women? Modelling the impact of autoinoculation from the gastrointestinal tract to the genital tract. BMC Infect Dis 15:200

De Clercq E, Kalmar I, Vanrompay D (2013) Animal models for studying female genital tract infection with *Chlamydia trachomatis*. Infect Immun 81(9):3060–3067

Dean D, Suchland RJ, Stamm WE (2000) Evidence for long-term cervical persistence of *Chlamydia trachomatis* by omp1 genotyping. J Infect Dis 182(3):909–916

Deka S, Vanover J, Dessus-Babus S, Whittimore J, Howett MK, Wyrick PB, Schoborg RV (2006) *Chlamydia trachomatis* enters a viable but non-cultivable (persistent) state within herpes simplex virus type 2 (HSV-2) co-infected host cells. Cell Microbiol 8(1):149–162

Deka S, Vanover J, Sun J, Kintner J, Whittimore J, Schoborg RV (2007) An early event in the herpes simplex virus type-2 replication cycle is sufficient to induce *Chlamydia trachomatis* persistence. Cell Microbiol 9(3):725–737

Dill BD, Dessus-Babus S, Raulston JE (2009) Identification of iron-responsive proteins expressed by *Chlamydia trachomatis* reticulate bodies during intracellular growth. Microbiology 155(Pt 1): 210–219

Dreses-Werringloer U, Padubrin I, Jürgens-Saathoff B, Hudson AP, Zeidler H, Köhler L (2000) Persistence of *Chlamydia trachomatis* is induced by ciprofloxacin and ofloxacin in vitro. Antimicrob Agents Chemother 44(12):3288–3297

Frazer LC, O'Connell CM, Andrews CW Jr, Zurenski MA, Darville T (2011) Enhanced neutrophil longevity and recruitment contribute to the severity of oviduct pathology during *Chlamydia muridarum* infection. Infect Immun 79(10):4029–4041

Geisler WM (2015) Diagnosis and management of uncomplicated *Chlamydia trachomatis* infections in adolescents and adults: summary of evidence reviewed for the 2015 Centers for Disease Control and Prevention Sexually Transmitted Diseases Treatment Guidelines. Clin Infect Dis 61(Suppl 8):S774–S784

Geisler WM, Lensing SY, Press CG, Hook EW 3rd (2013) Spontaneous resolution of genital *Chlamydia trachomatis* infection in women and protection from reinfection. J Infect Dis 207 (12):1850–1856

Geisler WM, Uniyal A, Lee JY, Lensing SY, Johnson S, Perry RC, Kadrnka CM, Kerndt PR (2015) Azithromycin versus doxycycline for urogenital *Chlamydia trachomatis* infection. N Engl J Med 373(26):2512–2521

Gieffers J, Rupp J, Gebert A, Solbach W, Klinger M (2004) First-choice antibiotics at subinhibitory concentrations induce persistence of *Chlamydia pneumoniae*. Antimicrob Agents Chemother 48(4):1402–1405

Golden MR, Whittington WL, Handsfield HH et al (2005) Effect of expedited treatment of sex partners on recurrent or persistent gonorrhea or chlamydial infection. N Engl J Med 352(7): 676–685

Gratrix J, Singh AE, Bergman J, Egan C, Plitt SS, McGinnis J, Bell CA, Drews SJ, Read R (2015) Evidence for increased Chlamydia case finding after the introduction of rectal screening among women attending 2 Canadian sexually transmitted infection clinics. Clin Infect Dis 60(3): 398–404

Hall JV, Sun J, Slade J, Kintner J, Bambino M, Whittimore J, Schoborg RV (2014) Host nectin-1 is required for efficient *Chlamydia trachomatis* serovar E development. Front Cell Infect Microbiol. 4:158

Harper A, Pogson CI, Jones ML, Pearce JH (2000) Chlamydial development is adversely affected by minor changes in amino acid supply, blood plasma amino acid levels, and glucose deprivation. Infect Immun 68(3):1457–1464

Hillis SD, Owens LM, Marchbanks PA, Amsterdam LF, Mac Kenzie WR (1997) Recurrent chlamydial infections increase the risks of hospitalization for ectopic pregnancy and pelvic inflammatory disease. Am J Obstet Gynecol 176(1 Pt 1):103–107

Hogan RJ, Mathews SA, Mukhopadhyay S, Summersgill JT, Timms P (2004) Chlamydial persistence: beyond the biphasic paradigm. Infect Immun 72(4):1843–1855

Hosenfeld CB, Workowski KA, Berman S, Zaidi A, Dyson J, Mosure D, Bolan G, Bauer HM (2009) Repeat infection with Chlamydia and gonorrhea among females: a systematic review of the literature. Sex Transm Dis 36(8):478–489

Igietseme JU, Portis JL, Perry LL (2001) Inflammation and clearance of *Chlamydia trachomatis* in enteric and nonenteric mucosae. Infect Immun 69(3):1832–1840

Jerchel S, Knebel G, König P, Bohlmann MK, Rupp J (2012) A human fallopian tube model for investigation of *C. trachomatis* infections. J Vis Exp 66:4036

Johnson FW, Hobson D (1977) The effect of penicillin on genital strains of *Chlamydia trachomatis* in tissue culture. J Antimicrob Chemother 3(1):49–56

Kahane S, Friedman MG (1992) Reversibility of heat shock in *Chlamydia trachomatis*. FEMS Microbiol Lett 76(1–2):25–30

Kavanagh K, Wallace LA, Robertson C, Wilson P, Scoular A (2013) Estimation of the risk of tubal factor infertility associated with genital chlamydial infection in women: a statistical modelling study. Int J Epidemiol 42(2):493–503

Kelver ME et al. (1996) Estrogen regulation of lactoferrin expression in human endometrium. Am J Reprod Immunol 36(5):243–247

Kessler M, Zielecki J, Thieck O, Mollenkopf HJ, Fotopoulou C, Meyer TF (2012) *Chlamydia trachomatis* disturbs epithelial tissue homeostasis in fallopian tubes via paracrine Wnt signaling. Am J Pathol 180(1):186–198

Kintner J, Lajoie D, Hall J, Whittimore J, Schoborg RV (2014) Commonly prescribed β-lactam antibiotics induce *C. trachomatis* persistence/stress in culture at physiologically relevant concentrations. Front Cell Infect Microbiol 4:44

Klöckner A, Otten C, Derouaux A et al (2014) AmiA is a penicillin target enzyme with dual activity in the intracellular pathogen *Chlamydia pneumoniae*. Nat Commun 5:4201

Kramer MJ, Gordon FB (1971) Ultrastructural analysis of the effects of penicillin and chlortetracycline on the development of a genital tract Chlamydia. Infect Immun 3(2):333–341

Land JA, Van Bergen JE, Morré SA, Postma MJ (2010) Epidemiology of *Chlamydia trachomatis* infection in women and the cost-effectiveness of screening. Hum Reprod Update 16(2): 189–204

Levanon K, Ng V, Piao HY et al (2010) Primary ex vivo cultures of human fallopian tube epithelium as a model for serous ovarian carcinogenesis. Oncogene 29(8):1103–1113

Lewis ME, Belland RJ, AbdelRahman YM et al (2014) Morphologic and molecular evaluation of *Chlamydia trachomatis* growth in human endocervix reveals distinct growth patterns. Front Cell Infect Microbiol. 4:71

Liechty ER, Bergin IL, Bassis CM, Chai D, LeBar W, Young VB, Bell JD (2015) The levonorgestrel-releasing intrauterine system is associated with delayed endocervical clearance of *Chlamydia trachomatis* without alterations in vaginal microbiota. Pathog Dis 73(8):ftv070

Low N, Egger M, Sterne JA, Harbord RM, Ibrahim F, Lindblom B, Herrmann B (2006) Incidence of severe reproductive tract complications associated with diagnosed genital chlamydial infection: the Uppsala Women's Cohort Study. Sex Transm Infect. 2(3):212–218

Macleod J, Salisbury C, Low N et al (2005) Coverage and uptake of systematic postal screening for genital *Chlamydia trachomatis* and prevalence of infection in the United Kingdom general population: cross sectional study. BMJ 330(7497):940

Marks E, Tam MA, Lycke NY (2010) The female lower genital tract is a privileged compartment with IL-10 producing dendritic cells and poor Th1 immunity following *Chlamydia trachomatis* infection. PLoS Pathog 6(11):e1001179

Marrazzo JM, White CL, Krekeler B, Celum CL, Lafferty WE, Stamm WE, Handsfield HH (1997) Community-based urine screening for *Chlamydia trachomatis* with a ligase chain reaction assay. Ann Intern Med 127(9):796–803

Matsumoto A, Manire GP (1970) Electron microscopic observations on the effects of penicillin on the morphology of *Chlamydia psittaci*. J Bacteriol 101(1):278–285

Menon S, Timms P, Allan JA, Alexander K, Rombauts L, Horner P, Keltz M, Hocking J, Huston WM (2015) Human and pathogen factors associated with *Chlamydia trachomatis*-related infertility in women. Clin Microbiol Rev 28(4):969–985

Morrison RP, Caldwell HD (2002) Immunity to murine chlamydial genital infection. Infect Immun 70(6):2741–2751

Morrison RP, Belland RJ, Lyng K, Caldwell HD (1989) Chlamydial disease pathogenesis. The 57-kD chlamydial hypersensitivity antigen is a stress response protein. J Exp Med 170(4): 1271–1283

Newman L, Rowley J, Vander Hoorn S et al (2015) Global estimates of the prevalence and incidence of four curable sexually transmitted infections in 2012 based on systematic review and global reporting. PLoS ONE 10(12):e0143304

Paavonen J, Puolakkainen M, Paukku M, Sintonen H (1998) Cost-benefit analysis of first-void urine *Chlamydia trachomatis* screening program. Obstet Gynecol 92(2):292–298

Patton DL, Askienazy-Elbhar M, Henry-Suchet J, Campbell LA, Cappuccio A, Tannous W, Wang SP, Kuo CC (1994) Detection of *Chlamydia trachomatis* in fallopian tube tissue in women with postinfectious tubal infertility. Am J Obstet Gynecol 171(1):95–101

Perfettini JL, Darville T, Dautry-Varsat A, Rank RG, Ojcius DM (2002) Inhibition of apoptosis by gamma interferon in cells and mice infected with *Chlamydia muridarum* (the mouse pneumonitis strain of *Chlamydia trachomatis*). Infect Immun 70(5):2559–2565

Perry LL, Su H, Feilzer K, Messer R, Hughes S, Whitmire W, Caldwell HD (1999) Differential sensitivity of distinct *Chlamydia trachomatis* isolates to IFN-gamma-mediated inhibition. J Immunol 162(6):3541–3548

Peters RP, Dubbink JH, van der Eem L (2014) Cross-sectional study of genital, rectal, and pharyngeal Chlamydia and gonorrhea in women in rural South Africa. Sex Transm Dis 41(9): 564–569

Phillips Campbell R, Kintner J, Whittimore J, Schoborg RV (2012) Chlamydia muridarum enters a viable but non-infectious state in amoxicillin-treated BALB/c mice. Microbes Infect 14(13): 1177–1185

Phillips DM, Swenson CE, Schachter J (1984) Ultrastructure of *Chlamydia trachomatis* infection of the mouse oviduct. J Ultrastruct Res 3:244–256

Phillips-Campbell R, Kintner J, Schoborg RV (2014) Induction of the Chlamydia muridarum stress/persistence response increases azithromycin treatment failure in a murine model of infection. Antimicrob Agents Chemother 58(3):1782–1784

Picard MD, Bodmer JL, Gierahn TM et al (2015) Resolution of *Chlamydia trachomatis* infection is associated with a distinct T-cell response profile. Clin Vaccine Immunol 22(11):1206–1218

Pospischil A, Borel N, Chowdhury EH, Guscetti F (2009) Aberrant chlamydial developmental forms in the gastrointestinal tract of pigs spontaneously and experimentally infected with *Chlamydia suis*. Vet Microbiol 135(1–2):147–156

Prusty Böhme L, Bergmann B, Siegl C, Krause E, Mehlitz A, Rudel T (2012) Imbalanced oxidative stress causes chlamydial persistence during non-productive human herpes virus co-infection. PLoS ONE 7(10):e47427

Ramsey KH, Miranpuri GS, Sigar IM, Ouellette S, Byrne GI (2001) Chlamydia trachomatis persistence in the female mouse genital tract: inducible nitric oxide synthase and infection outcome. Infect Immun 69(8):5131–5137

Rank RG, Yeruva L (2014) Hidden in plain sight: chlamydial gastrointestinal infection and its relevance to persistence in human genital infection. Infect Immun 82(4):1362–1371

Raulston JE (1997) Response of *Chlamydia trachomatis* serovar E to iron restriction in vitro and evidence for iron-regulated chlamydial proteins. Infect Immun 65(11):4539–4547

Raulston JE, Miller JD, Davis CH, Schell M, Baldwin A, Ferguson K, Lane H (2007) Identification of an iron-responsive protein that is antigenic in patients with *Chlamydia trachomatis* genital infections. FEMS Immunol Med Microbiol 51(3):569–576

Riley MM, Zurenski MA, Frazer LC, O'Connell CM, Andrews CW Jr, Mintus M, Darville T (2012) The recall response induced by genital challenge with *Chlamydia muridarum* protects the oviduct from pathology but not from reinfection. Infect Immun 80(6):2194–2203

Savy M, Hennig BJ, Doherty CP et al (2010) Haptoglobin and sickle cell polymorphisms and risk of active trachoma in Gambian children. PLoS ONE 5(6):e11075

Scott Lamontagne D, Baster K, Emmett L et al (2007) Incidence and reinfection rates of genital chlamydial infection among women aged 16-24 years attending general practice, family planning and genitourinary medicine clinics in England: a prospective cohort study by the Chlamydia Recall Study Advisory Group. Sex Transm Infect. 83(4):292–303

Shemer Y, Sarov I (1985) Inhibition of growth of *Chlamydia trachomatis* by human gamma interferon. Infect Immun 48(2):592–596

Slade J, Hall JV, Kintner J, Schoborg RV (2016) Chlamydial pre-infection protects from subsequent herpes simplex virus-2 challenge in a murine vaginal super-infection model. PLoS ONE 11(1):e0146186

Stephens RS (2003) The cellular paradigm of chlamydial pathogenesis. Trends Microbiol 11(1): 44–51

Tan C, Hsia RC, Shou H, Carrasco JA, Rank RG, Bavoil PM (2010) Variable expression of surface-exposed polymorphic membrane proteins in in vitro-grown *Chlamydia trachomatis*. Cell Microbiol 12(2):174–187

Tanami Y, Yamada Y (1973) Miniature cell formation in *Chlamydia psittaci*. J Bacteriol 114(1):408–412

Thompson CC, Carabeo RA (2011) An optimal method of iron starvation of the obligate intracellular pathogen, *Chlamydia trachomatis*. Front Microbiol 2:20

Torrone E, Papp J, Weinstock H, Centers for Disease Control and Prevention (CDC) (2014) Prevalence of *Chlamydia trachomatis* genital infection among persons aged 14-39 years–United States, 2007-2012. MMWR Morb Mortal Wkly Rep 63(38):834–838

Trebach JD, Chaulk CP, Page KR, Tuddenham S, Ghanem KG (2015) Neisseria gonorrhoeae and *Chlamydia trachomatis* among women reporting extragenital exposures. Sex Transm Dis 42 (5):233–239

van Liere GA, Hoebe CJ, Wolffs PF, Dukers-Muijrers NH (2014) High co-occurrence of anorectal chlamydia with urogenital chlamydia in women visiting an STI clinic revealed by routine universal testing in an observational study; a recommendation towards a better anorectal chlamydia control in women. BMC Infect Dis 14:274

van Valkengoed IG, Morré SA, van den Brule AJ, Meijer CJ, Bouter LM, Boeke AJ (2004) Overestimation of complication rates in evaluations of *Chlamydia trachomatis* screening programmes—implications for cost-effectiveness analyses. Int J Epidemiol 33(2):416–425

Vanover J, Sun J, Deka S, Kintner J, Duffourc MM, Schoborg RV (2008) Herpes simplex virus co-infection-induced *Chlamydia trachomatis* persistence is not mediated by any known persistence inducer or anti-chlamydial pathway. Microbiology 154(Pt 3):971–978

Vanover J, Kintner J, Whittimore J, Schoborg RV (2010) Interaction of herpes simplex virus type 2 (HSV-2) glycoprotein D with the host cell surface is sufficient to induce *Chlamydia trachomatis* persistence. Microbiology 156(Pt 5):1294–1302

Vardhan H, Bhengraj AR, Jha R, Singh Mittal A (2009) *Chlamydia trachomatis* alters iron-regulatory protein-1 binding capacity and modulates cellular iron homeostasis in HeLa-229 cells. J Biomed Biotechnol. 2009:342032

Versteeg B, van Rooijen MS, Schim van der Loeff MF, de Vries HJ, Bruisten SM (2014) No indication for tissue tropism in urogenital and anorectal *Chlamydia trachomatis* infections using high-resolution multilocus sequence typing. BMC Infect Dis 14:464

Walker J, Tabrizi SN, Fairley CK et al (2012) *Chlamydia trachomatis* incidence and re-infection among young women—behavioural and microbiological characteristics. PLoS One 7(5): e37778

Wallace LA, Scoular A, Hart G, Reid M, Wilson P, Goldberg DJ (2008) What is the excess risk of infertility in women after genital chlamydia infection? A systematic review of the evidence. Sex Transm Infect. 84(3):171–175

Wolf K, Fischer E, Hackstadt T (2000) Ultrastructural analysis of developmental events in *Chlamydia pneumoniae*-infected cells. Infect Immun 68(4):2379–2385

Wyrick PB (2000) Intracellular survival by Chlamydia. Cell Microbiol 2(4):275–282

Wyrick PB (2010) *Chlamydia trachomatis* persistence in vitro: an overview. J Infect Dis 201 (Suppl 2):S88–S95

Wyrick PB, Knight ST (2004) Pre-exposure of infected human endometrial epithelial cells to penicillin in vitro renders *Chlamydia trachomatis* refractory to azithromycin. J Antimicrob Chemother 54(1):79–85

Xu F, Stoner BP, Taylor SN, Mena L, Tian LH, Papp J, Hutchins K, Martin DH, Markowitz LE (2011) Use of home-obtained vaginal swabs to facilitate rescreening for *Chlamydia trachomatis* infections: two randomized controlled trials. Obstet Gynecol 118(2 Pt 1):231–239

Yeruva L, Spencer N, Bowlin AK, Wang Y, Rank RG (2013a) Chlamydial infection of the gastrointestinal tract: a reservoir for persistent infection. Pathog Dis 68(3):88–95
Yeruva L, Melnyk S, Spencer N, Bowlin A, Rank RG (2013b) Differential susceptibilities to azithromycin treatment of chlamydial infection in the gastrointestinal tract and cervix. Antimicrob Agents Chemother 57(12):6290–6294
Yoshimura K, Yoshimura M, Kobayashi T, Kubo T, Hachisuga T, Kashimura M (2009) Can bacterial vaginosis help to find sexually transmitted diseases, especially chlamydial cervicitis? Int J STD AIDS 20(2):108–111
Zhang Q, Huang Y, Gong S, Yang Z, Sun X, Schenken R, Zhong G (2015) In vivo and ex vivo imaging reveals a long-lasting chlamydial infection in the mouse gastrointestinal tract following genital tract inoculation. Infect Immun 83(9):3568–3577

Immunopathogenesis of Chlamydial Infections

Ashlesh K. Murthy, Weidang Li and Kyle H. Ramsey

Abstract Chlamydial infections lead to a number of clinically relevant diseases and induce significant morbidity in human populations. It is generally understood that certain components of the host immune response to infection also mediate such disease pathologies. A clear understanding of pathogenic mechanisms will enable us to devise better preventive and/or intervention strategies to mitigate the morbidity caused by these infections. Over the years, numerous studies have been conducted to explore the immunopathogenic mechanisms of *Chlamydia*-induced diseases of the eye, reproductive tract, respiratory tract, and cardiovascular systems. In this article, we provide an overview of the diseases caused by *Chlamydia*, animal models used to study disease pathology, and a historical context to the efforts to understand chlamydial pathogenesis. Furthermore, we discuss recent findings regarding pathogenesis, with an emphasis on the role of the adaptive immune response in the development of chlamydial disease sequelae. Finally, we summarize the key insights obtained from studies of chlamydial pathogenesis and avenues that remain to be explored in order to inform the next steps of vaccine development against chlamydial infections.

Ashlesh K. Murthy and Weidang Li—Contributed equally.

A.K. Murthy (✉) · W. Li
Department of Pathology, Midwestern University, 555, 31st Steet, Downers Grove, IL 60515, USA
e-mail: amurth@midwestern.edu

K.H. Ramsey
Department of Microbiology and Immunology, Midwestern University, Downers Grove, IL 60515, USA

Current Topics in Microbiology and Immunology (2018) 412:183–216
DOI 10.1007/82_2016_18

Published Online: 02 July 2016

Contents

1 Introduction

The genus *Chlamydia* consists of various species of *chlamydiae* that are obligate intracellular pathogens and infect humans with a tropism for the epithelial linings of conjunctiva, respiratory tract, and genitourinary tract. The initial infection is typically resolved subsequent to the induction of a robust adaptive immune response, but such immunity only offers partial protection against reinfection (Batteiger et al. 2010). The majority of chlamydial infections tend to be initially asymptomatic and therefore go untreated (Brunham and Rey-Ladino 2005). When the initial infection is symptomatic and identified based on the detection of chlamydial organisms and acute inflammation, treatment with antimicrobial agents is usually efficacious in resolving the infection and inflammation (Geisler 2010). However, most infections caused by *Chlamydia* linger for weeks to months in humans, and the chronic low-grade inflammation during this period gives rise to fibrosis and scarring (Paavonen et al. 2008). Another factor contributing to pathology is the high prevalence of repeat infections with the same or different serovars of *Chlamydia* (Bebear and Barbeyrac 2009). Chronic inflammation can occur at the sites of initial infection such as the conjunctiva, respiratory epithelium, and genitourinary epithelium, or at distant sites such as vascular endothelium and synovial membranes (Stephens 2003). Such chronic inflammation leads to clinically important disease sequelae, remnants of the infection which last beyond the clearance of the pathogen, and affects a small subset of all infected people (Oakeshott et al. 2010). These sequelae at the sites of infection may be in the form of blinding trachoma, exacerbation of asthma, pelvic inflammatory disease and infertility in women, and at distant sites in the form of reactive arthritis and exacerbation of atherosclerosis (Stephens 2003; Campbell and Rosenfeld 2015). There is a wide variety of sequelae caused by infection with different species of *Chlamydia,* and these have been investigated using a correspondingly diverse set of conditions and animal models. The vast majority of insights come from studies of trachoma and female reproductive tract disease, and relatively few come from studies of atherosclerosis, asthma, and arthritis. Recently, issues related to immunopathogenesis of trachoma (Taylor et al. 2014; Derrick et al. 2015) and genital tract infections (O'Meara et al. 2014a) have been comprehensively reviewed. We will draw upon literature from multiple *Chlamydia* disease models and discuss the role of immune responses in pathogenesis of *Chlamydia*-induced disease.

2 Diseases Caused by *Chlamydia* in Humans

Infection of *Chlamydia trachomatis* serotypes A to C causes chronic inflammation of the conjunctiva or active trachoma, which is still endemic in many of the poorest or remote countries including Africa, Asia, Australia, and the Middle East (Taylor et al. 2014). The World Health Organization (WHO) classes 53 countries as endemic for blinding trachoma, which is responsible for the visual impairment of about 2.2 million people, including irreversible blindness in 1.2 million people. There are a number of classification systems for the clinical signs of trachoma. Under the WHO-simplified grading system, the presence of five or more follicles on the conjunctival surface of a single eye is classified as trachomatous inflammation follicular (TF). Repeated *C. trachomatis* infection in endemic communities can trigger chronic conjunctival inflammation (trachomatous inflammation intense, TI) in some individuals, causing conjunctival fibrosis (trachomatous scarring, TS). Progressive fibrosis may lead to entropion, inward turning of the lid, or misdirected lashes (trachomatous trichiasis, TT), all of which abrade the corneal surface. This abrasive damage may lead to corneal opacity (CO) and blindness. Not all cases of active trachoma develop conjunctival scarring; the key to trachoma is that repeated episodes of reinfection and inflammation lead to the blinding complications. In this regard, there is accumulating evidence of the importance of lymphoid follicles as local stores of protective T lymphocytes within a mucosal site (Leslie 2016; Mueller and Mackay 2016), and therefore, it is arguable that lymphoid follicles are pathological in context of trachoma.

C. trachomatis serotype D to K infects the endocervical epithelia of women and the urethral epithelia in both sexes and is the leading cause of bacteria sexually transmitted infections in humans (Stamm and Batteiger 2010). In 2014, more than 1.4 million cases of *Chlamydia* were reported to Centers for Disease Control USA, but an estimated 2.86 million infections occur annually (Centers for Disease Control and Prevention 2014). Each year, there are estimated 357 million new infections with 1 of 4 STIs: *Chlamydia* (131 million), gonorrhea (78 million), syphilis (5.6 million), and trichomoniasis (143 million). The infection rate of *Chlamydia* has been increasing steadily. Individuals with genital *Chlamydia* infection often do not exhibit any symptom (75–90 % of woman; 30–50 % of men); however, they still can transmit infection (Stamm and Holmes 1990). Among untreated women, 20–40 % have involvement of fallopian tubes and pelvic inflammatory disease (PID) (WHO 2006). They also may develop severe sequelae, such as ectopic pregnancy and infertility (Westrom and Mardh 1990; Moore and Cates 1990; Wolner-Hanssen et al. 1990). Neonatal infection also can occur during childbirth. C. *trachomatis* infections in neonates cause conjunctivitis and pneumonitis (Stamm and Batteiger 2010). Chlamydial pneumonitis may have long-lasting effects on respiratory function that last into adulthood and may exacerbate asthma (Hansbro et al. 2004).

Among men with chlamydial urogenital infection, at least 50 % are asymptomatic. Chlamydial urethritis is the primary presentation for men. When left untreated, it can lead to complications such as epididymitis and prostatitis, but neither has been typically associated with long-term sequelae (Berger 1990). It is interesting to note that there are scant reports of prior chlamydial infection resulting in male factor infertility (Adams et al. 2004; Chen and Donovan 2003).

The more invasive serovars L1, L2, L2a, or L3 of *C. trachomatis* primarily infect lymphatics and lymph nodes of human and cause lymphogranuloma vernereum (LGV) (Stoner and Cohen 2015). The agent gains entrance through breaks in the skin, or crosses the epithelial cell layer of mucous membranes. LGV is endemic in Africa, Asia, Europe, South America, and the Caribbean, with men affected more commonly than women. As is common to chlamydial infections, chronic LGV causes potentially severe infections with possibly irreversible sequelae (e.g., lymphatic scarring, edema, genital elephantiasis) if adequate treatment is not begun promptly.

Chlamydophila pneumoniae mostly causes upper respiratory tract infections but is also a cause of community-acquired pneumonia (Grayston et al. 1993, 1986). It is very common throughout the world, and it easily spreads in groups of people by inhaling aerosols containing bacteria. It is estimated that about 70 % of *C. pneumoniae* respiratory tract infections are asymptomatic or with minimal symptoms. About 20 % of infected patient are symptomatic upper respiratory tract infections, and the remaining 10 % are pneumonia cases (Choroszy-Krol et al. 2014). As with nearly all chlamydial agents, *C. pneumoniae* also has the ability to induce a chronic inflammatory response. In the respiratory tree, this response has been associated with chronic obstructive pulmonary disease (COPD) and asthma (Hansbro et al. 2004; von Hertzen et al. 1997; Hahn et al. 1991).

Forty to seventy percent of population has been found to have the presence of specific antibodies against *C. pneumoniae,* and a higher incidence of antibodies to *C. pneumoniae* has observed in patients with ischemic heart disease, prior myocardial infarction, and atherosclerosis (Player et al. 2014; Sakurai-Komada et al. 2014; Deniset et al. 2010). Interestingly, the organism can be detected in fatty streaks and atherosclerotic plaques, but not in normal vessels (Campbell and Kuo 2002; Campbell et al. 1992; Erkkila et al. 2002). Whereas an association between *C. pneumoniae* and exacerbation of atherosclerosis has clearly been documented based on multiple lines of evidence in human studies (Campbell and Rosenfeld 2015; Player et al. 2014; Honarmand 2013), a cause-and-effect relationship has yet to be conclusively determined. Two large antibiotic treatment trials failed to reduce the risk of secondary coronary events (Honarmand 2013; Campbell and Rosenfeld 2014), but a lead investigator of at least one of those trials, and others, has been careful to point out that the studies did not exclude a role for *C. pneumoniae* in atherosclerosis initiation or progression (Grayston et al. 2015). However, in rabbits or mice fed a hyperlipidemic diet, exacerbation of atherosclerosis can clearly be induced following intravascular or intranasal *C. pneumoniae* infection, respectively (Muhlestein 2000; Saikku et al. 1998). In summary, a definitive role for *C. pneumoniae* in atherosclerosis initiation or progression is worthy of further exploration. If eventually confirmed, this will no doubt add to the growing list of chronic inflammatory and scarring diseases, of chlamydial etiology.

In summary, there are a few common features of chlamydial infections and disease development:

1. Chlamydial infections tend to affect large numbers of individuals globally.
2. Most of such infections are asymptomatic and go untreated.
3. When symptomatic, the acute infection causes inflammation, and at this stage, majority of infections can be identified and treated efficaciously.
4. When the infection remains untreated or with repeated infection episodes, fibrotic scarring and disease sequelae such as blinding trachoma, infertility, and cardiovascular disease ensue in a subset of individuals.

Our review will focus primarily around the last point, and in this context, we will use the terms "pathology," "pathogenesis," and "disease" to mean the chronic disease sequelae, not the inflammatory response that accompanies acute infections, although the acute inflammation may culminate in the disease sequelae. Most human chlamydial studies have provided only correlative evidence, as it is understandably difficult to design prospective studies to study chlamydial disease sequelae when treatments are readily available to eradicate known acute infections. Therefore, a variety of animal models have been used to study chlamydial disease development and obtain definitive and mechanistic data. Each model reflects some aspect(s) of human disease, but no model completely mirrors the human infection and disease development.

3 Animal Models of Chlamydial Pathogenesis

Trachoma Models of trachoma have been developed in non-human primates (NHP; pig-tailed macaque, rhesus, cynomolgus, and owl monkey) using *C. trachomatis* serovars A, B, or clinical isolates and in guinea pigs using *Chlamydia caviae* (guinea pig inclusion conjunctivitis agent or GPIC) (Taylor 1985; Rank and Whittum-Hudson 1994; Howard et al. 1976). These ocular models in NHP can appropriately mimic the acute aspects of human trachoma infection and ensure that infection exposure and disease are not related to reinfection (Taylor et al. 1981, 1982). In the cynomolgus model, the primary ocular infection leads to an acute, self-limiting conjunctivitis with complete resolution within 10–14 weeks. Monkeys display high levels of bacterial shedding in the initial 4–5 weeks after inoculation, whereas later time periods (6–10 weeks) are characterized by fluctuating periods of culture positivity and negativity. However, the follicular and inflammatory clinical signs remain during this period of low infectious burden. Rechallenged monkeys can show significantly less chlamydial shedding for a much shorter duration and display attenuated clinical signs (Taylor et al. 1984). Resistance to reinfection suggests that monkeys acquire partial immune protection following the primary infection. Similar results have been obtained from the owl monkeys, as well as human volunteers (Mabey et al. 2014), or using the GPIC agent in guinea pigs (Howard et al. 1976; Rank and Barron 1987).

Although scarring per se has not been modeled, the chronic inflammation similar to that leading to scarring in human trachoma can be induced in monkey models using repeated exposure to live *Chlamydia* infection (Taylor et al. 1982). In the cynomolgus monkey model (Taylor et al. 1981), *C. trachomatis* can be detected within one week of a challenge inoculation as also seen after primary inoculation. Even with continuation of weekly inoculations, *C. trachomatis* cannot be identified after a period of time depending on the sensitivity of the test. However, the follicular and inflammatory response persists for as long as inoculations are continued and takes nearly 3 months to resolve once inoculation is stopped. These observations are highly consistent with human trachoma disease. Both have a period in which clinical signs persist and *C. trachomatis* cannot be detected.

Genital tract Chlamydia Infection Several animal models have been used to model *C. trachomatis* genital tract infections in humans, including mouse, guinea pig, pig, non-human primate, rabbit, and sheep (Rank 1994).

The mouse is still the most commonly used animal in studies of *Chlamydia* genital infection because of several considerations: the ease of handling, small size, relatively low cost, the availability of many defined genetically modified mouse strains, and a plethora of mouse-specific reagents (O'Meara et al. 2014a). More importantly, and as we shall see, the mouse model mimics many aspects of *C. trachomatis* infection in women.

There are two established mouse models: the *C. trachomatis* mouse model and the *C. muridarum* mouse model. Infection in both models is enhanced by pretreatment mice with long-acting progestins such as medroxyprogesterone acetate (P4), which halts the otherwise rapid estrus cycle and enriches the number of target epithelium cells and thus enhances initial infection (Brunham and Rey-Ladino 2005; Morrison and Caldwell 2002). In the absence of P4 pretreatment, infection is erratic and inconsistent with *C. muridarum.* Without P4 pretreatment, mice are highly resistant to *C. trachomatis* infection.

Chlamydial infection in mice mimics that in humans in many ways. For example, mice can be genitally infected via intravaginal inoculation with either *C. muridarum* or most human *C. trachomatis* serovars. Intravaginal inoculation with *C. trachomatis* typically produces a mild genital tract infection that resolves relatively quickly and is not able to ascend to the upper genital tract with high frequency. Higher doses of infectious EB are required to establish infection with

C. trachomatis than with *C. muridarum,* but the bacteria shedding from the genital tract are much lower compared to *C. muridarum* infection. There is also less upper genital tract pathology and minimal complications after vaginal *C. trachomatis* inoculation (O'Meara et al. 2014a). However, if high doses of EB are inoculated directly into the mouse uterus, uterine horns, or ovarian bursa, *C. trachomatis* infection can cause severe upper genital sequelae, such as hydrosalpinx and infertility, which is also dependent on the mouse strain (Tuffrey et al. 1986). It should also be noted that careful *C. trachomatis* strain selection can yield an infection that routinely ascends into the upper genital tract to induce chronic inflammatory processes (Sturdevant et al. 2010). Whether these inflammatory changes are permanent (yielding infertility for example) or reversible has not yet been determined. Clearly, this could become an interesting new twist on the mouse model.

C. muridarum, a natural pathogen of the mouse, was originally isolated from the lung of mice (Barron et al. 1981). While it has never been isolated from any animal but laboratory mice and hamsters (Zhang et al. 1993), there is evidence of rodent chlamydial infection in nature (Ramsey et al. 2016). Intravaginal inoculation with *C. muridarum* resembles an acute genital *C. trachomatis* infection in women. The primary infected cell is the cervical epithelium, but under the influence of P4, the vaginal epithelium can also be infected (O'Meara et al. 2014a). The infection ascends quickly to the upper genital tract (uterine horns by day 4–7 and oviducts by 10–14). The infection resolves within 30 days in most, and this is frequently followed by the development of hydrosalpinx, fibrosis, and infertility, 30–90 days post-infection, which in at least some ways mirrors common sequelae in woman after infection. The observation that mice pretreated with P4 and infected with *C. muridarum* develop disease sequelae after primary infection is a significant difference from the development of such sequelae in women. Women rarely develop these sequelae after a single primary infection but most often after repeated episodes of natural infection (Darville and Hiltke 2010). That said, the pathology in mice worsens with repeated infections similar to that in natural genital chlamydial infections in humans (Igietseme et al. 2009; Murthy et al. 2011a). Due to these reasons, the mouse model of *C. muridarum* infection lends itself well for the studies of chlamydial disease development in the genital tract. Using many well-defined inbred and knockout mouse models, the role of immune cells, cytokines, and pathology after *Chlamydia* infection is fully studied. Many of the insights into innate and adaptive immunity against chlamydial infection have resulted from mouse model of *C. muridarum* infection and have, in some cases, guided or corroborated similar assessments and corollaries in humans (O'Meara et al. 2014a).

Another model for chlamydial genital infections is the guinea pig infected with the *Chlamydia caviae* GPIC. This guinea pig genital tract infection closely resembles a genital infection with *C. trachomatis* in human, and it also frequently develops the pathology in the endometrium and oviduct (Rank et al. 1982). An important advantage of this model includes the ability to study chlamydial sexual transmission (Rank et al. 2003). Additionally, the guinea pig is a good model for hormonal research and its influence on chlamydial infection since humans and guinea pigs have comparable estrous cycles (19 days in guinea pigs), as opposed to the much shorter 4–5 day cycling in mice. Immunity to reinfection that occurs in the guineas is short lasting, which is also analogous to humans. Therefore, this model may be suitable to evaluate potential vaccine candidates. Unfortunately, studying immune responses in detail represents a greater challenge in this model where few genetic knockout or transgenic strains exist and immunological reagents are limited.

The pig as a large animal model has also been used for chlamydial research. They are not only physiologically and genetically more closely related to humans, but also the immune system between pigs and human is more similar than between mice and humans. Pigs are naturally infected with *Chlamydophila abortus* and *Chlamydia suis,* but *Chlamydophila psittaci, Chlamydophila pecorum,* and *C. trachomatis* are also able to infect pigs. The pig model has been used successfully to investigate recombinant protein-based and DNA-based vaccine candidates (Harkinezhad et al. 2009; Schautteet et al. 2012). However, the natural pathogen of pigs *C. suis* does not induce tubal infertility and PID. Therefore, the pig model may be more appropriate for investigating putative vaccine candidates and less so for studies of human urogenital pathology. Additionally, pigs are more expensive and complicated than using rodents in the laboratory.

Several non-human primates have been used as potential models to study genital C. *trachomatis* infections, including the marmoset, grivet and baboon, and pigtailed macaque. The pigtailed macaque model was initially developed by Patton and colleagues; it has been the most frequently used primate model for genital *Chlamydia* research (Ripa et al. 1979; Bell et al. 2011; De et al. 2013). *C. trachomatis* can naturally infect this macaque species without hormonal pretreatment, and the infected macaques develop cervicitis and salpingitis, which are highly similar to genital tract inflammation in humans. Repeated infection of macaques leads to cause extensive tubal scaring, chronic salpingitis, and distal tubal obstruction, like the development of PID in women and what is seen in the *C. muridarum* mouse model. Therefore, this model is ideal to study the histopathology and immunopathology of *C. trachomatis*-induced salpingitis. Certainly, macaques are also very good model for vaccine and immune response studies. However, the high-cost, limited resources, the need for extensive adequate facilities, and rarely available expertise limit their use.

Pneumonia and chronic disease: The mouse, rat, hamster, rabbit, and monkey have been used to study *C. pneumoniae* infection (including lung infection), *C. pneumoniae*-induced atherosclerosis, and cardiovascular infection (Campbell and Kuo 2002; Saikku et al. 1998). Recently, *C. pneumoniae* has been identified as a zoonotic pathogen, and it can infect a wide range of host species, such as the koala, frogs, and reptiles (Roulis et al. 2013; Waugh et al. 2015). The mouse model is used extensively in the investigation of a possible causal link between respiratory *Chlamydia pneumoniae* infection and asthma, COPD, and atherosclerosis and for the evaluation of immunopathogenic mechanisms (Campbell et al. 2005a; Campbell and Kuo 1999; Chen et al. 2010a; Zafiratos et al. 2015). It also has been used to screen vaccine candidates (Waugh et al. 2015).

***C. muridarum* infections in mice**: At this juncture, it is pertinent to make a special mention of the *C. muridarum* model of chlamydial infection. Significant advances have been made in our understanding of protective immunity and pathogenesis using this mouse model. *C. muridarum* infects the columnar epithelial cells in the genital tracts of female and male mice, and lower tract infection closely mimics acute genital tract infection in men and women (O'Meara et al. 2014a). *C. muridarum* also infects respiratory tract and causes pharyngitis, bronchitis, and pneumonitis in mice (Barron et al. 1981). Therefore, this mouse chlamydial pathogen has been used as a model organism for the study of human *C. trachomatis* urogenital and respiratory tract infections. Following intravaginal infection, the infected mice shed high numbers of bacteria from the vagina during the first week and progressively clear the infection by a month after challenge. Beginning as soon as 28 days and up to 50 days after inoculation, mice begin to display sequelae in the upper genital tract and develop hydrosalpinx (fluid-filled oviducts). A significant number of female mice are rendered infertile by one or more infections of *C. muridarum,* and hydrosalpinx has been used as a surrogate marker of infertility (O'Meara et al. 2014a). There is strong correlation between scarred oviducts and the formation of hydrosalpinx (Shah et al. 2005). Although some strains of mice are more resistant to hydrosalpinx than others (Chen et al. 2014), the overall finding of hydrosalpinx in women is not thought to be as common in women as in mice. Although the basis for this difference is not completely understood, the use of P4 in the mouse model may offer a partial explanation. P4 is often used in the mouse model to make the female mice more susceptible to infection and pathology; mice infected without this treatment display considerable variation in infectivity and shedding patterns (Vasilevsky et al. 2014). Conversely, women in general have lower frequency of hydrosalpinx, but those who use P4 have higher incidence of infection and PID (Darville and Hiltke 2010). Additionally, following the identification of different downstream mechanisms of IFN-γ mediated clearance of *C. trachomatis* and *C. muridarum* in their respective natural hosts (Nelson et al. 2005), there has been cautious uncertainty of the relevance of data acquired using this model to human infections. Despite these differences, in the sections below, we will discuss how the bulk of available evidence suggests that mechanistic findings made using the *C. muridarum* mouse model have largely been supported by correlative evidence from human studies and other animal models, dispelling undue fears about the usage of this model.

4 Chlamydial Immunopathogenesis

A number of host and pathogen factors appear to determine the disease outcomes following chlamydial infections, and these have been discussed in context of trachoma, infertility, and atherosclerosis in detail in recent review articles (Campbell and Rosenfeld 2015; Taylor et al. 2014; Derrick et al. 2015; O'Meara et al. 2014a; Menon et al. 2015; Sessa et al. 2014). We will focus our discussion to emphasize the literature pertaining to the role of adaptive immunity in immunopathogenesis of chlamydial infections.

A discussion regarding immunopathogenesis of chlamydial infections has centered around two hypotheses: the "immunological hypothesis" implicating adaptive immune cells in causing pathology (Brunham and Rey-Ladino 2005) and the "cellular hypothesis" implicating the infected cell as a key inducer and regulator of pathology (Stephens 2003). The historical perspective on how the immunological and cellular hypothesis was proposed was elegantly discussed in 2003 by Stephens (2003), the original proponent of the cellular hypothesis. To lay a platform for our discussion, we briefly restate that historical perspective here.

The immunological paradigm of chlamydial pathogenesis was initially proposed based on several observations. Scarring trachoma occurs only after repeated episodes of infection, and in trachoma vaccine trials in monkeys, reinfection often produced more severe clinical disease (Mabey et al. 2014). Since repeat infection can occur with the same or different serovars, adaptive immune response to a chlamydial antigen shared between different serovars of *Chlamydia* was considered an important player in pathogenesis (Grayston et al. 1985). T lymphocytes were implicated because guinea pigs which had resolved an infection demonstrated delayed-type hypersensitivity (DTH) reaction following either a challenge with high dose of chlamydial organisms or with a triton X-100 extract, not with the triton X-100 buffer alone (Watkins et al. 1986). Subsequent experiments in cynomoglus monkeys supported that DTH could be induced in the eyes of previously infected, not naïve, monkeys with the triton X-100 extract (Taylor et al. 1987). The triton X-100 buffer itself induced inflammation after 3 days of instillation leading to the speculation whether the disease was induced by the buffer itself. However, inflammation was observed as early as 24 h after instillation of chlamydial extract, not buffer, and the lack of similar responses to buffer or extract in naïve monkeys suggested that a chlamydial component was involved (Taylor et al. 1987). Additionally, these studies suggested that the pathogenic chlamydial component was not expressed on the chlamydial surface and was not LPS, but probably a subsurface component of *Chlamydia*. Subsequent studies indicated that the potential offender could be a soluble 57,000 m.w protein (Morrison et al. 1989a), which later was concluded to be the chlamydial heat-shock protein 60 (Hsp60) based on its ease of extraction by detergents (Bavoil et al. 1990; Morrison et al. 1989b). A subsequent study used cloned chlamydial Hsp60 to subcutaneously prime guinea pigs and subjected those animals to ocular challenge with GPIC, but did not find enhancements in disease severity (Rank et al. 1995). This further raised the speculation whether the triton X-100 buffer induced inflammation was a confounding factor in the guinea pig and monkey experiments conducted previously (Stephens 2003). However, studies using detergent-free preparations have not been pursued further in animal models. Correlative clinical studies in humans using anti-Hsp60 responses based on serology in trachoma, salpingitis, and *C. pneumoniae* cardiovascular disease yielded supportive evidence initially (Stephens 2003; Brunham et al. 1985), but some recent large studies have failed to show an association (Lu et al. 2012a; Ness et al. 2008). Given that the guinea pig studies by

Rank et al. (1995) had not only failed to show exacerbation of disease, but demonstrated the induction of protection against the challenge infection, the correlations of anti-Hsp60 antibody response to disease in individuals with repeated infection may be ascribed to the increased exposure of this population to the infection. Thus, the role of Hsp60 in DTH and chlamydial pathogenesis has yet to be conclusively determined.

An alternative hypothesis involving autoimmunity was also proposed because chlamydial Hsp60 and human Hsp60 share at least some antibody-binding epitopes (Yi et al. 1993), and a subset of *Chlamydia* seropositive individuals display such antibodies (Domeika et al. 1998). T cells reactive to chlamydial Hsp60 have been found in mice and humans, and these cells predominantly produce IL-10 and presumably down regulate Th1 responses, but were not tested for cross-reactivity against human Hsp60 (Beatty and Stephens 1992; Witkin et al. 1994; Kinnunen et al. 2002). Thus, the bulk of evidence implicating autoimmunity involving chlamydial Hsp60 as a mechanism of chlamydial pathogenesis is correlative. In summary, conclusive evidence was not available from studies of chlamydial Hsp60 to support the immunological hypothesis as a mechanism of chlamydial pathogenesis, and there seemed to be no breakthroughs to suggest a route forward in that direction.

Based on evidence in vitro wherein chlamydial infection of cell cultures induces a variety of inflammatory mediators (Rasmussen et al. 1997), Stephens proposed the cellular hypothesis in 2003 (Stephens 2003) as an alternate way of approaching the problem of chlamydial pathogenesis. The essence of this hypothesis is that:

(A) infection of non-immune cells such as epithelial and vascular endothelial cells is the primary driver of *Chlamydia*-induced inflammation;
(B) the infection induces production of chemokines, cytokines, and growth factors, and much of that response is dependent upon chlamydial growth or persistence in the affected cell;
(C) this inflammatory milieu would further recruit immune cells, including T cells, which also would produce inflammatory mediators; and
(D) the collective inflammatory environment thus lays the framework for a persisting inflammatory response and/or repeated bouts of inflammation, which is eventually responsible for chlamydial disease manifested as chronic inflammatory infiltrates and, as often seen, scarring in affected tissues.

Thus, the cellular hypothesis allowed for a pathogenic role for T cells, albeit secondary to the infection itself. Additionally, it was hypothesized that during repeat infection, the adaptive response is robust and even if short-lived could induce significant inflammatory damage leading to long-term disease sequelae. Therefore, the cellular and immunological hypotheses are not mutually exclusive, but primarily differ in the nature and extent of involvement of adaptive immune responses in chlamydial pathogenesis. Since the proposal of this hypothesis, numerous studies have been conducted and found a number of pro-acute or innate inflammatory mediators that correlate with or contribute to chlamydial pathogenesis and support the cellular hypothesis.

5 Role of Components of Innate Immune System in Chlamydial Pathogenesis

The contribution of a number of innate immune mediators has been evaluated in the context of chlamydial pathogenesis. These have been recently reviewed in detail (Derrick et al. 2015; O'Meara et al. 2014a; Menon et al. 2015).

The role of pattern recognition receptors (PRR) including Toll-like receptors (TLR) 2 and TLR 4, and cytosolic PRRs including nucleotide oligomerization domain 1 (NoD1) in chlamydial pathogenesis has been evaluated. It was reported initially that Toll-like receptor (TLR) 2-deficient mice display comparable kinetics of chlamydial shedding, but significantly reduced oviduct pathology following *C. muridarum* infection (Darville et al. 2003). However, a later study demonstrated that while TLR2-deficient mice may display a trend toward a reduction in oviduct pathology at day 35 after infection which represents acute/ongoing inflammation, chronic sequelae measured at day 60–80 after challenge in these mice do not show any significant differences in hydrosalpinx (Dong et al. 2014). These results were supported by the observation that mice deficient in MyD88, a critical adaptor molecule for TLR2, displayed more severe infection, compared to wild-type animals (Nagarajan et al. 2005). Additionally, another study in MyD88-deficient mice reported the induction of a TH2-dominant response and severe pathology in the upper genital tract following *C. muridarum* infection (Chen et al. 2010b). In summary, the predominant evidence suggests against a significant role for TLR2/MyD88 pathway in induction of chlamydial pathologies.

Among pro-inflammatory cytokines, IL-1β has been shown to play a modest role in chlamydial clearance, but contributes significantly to oviduct pathology in mice (Prantner et al. 2009). Caspase-1 cleaves pro-IL-1β to the biologically active form, and mice deficient in caspase-1 also display comparable kinetics of infection but significant reduction in oviduct pathology (Cheng et al. 2008). The process by which pro-caspase-1 is converted to mature and biologically active caspase-1 is known to involve Nod-1 or the formation of the inflammasome involving NoD-like receptor P3 (NLRP3) and the adaptor molecule apoptosis-associated speck-like (ASC) protein. Mice deficient in either NLRP3, NLRC4, or ASC do not display reductions in chlamydial oviduct pathology (Nagarajan et al. 2012). On the other hand, it has been demonstrated that the cytosolic PRR NoD1, not the NLRP3/ASC inflammasome, contributes to IL-1β secretion in human trophoblasts after sensing *C. trachomatis* (Kavathas et al. 2013). NoD1 also has been shown to induce IL-8, an important chemokine responsible for the recruitment of inflammatory cells, during *C. trachomatis* infection (Buchholz and Stephens 2008), and the IL-8 production was shown to occur independently of TLR2/MyD88 pathway. Collectively, in vitro evidence suggests that NoD1 is important in the activation of pro-caspase-1 to caspase-1 and subsequent induction of IL-1β and IL-8, both of which contribute to pathogenesis. NoD1 signaling also has been shown to induce Type 1 IFNs, especially IFN-β during chlamydial infections which has been shown to contribute significantly to oviduct pathology following *C. muridarum* infection (Nagarajan et al. 2008). NoD1 functional polymorphisms have been shown to correlate with *C. trachomatis* infection/tubal factor infertility (Brankovic et al. 2015), as well as *C. pneumoniae* infection/stroke (Tiszlavicz et al. 2009). However, mice deficient in NoD1 do not display differences in cytokine induction, infection course, or pathology following C. muridarum infection when compared to wild-type animals (Welter-Stahl et al. 2006), suggesting possible compensation from other signaling pathways.

Notwithstanding the upstream mechanisms, it is clear that caspase-1 is a key player in chlamydial pathologies. Caspase-3, along with caspase-1, and presumably other caspases were recently shown to be involved in the development of chlamydial pathologies (Igietseme et al. 2013). In this study, caspases were shown to degrade Dicer, a fertility-promoting ribonuclease II enzyme, and lead to alteration in critical miRNAs that regulate growth, differentiation, and development including mir-21 (Igietseme et al. 2013). Interestingly, uninfected mice deficient in Dicer display oviduct abnormalities, ectopic pregnancy, and infertility (Luense et al. 2009), which are strikingly similar to chlamydial pathologies in human. A more recent study by this group further demonstrated caspase-mediated alteration of a number of microRNAs involved in epithelial–mesenchyme transition, fibrosis, and fertility-related epithelial dysfunction (Igietseme et al. 2015a).

Tumor necrosis factor-α (TNF-α) is another pro-inflammatory acute phase cytokine implicated in chlamydial pathogenesis. We have demonstrated the mice deficient in TNF-α, TNF receptor 1 and/or TNF receptor 2, display minimal oviduct pathology following *C. muridarum* infection (Manam et al. 2015). The contribution of TNFR1 to pathogenesis of *C. muridarum*/oviduct pathology (Dong et al. 2014) and *C. pneumoniae*/atherosclerosis (Campbell et al. 2005b) in mice has been demonstrated by independent groups. Igietseme et al. (2015a) also suggested recently that TNF-α would lead to downstream activation of caspases and inactivation of Dicer leading to chlamydial pathologies. This proposed connection between TNF-α and caspases in chlamydial pathogenesis is a distinct possibility but one that remains to be definitively proven.

Aside from epithelial cells which get infected by *Chlamydiae* and participate in pathogenesis via the mechanisms described above, leukocytes including macrophages and neutrophils are capable, perhaps more so than epithelial cells, in producing the plethora of inflammatory mediators implicated in pathogenesis. In this regard, we have previously provided multiple lines of evidence implicating neutrophils in chlamydial immunopathologies. Specifically, mice deficient in CXC chemokine receptor 2 (CXCR2), matrix metalloprotease-9 (MMP-9), or phagocyte oxidase display significantly reduced chlamydial UGT pathology (Lee et al. 2010a; Imtiaz et al. 2007; Ramsey et al. 2001). CXCR2 is involved in chemotaxis inflammatory cells, MMP-9 induced degradation of extracellular matrix and inflammation, and phagocyte oxidase is a membrane-bound complex that is used to engulf microorganisms, and all are important components of neutrophil function. Additionally, depletion of neutrophils using anti-Ly6 depleting antibodies induces partial reduction of chlamydial UGT pathology (Lee et al. 2010b). The full extent of neutrophil involvement could not be studied using depleting antibodies because upon antibody-mediated depletion, band cells with partial neutrophil function populate peripheral tissues including the genital tract (Frazer et al. 2011). It is important to note many of the mediators described above also can be produced by macrophages, suggesting a possible pathogenic role for this cell type. However, definitive evidence to this end has yet to be attained.

Collectively, a number of components of the innate immune system have been described as key players in chlamydial pathogenesis. It is to be noted that much of the definitive evidences have come from the mouse model of *C. muridarum* infection. Additionally, the available evidence suggests a complex meshwork of events, rather than individual mediators/pathways acting in isolation, in causation of the chronic disease sequelae following chlamydial infections.

6 Role of Components of Adaptive Immune System in Chlamydial Pathogenesis

Whereas accumulating evidence suggests a plethora of innate immunological mediators may contribute to chlamydial disease, the immunological hypothesis is important primarily for two reasons: (A) the exacerbation of ocular disease in vaccinated monkeys of and in the human trachoma vaccine trials suggested the importance of avoiding a deleterious antigen-specific response, if one were to exist (and to be sure, we do not have firm data that it does) (Mabey et al. 2014), and (B) antigen-specific immune responses would make better biomarkers of impending disease and also better targets for the prevention/treatment of disease when compared to innate immune responses. New evidence continues to support a prominent role for adaptive immune responses in the disease induction process. For example, O'Meara et al. (2014b) demonstrated that even when upper genital tract chlamydial infection was not detectable, oviduct pathology occurred at wild-type levels. Johnson et al. (2012) have demonstrated that unmanipulated splenocytes from *Chlamydia*-immune mice can activate specific protective clones $CD4^+$ T cells, and such antigen-presenting cell effects were enhanced at 6 months compared to three week following infection. A similar process could be envisioned for ongoing stimulation or targeting of pathogenic T cell responses to sites of sequelae well after clearance of the infection. Support for this line of thought also comes from a recent trachoma study where scarring and clinical inflammation continued to progress in the absence of detectable infection over a 2-year period, and there was an association with clinical inflammation, not scarring progression, of multiple innate immune markers such as S100A7, IL1B, IL17A, CXCL5, CTGF, CEACAM5, MMP7, CD83, and reduced SPARCL1 (Burton et al. 2015). These results support the possibility of a *Chlamydia*-specific adaptive immune response in chlamydial pathogenesis.

The role of specific components of the adaptive immune response has been evaluated for their contribution to chlamydial pathogenesis.

6.1 B Cells

Although a Th2 cytokine profile has been associated with a robust antibody response, including mucosal immunoglobulin A, as well as chlamydial pathologies, B cells and antibody themselves have for the most part been associated with protective immunity, particularly to secondary or "challenge" infections rather than pathogenesis (Farris et al. 2010; Su et al. 1997; Moore et al. 2002; Yang and Brunham 1998), and we have reported that the absence of B cells enhances oviduct pathology (Murthy et al. 2009). A recent study further demonstrated the importance of B cells in preventing dissemination of *Chlamydia* into the peritoneal cavity, thus supporting a protective role for these mediators in chlamydial infections (Li and McSorley 2013).

6.2 T Helper Cells

In context of $CD4^+$ T cells, the bulk of evidence from the mouse model of *C. muridarum* and *C. trachomatis* infections and data from human studies including those in HIV-seropositive women suggest a role for Th1-type $CD4^+$ T cells in protection against infection and reduction of chronic disease (O'Meara et al. 2014a; Kimani et al. 1996). To this end, supportive evidence for the immunological hypothesis comes from the observations in humans and animal models of trachoma, salpingitis, lung infection, and reactive arthritis wherein a Th1 cytokine profile (IL-2, IL-12, and IFN-γ) correlates with protection against chlamydial infection and disease, whereas a Th2 cytokine profile (IL-4, IL-5, IL-10, IL-13) correlates with persistence and disease (Stephens 2003). Persistence of *Chlamydia* is a viable but non-cultivable state of the organism brought about due to a submicrobicidal level of various stressors such as downstream IFN-γ effectors, hypoxia, and antimicrobials, which do not kill the organism but drive it into an aberrant resting state (Bavoil 2014). Upon removal of the stressor, there is evidence that the organism may return to its replicating state. For the most part, evidence has suggested that a potent Th1 cytokine environment is essential to curtail the infection (Derrick et al. 2015; O'Meara et al. 2014a; Menon et al. 2015). Mice deficient in interleukin-10, a Th2 cytokine displayed superior clearance of lung *C. trachomatis* infection and a robust Th1-type DTH response and these changes could be reversed by local delivery of recombinant IL-10 (Yang et al. 1999). Additionally, IL-10 knockout mice displayed accelerated clearance of *C. pneumoniae* respiratory infection and enhanced splenic antigen-specific cell proliferation as well as pulmonary pro-inflammatory cytokine production (Penttila et al. 2008). Although the lung infection model in either study only addressed inflammation and antigen-specific response during acute infection, not chronic pathogenesis, these results were interpreted to mean that a balance between Th1 and Th2 cytokine profiles directly affects bacterial clearance or persistence; thus, pathogenesis was linked to the duration of bacterial presence and resulting prolonged inflammation. One could envision that during a reduction or even absence of an otherwise protective Th1 response, prolonged infection or persistence would occur with concomitant prolonged inflammation, a fibrogenic tissue remodeling response, and this would lead to enhanced disease. This argument appeared to further support only a secondary/indirect role for adaptive immunity in chlamydial pathogenesis.

6.3 Regulatory T Cells

Whereas an IL-10 response was considered a Th2 cytokine profile in earlier studies, it later began to be associated with the then newly characterized regulatory T cell subset ($CD4^+$ $CD25^+$ $FoxP3^+$ Tregs). This cell subset, capable of producing IL-10 and TGF-β, was reported in several disease models to be involved in the induction of immunological tolerance (Sakaguchi et al. 2010). Human studies in infertile women had demonstrated the presence of T cells that were reactive to chlamydial Hsp60 and produced IL-10 (Kinnunen et al. 2002), suggesting a pathogenic role of Treg cells. Conjunctival IL-10 and Foxp3 transcripts were reported to be elevated in patients with conjunctival chlamydial infection, with or without disease, and the Foxp3 transcript was elevated in patients where clinical signs of disease were present without detectable infection (Faal et al. Faal et 2006). One study using a human genital tract isolate of *C. trachomatis* serovar D displayed a protective role of Tregs against immunopathology using mice deficient in inducible costimulatory molecule (ICOS), a molecule expressed on a subset of Tregs that depend on IL-10 production for the suppression of Th1 responses (Marks et al. 2007). ICOS KO mice displayed greatly augmented Th1 effector cells and impaired Treg responses, along with sterilizing immunity against reinfection, but moderately enhanced immunopathology. However, the study directly addressed only the role of ICOS, not that of Tregs. Nevertheless, the study somewhat supported the conclusion that in the absence of IL-10, a robust Th1 response enhances chlamydial clearance and reduces pathology. An effector role of IL-10 in inducing chlamydial pathogenesis in the female upper reproductive tract came under further question with the demonstration that the lower genital tract is dominated by an IL-10-producing dendritic cells and poor Th1 cell response, whereas the upper genital tract is dominated by a Th1 $CD4^+$ T cell response following *C. trachomatis* serovar D infection (Marks et al. 2010).

While a plethora of damaging innate immune effectors had been identified at this stage, the research field had yet to find evidence of offending adaptive immune response component(s) that overtly caused pathology. Again, we feel it prudent to emphasize that the lung infection model and the *C. trachomatis* genital infection model are reasonable models to study acute chlamydial infections and protective immunity, not well-suited for mechanistic investigation of chronic pathogenesis. Where they were used for that purpose early on, the main interpretation that could be made was that pathology correlated with a longer duration of infection or inflammation.

Subsequently, the mouse model of genital *C. muridarum* infection model began to be used widely (Barron et al. 1981). Not widely embraced at first, this model grew from the seminal work of Rank and colleagues, exploring mechanisms of protective immunity in the 1980s and 1990s. These studies showed that immunity in the *C. muridarum* model is primarily T cell-mediated. While the model was primarily used to assess factors that influence lower genital tract shedding during primary infection, it should be noted, however, that these investigations laid the framework for mechanistic studies of pathogenesis pertaining to the long-term disease sequelae such as hydrosalpinx and infertility. Many of the initially identified mediators were those elicited via the innate immune response as discussed above and eventually others in the adaptive immune response.

In this model, Moniz et al. demonstrated that depletion of pDC from mice resulted in significantly reduced oviduct dilatation and fibrosis scores (Moniz et al. 2010). In addition, they found that reduction in pathology correlated with a modest reduction in the ratio of splenic Treg to Th1 cells, as well as significant (fourfold to sixfold) enhancements in IFN-γ-producing T cells. This underscored a role for pDC in chlamydial pathogenesis and indicated a potential pathogenic role of Tregs. Direct evidence came more recently in a study from Moore-Connors et al. (2013), wherein depletion of Tregs using anti-CD25 treatment prior to *C. muridarum* genital infection resulted in significantly attenuated inflammation, neutrophil recruitment, and oviduct pathology. An interesting finding of this study was that Tregs were shown to induce conversion of naïve $CD4^+$ T cells, as well as themselves, into Th17 T cells. Additionally, depletion of Tregs resulted in significant reduction of Th17, not Th1, $CD4^+$ T cell response (Moore-Connors et al. 2013). These results provided strong support for a role of Tregs in chlamydial pathogenesis. In a recent study addressing mechanisms of protective immunity against genital *C. trachomatis* challenge, it was found that an immunization regimen successful in inducing early resolution of challenge infection and reducing chronic pathology activated immunogenic CD103-dendritic cells and a Th1 $CD4^+$ T cell response (Stary et al. 2015). Conversely in the same study, an immunization regimen which did not efficaciously reduce chlamydial burden or oviduct pathology upregulated expression of anti-inflammatory markers including PD-L2 and IL-10 on a tolerogenic $CD103^+$ dendritic cell subset. Although Tregs were not evaluated directly, these results support a pathogenic role for Tregs in chlamydial infection. On the other hand, a regulatory subset of $CD8^+$ T cells ($CD8^+$ $CXCR5^+$) expressing Treg markers Foxp3 and CD25 has been reported to reduce the severity of oviduct dilatation following genital *C. muridarum* infection when adoptively transferred into CXCR5 knockout mice (Jiang et al. 2013). In summary, the role of Tregs in pathogenesis may be complex and involve multiple subsets of T cells, but the effector mechanism by which these cells contribute to pathogenesis has yet to be determined.

6.4 Th 17 Cells

One of the intriguing findings by Moore-Connor et al. study (2013) was the role of Tregs in activation of Th17 $CD4^+$ T cell responses. Th17 cells produce IL-17 that recruits neutrophils and possibly other pro-inflammatory cells to sites of infection; therefore, this response is thought of as a bridge between innate and adaptive immune response (Khader et al. 2009). The role of Th17 $CD4^+$ T cells in chlamydial pathogenesis has been addressed by several studies (O'Meara et al. 2014a), and an association between IL-17 and chlamydial disease has been suggested in studies from animal models as well as humans (Masson et al. 2015). Early studies of *C. muridarum* respiratory infection demonstrated a role for IL-17A in the recruitment of inflammatory cells to sites of infection and protection against mortality from infection (Zhou et al. 2009). Additionally, it was observed that in vivo neutralization of IL-17A during respiratory *C. muridarum* infection significantly reduced Th1 response and enhanced Th2 responses (Bai et al. 2009). However, neither of these studies evaluated the chronic disease sequelae. Using IL-17A knockout mice on a C57BL/6 wild-type background, IL-17A was found to be pro-atherogenic in a high-fat diet-induced *C. pneumoniae*-accelerated atherosclerosis in mice (Chen et al. 2010a), providing evidence for a pathogenic role of Th 17 cells in chronic disease sequelae. This was supported by evidence from studies using the genital infection model wherein IL-17A knockout mice on either a BALB/c or C57BL/6 wild-type background also displayed reduced infection clearance as well as reduced oviduct pathology (Andrew et al. 2013; Arkatkar et al. 2015). Additionally, mice immunized intranasally live *C. muridarum* elementary bodies (EB) induced robust protection against both chlamydial burden and oviduct pathology following genital *C. muridarum* challenge, and this correlated with high IFN-γ and low IL-17 production from T cells (Lu et al. 2012b). In the same study, mice immunized with UV-inactivated chlamydial EB induced a low IFN-γ and high IL-17 response from T cells and did not protect against oviduct pathology. These studies suggested a pathogenic role for IL-17 in chlamydial infections. Furthermore, O'meara et al. (2014b) found that among two vaccination regimens they were using, MOMP with cholera toxin and CpG as adjuvants prevented ascent of *Chlamydia* to upper genital tract, but not oviduct pathology; on the other hand, MOMP with CTA1-DD as adjuvant reduced oviduct pathology, not chlamydial shedding. They explored the IL-17 receptor signaling pathways and found that the regimen that protected against infection, not oviduct pathology, displayed an upregulation of IL-17 receptor signaling, whereas protection against oviduct pathology, not infection, correlated with downregulation of IL-17 receptor signaling. Based on this, the authors suggested that IL-17 signaling may play a role in both protection and pathogenesis based on the balance of downstream receptors that are activated and that protection against chronic chlamydial disease involved reduced induction of IL-17. IL-17 receptor A knockout mice displayed reduced neutrophil recruitment and Th1 response, but the course of infection and oviduct pathology remained unaltered (Scurlock et al. 2011). A compensatory influx of macrophages and TNF-α production was found in the IL-17RA KO mice, and this was ascribed to compensate for the deficient IL-17 signaling and neutrophil recruitment toward induction of pathology in these animals. However, mice deficient in IL-23, required for activation of IL-22 and Th17 $CD4^+$ T cell response, also displayed reduced Th17 but unaltered Th1 $CD4^+$ T cell response, and comparable resolution of infection and only a trend toward reduction of oviduct pathology when compared to wild-type animals (Frazer et al. 2013). Overall, the role of Th17 responses in chlamydial pathogenesis appears to be complex and continues to be explored, with strong suggestions that they contribute to pathogenesis.

6.5 $CD8^+$ T Cells

$CD8^+$ T cells are the other important T cell subsets have been studied extensively in context of protective immunity against chlamydial infections. $CD8^+$ T cells are recruited in considerable numbers to sites of chlamydial infection, but evidence for a role in protective immunity for this cell type has been sparse. Some clones of $CD8^+$ T cells have been shown to induce protective immunity against chlamydial infection, but they do so based on their ability to secrete IFN-γ, not cytolysis (Starnbach et al. 1994; Igietseme et al. 1994). It has been considered counterintuitive that $CD8^+$ T cells, known for their ability to use cytolytic mechanisms and protect against intracellular viral infection, seem to have a relatively minimal role in protection against a primary or secondary chlamydial infection. In this regard, *Chlamydia* is a vacuolar pathogen and so far it seems relatively few chlamydial components access the host cytosol, which may partly explain the relatively small role for $CD8^+$ T cells in cytolysis. Chlamydial infection also has been demonstrated to induce downregulation of MHC I on infected cells, providing another possible mechanism of evading $CD8^+$ T cell-mediated cytolysis (Zhong et al. 2000; Ibana et al. 2011). It has been shown that a polyclonal $CD8^+$ T cell response against chlamydial antigens primarily is induced against soluble chlamydial antigens secreted out of the bacterium, not to integral antigens in the chlamydial EB or RB (Johnson et al. 2014). It is also possible that chlamydial proteins that reach the host cytosol in substantial quantities typically activate a $CD8^+$ T cell response very late in the intracellular developmental cycle and cannot prevent the reticulate body to elementary body reconversion and therefore cannot contain infection. Conversely, antigen-specific $CD8^+$ T cells that recognize the chlamydial protein CrpA, which is an inclusion membrane protein and enters the MHC I pathway, have been demonstrated to respond to genital *C. trachomatis* infection (Fling et al. 2001; Starnbach et al. 2003). A T cell receptor transgenic mouse in which all $CD8^+$ T cells recognize CrpA was shown to display partial protective immunity against an intravenous *C. trachomatis* challenge, although the relevance of this model of infection is arguable (Starnbach et al. 2003). Additionally, one recent study in an ocular infection monkey model demonstrated that monkeys prevaccinated with plasmid-deficient *Chlamydiae* and determined to be solidly protected against infectious challenge with virulent *Chlamydia* were unable to control a subsequent challenge infection when $CD8^+$ T cells were depleted using neutralizing antibodies (Olivares-Zavaleta et al. 2014). This may suggest that multiple vaccinations may generate high enough numbers of particular antigen-specific clones of $CD8^+$ T cells and/or populate them at sites of infection as tissue-resident memory cells (Johnson and Brunham 2016). Alternatively, chlamydial infection has been shown to upregulate molecules such as PD-L1 at sites of infection which dampen the activation of antigen-specific $CD8^+$ T cell response. Deletion or inhibition of PD-L1 has been shown to allow activation and enhance the clearance of *C. trachomatis* infection by $CD8^+$ T cells (Fankhauser and Starnbach 2014). It has been proposed that immunization with a plasmid-deficient *Chlamydia* perhaps lacks the ability to induce such dampening response and leads to activation of protective $CD8^+$ T cell responses (Porcella et al. 2015). Although a subject of high interest for several years, the role of $CD8^+$ T cells in protective immunity against chlamydial infections remains to be clarified.

On the other hand, multiple lines of evidence from various chlamydial infection models implicate $CD8^+$ T cells in chlamydial pathogenesis. A study of 302 sex workers in Kenya indicated that HLA-A31 was significantly associated with *C. trachomatis* pelvic inflammatory disease (Kimani et al. 1996). In a Gambian study of trachoma, the MHC I allele HLA-A28 was found to be associated with scarring trachoma, whereas the MHC class II genes, HLA-DRB1 or HLA-DQB1, were not (Conway et al. 1996). In other studies involving Tanzanain and Gambian populations, other MHC class I genes including HLA-B*07 or HLA-B*08 were associated with TS (Abbas et al. 2009; Roberts et al. 2014). The Tanzanian study also indicated an association of HLA-DRB1*11 (an MHC class II gene) in women with less TS (Abbas et al. 2009). Following repeated *C. trachomatis* infection, fallopian tubes of female macaques also displayed $CD8^+$ T cells as the majority (nearly 62 %) of T cells infiltrating sites of infection and these cells produced Th1-type cytokines (Van Voorhis et al. 1996, 1997). Igietseme et al. demonstrated a significant protection against infertility in CD8 knockout mice compared to WT animals, following four episodes of vaginal *C. muridarum* infection (Igietseme et al. 2009). We have demonstrated that following primary *C. muridarum* infection, a deficiency of $CD8^+$ T cells (in three different models of deficiency) resulted in unaltered kinetics of vaginal chlamydial shedding, but significantly reduced oviduct pathology (Murthy et al. 2011b). Reconstitution of CD8 KO mice with wild-type $CD8^+$ T cells at the time of infection restored pathology to wild-type levels. We also found that mice deficient in TNF-α or perforin displayed the same phenotype. Reconstitution of CD8 KO mice with wild-type or perforin KO, not TNF-α KO, $CD8^+$ T cells restored pathology to wild-type levels (Murthy et al. 2011b). A recent study using the genital *C. trachomatis* serovar D infection induces infertility in wild type, not TNF-α KO female mice (Igietseme et al. 2015b). In that study, reconstitution of TNF-α KO mice with wild-type T cells restored infertility to wild-type levels following genital *C. trachomatis* infection. These results suggest that $CD8^+$ T cells cause genital chlamydial pathogenesis and implicate TNF-α production as a pathogenic mechanism. We also demonstrated recently that high-fat diet-fed CD8 KO mice displayed significant reduction in atherosclerosis development following intranasal *C. pneumoniae* infection (Zafiratos et al. 2015). Additionally, repletion of CD8 KO mice with wild-type $CD8^+$ T cells restored the development of atherosclerotic pathology to wild-type levels. These results from a different infection model using a human pathogen *C. pneumoniae* further support the pathogenic role of $CD8^+$ T cells; however, whether or not $CD8^+$ T cells induce diseases in different organ systems using similar mechanisms remains to be determined.

We have further characterized that both TNF receptor 1 and TNF receptor 2 are required for *Chlamydia*-induced oviduct pathology, not chlamydial clearance. Moreover, TNF receptor 2, not TNF receptor 1, on $CD8^+$ T cells was important for the activation of *Chlamydia*-specific $CD8^+$ T cells and causation of oviduct pathology (Manam et al. 2015). TNFR 1 is expressed on all nucleated cells of the body, whereas TNF receptor 2 has a more limited distribution of hematopoietic cells. Therefore, our results collectively suggest that pathogenic TNF^+, $TNFR2^+$, $CD8^+$ T cells, and $TNFR1^+$ non-CD8 cells mediate chlamydial pathogenesis. While $CD8^+$ T cells are an adaptive immune cell type, there has been evidence for roles of non-antigen-specific $CD8^+$ T cells in other disease processes (Chen et al. 2005; Sobottka et al. 2009). When we characterized genital *C. muridarum* infection in OT-1 transgenic mice, wherein 100 % of $CD8^+$ T cells recognize an irrelevant ovalbumin peptide and therefore do not recognize chlamydial antigens, we found that vaginal chlamydial shedding remained unaltered, whereas oviduct pathology was significantly reduced (Manam et al. 2013). Repletion of OT-1 mice with wild-type $CD8^+$ T cells restored the ability of these mice to generate *Chlamydia*-specific $CD8^+$ T cell response and to induce oviduct pathology at wild-type levels (Vlcek et al. 2016). In summary, we have demonstrated compelling evidence in the mouse model using *C. muridarum*/oviduct pathology and *C. pneumoniae*/atherosclerosis for a pathogenic role of $CD8^+$ T cells as well as the antigen-specific nature of this phenomenon.

In the recent ocular challenge study with virulent *C. trachomatis* in monkeys prevaccinated with plasmid-deficient *C. trachomatis*, depletion of $CD8^+$ T cells abrogated the protective immunity and promoted high chlamydial conjunctival burden following challenge (Olivares-Zavaleta et al. 2014). At the outset, it may seem to argue against the role of $CD8^+$ T cells in chronic chlamydial pathogenesis; however, as also discussed by the authors, scarring sequelae were not evaluated in this study and two of the three monkeys depleted of $CD8^+$ T cells displayed minimal inflammatory changes despite the high ocular chlamydial load. Collectively, multiple lines of evidence strongly suggest a role for $CD8^+$ T cells in pathogenesis.

7 Summary

Since the proposal of the cellular hypothesis of chlamydial pathogenesis, numerous studies have unearthed a wealth of information and insights into mechanisms of chlamydial disease sequelae. There are a few key insights that we have gained from these results:

1. **The mouse model of chlamydial infection is well-suited for mechanistic studies of chlamydial pathogenesis**. Much progress has been made using the genital *C. muridarum* and oviduct pathology or *C. pneumoniae* and atherosclerosis/asthma model in mice. For one, it allows the study of a true chronic disease process, rather than extrapolating results of acute inflammation during infection to manifestations of chronic disease. Additionally, the availability of various whole body or conditional gene knockout or knock-in mice including as well as transgenic mice allows studies of pathogenic mechanisms to an extent that is practically impossible in other animal models or humans. Other animal models including the guinea pig and monkeys are available, but are highly restrictive with respect to reagents, access, and cost. In the last decade, over a dozen immunological mediators of chlamydial pathogenesis have been identified and characterized using the mouse model, and to a large extent, these findings have been corroborated in human studies.
2. **Protection against infection may involve different mechanism(s) compared to protection against pathology**. At the outset, it would seem that if infection was prevented, pathology is automatically avoided. That is true; however, reinfections are common and thus even a natural chlamydial infection does not provide 100 % resistance to reinfection. Therefore, absolute resistance to infection may not be a realistic goal for an anti-*Chlamydia* vaccine. If we can only achieve partial protection against infection, there would still be room for a shortened infection to activate a sequence of immunopathogenesis. On the contrary, multiple lines of evidence have demonstrated that reduction in pathology can be achieved by altering certain immune components with minimal or no changes in kinetics of clearance of infection. Therefore, it could theoretically be possible to design a vaccine that directly targets the avoidance of a pathogenic immune response following infection, rather than enhanced clearance of the bacterium. We (Murthy et al. 2007) and others (O'Meara et al. 2014b) have described vaccine regimens that prevent pathology with only a moderate effect on reduction of infection.
3. **Multiple adaptive immune mechanisms play a role in chlamydial pathogenesis**. From the days of Th1/Th2 balance, this research field has come a long way and now identified the roles of various T cell populations including regulatory T cells, Th17 cells, and $CD8^+$ T cells in chlamydial pathogenesis. A key question that remains to be answered conclusively is to whether adaptive

immune responses contribute in an antigen-specific fashion to pathogenesis? The role of *Chlamydia*-specific $CD8^+$ T cells in pathogenesis supports this line of thought.

4. **Mechanisms of chlamydial immunopathogenesis appear to work in series.** Multiple immunological knockout mice including mice deficient in caspase-1, neutrophils, metalloproteinases, TNF-α, TNF receptor 1, TNF receptor 2, and $CD8^+$ T cells display comparable bacterial shedding to wild-type mice, with significantly reduced oviduct pathology. This suggests that multiple innate and adaptive components work in series, not parallel, toward induction of chlamydial disease sequelae. Although a number of innate immune mediators have been shown to play roles, a strong interaction of innate and adaptive immune response components in chlamydial pathogenesis is emerging.
5. **Adaptive immunopathogenic mechanisms appear to modulate pro-inflammatory mediators.** Traditionally, it is thought that an infection induces an innate immune response followed by adaptive immune response. A number of innate immune factors including neutrophils and TNF-α have found to play a role in chlamydial pathogenesis. That said, studies have also shown these innate immune factors to be induced/modulated by components of the adaptive immune response. For example, Th17 cells induce neutrophil recruitment, and $CD8^+$ T cells induce pathology via TNF-α production while mediating chlamydial pathogenesis. Therefore, components of innate immune system may be induced directly by infection and/or by the adaptive immune response and may contribute to pathogenesis in both capacities.

8 Outlook for Future

Based on the state of the art, we are now poised with important issues pertaining to mechanisms of chlamydial immunopathogenesis. One important question is "how do multiple components of the immune system interface with each other to culminate in disease pathology?" In this context, we propose that a "*Chlamydia* immunopathogenesis sequence/network" would be a more reasonable hypothesis than classical and somewhat more restrictive "immunological" or "cellular" hypothesis. Another important question: "Is a pathogenic response determined by particular chlamydial antigens or is it based on skewing of a polyclonal response toward a pathogenic phenotype?" The answer to this question will have a direct bearing on anti-chlamydial vaccine development.

The last decade has brought abundant and important insights into the significant contribution of adaptive immune responses to chlamydial pathogenesis. Given the inherent advantages of targeting an antigen-specific response for biomarker or therapy discovery, or for developing safe vaccines, future studies should focus on bringing clarity to this arena.

Acknowledgements This work was supported by Midwestern University Faculty Start-up Fund, National Institutes of Health (NIH) Grant 1R15AI101920, and American Heart Association (AHA) Midwest Affiliate Scientist Development Grant 13SDG17310011 to AKM. The content in this manuscript is solely the responsibility of the authors and does not represent the official views of any of the funding agencies. The authors declare no conflict of interest.

The authors declare no conflict of interest.

References

Abbas M, Bobo LD, Hsieh YH, Berka N, Dunston G, Bonney GE, Apprey V, Quinn TC, West SK (2009) Human leukocyte antigen (HLA)-B, DRB1, and DQB1 allotypes associated with disease and protection of trachoma endemic villagers. Invest Ophthalmol Vis Sci 50:1734–1738

Adams EJ, Charlett A, Edmunds WJ, Hughes G (2004) *Chlamydia trachomatis* in the United Kingdom: a systematic review and analysis of prevalence studies. Sex Transm Infect 80:354–362

Andrew DW, Cochrane M, Schripsema JH, Ramsey KH, Dando SJ, O'Meara CP, Timms P, Beagley KW (2013) The duration of *Chlamydia muridarum* genital tract infection and associated chronic pathological changes are reduced in IL-17 knockout mice but protection is not increased further by immunization. PLoS One 8:e76664

Arkatkar T, Gupta R, Li W, Yu JJ, Wali S, Neal GM, Chambers JP, Christenson LK, Arulanandam BP (2015) Murine MicroRNA-214 regulates intracellular adhesion molecule (ICAM1) gene expression in genital *Chlamydia muridarum* infection. Immunology 145: 534–542

Bai H, Cheng J, Gao X, Joyee AG, Fan Y, Wang S, Jiao L, Yao Z, Yang X (2009) IL-17/Th17 promotes type 1 T cell immunity against pulmonary intracellular bacterial infection through modulating dendritic cell function. J Immunol 183:5886–5895

Barron AL, White HJ, Rank RG, Soloff BL, Moses EB (1981) A new animal model for the study of *Chlamydia trachomatis* genital infections: infection of mice with the agent of mouse pneumonitis. J Infect Dis 143:63–66

Batteiger BE, Xu F, Johnson RE, Rekart ML (2010) Protective immunity to *Chlamydia trachomatis* genital infection: evidence from human studies. J Infect Dis 201(Suppl 2):S178–S189

Bavoil PM (2014) What's in a word: the use, misuse, and abuse of the word "persistence" in Chlamydia biology. Front Cell Infect Microbiol 4:27

Bavoil P, Stephens RS, Falkow S (1990) A soluble 60 kiloDalton antigen of Chlamydia spp. is a homologue of Escherichia coli GroEL. Mol Microbiol 4:461–469

Beatty PR, Stephens RS (1992) Identification of *Chlamydia trachomatis* antigens by use of murine T-cell lines. Infect Immun 60:4598–4603

Bebear C, de Barbeyrac B (2009) Genital *Chlamydia trachomatis* infections. Clin Microbiol Infect 15:4–10

Bell JD, Bergin IL, Schmidt K, Zochowski MK, Aronoff DM, Patton DL (2011) Nonhuman primate models used to study pelvic inflammatory disease caused by *Chlamydia trachomatis*. Infect Dis Obstet Gynecol 2011:675360

Berger RE (1990) Acute epididymitis. In: Holmes KK, Mardh PA, Sparling PF, Weisner PJ (eds) Sexually transmitted diseases. NY, McGraw-Hill, New York, pp 641–653

Brankovic I, van Ess EF, Noz MP, Wiericx WA, Spaargaren J, Morre SA, Ouburg S (2015) NOD1 in contrast to NOD2 functional polymorphism influence *Chlamydia trachomatis* infection and the risk of tubal factor infertility. Pathog Dis 73:1–9

Brunham RC, Rey-Ladino J (2005) Immunology of *Chlamydia* infection: implications for a *Chlamydia trachomatis* vaccine. Nat Rev Immunol 5:149–161
Brunham RC, Maclean IW, Binns B, Peeling RW (1985) *Chlamydia trachomatis*: its role in tubal infertility. J Infect Dis 152:1275–1282
Buchholz KR, Stephens RS (2008) The cytosolic pattern recognition receptor NOD1 induces inflammatory interleukin-8 during *Chlamydia trachomatis* infection. Infect Immun 76:3150–3155
Burton MJ, Rajak SN, Hu VH, Ramadhani A, Habtamu E, Massae P, Tadesse Z, Callahan K, Emerson PM, Khaw PT, Jeffries D, Mabey DC, Bailey RL, Weiss HA, Holland MJ (2015) Pathogenesis of progressive scarring trachoma in Ethiopia and Tanzania and its implications for disease control: two cohort studies. PLoS Negl Trop Dis 9:e0003763
Campbell LA, Kuo C (1999) Mouse models of *Chlamydia pneumoniae* infection and atherosclerosis. Am Heart J 138:S516–S518
Campbell LA, Kuo CC (2002) *Chlamydia pneumoniae* pathogenesis. J Med Microbiol 51:623–625
Campbell LA, Rosenfeld ME (2014) Persistent *C. pneumoniae* infection in atherosclerotic lesions: rethinking the clinical trials. Front Cell Infect Microbiol 4:34
Campbell LA, Rosenfeld ME (2015) Infection and atherosclerosis development. Arch Med Res 46:339–350
Campbell LA, Perez MM, Hamilton DJ, Kuo CC, Grayston JT (1992) Detection of *Chlamydia pneumoniae* by polymerase chain reaction. J Clin Microbiol 30:434–439
Campbell LA, Nosaka T, Rosenfeld ME, Yaraei K, Kuo CC (2005a) Tumor necrosis factor alpha plays a role in the acceleration of atherosclerosis by *Chlamydia pneumoniae* in mice. Infect Immun 73:3164–3165
Campbell LA, Nosaka T, Rosenfeld ME, Yaraei K, Kuo CC (2005b) Tumor necrosis factor alpha plays a role in the acceleration of atherosclerosis by *Chlamydia pneumoniae* in mice. Infect Immun 73:3164–3165
Centers for Disease Control and Prevention (2015) Sexually transmitted disease surveillance 2014. Department of Health and Human Services, Atlanta
Chen MY, Donovan B (2003) Screening for genital *Chlamydia trachomatis* infection: are men the forgotten reservoir? Med J Aust 179:124–125
Chen AM, Khanna N, Stohlman SA, Bergmann CC (2005) Virus-specific and bystander CD8 T cells recruited during virus induced encephalomyelitis. J Virol 79:4700–4708
Chen S, Shimada K, Zhang W, Huang G, Crother TR, Arditi M (2010a) IL-17A is proatherogenic in high-fat diet-induced and *Chlamydia pneumoniae* infection-accelerated atherosclerosis in mice. J Immunol 185:5619–5627
Chen L, Lei L, Chang X, Li Z, Lu C, Zhang X, Wu Y, Yeh IT, Zhong G (2010b) Mice deficient in MyD88 develop a Th2-dominant response and severe pathology in the upper genital tract following *Chlamydia muridarum* infection. J Immunol 184:2602–2610
Chen J, Zhang H, Zhou Z, Yang Z, Ding Y, Zhou Z, Zhong E, Arulanandam B, Baseman J, Zhong G (2014) Chlamydial induction of hydrosalpinx in 11 strains of mice reveals multiple host mechanisms for preventing upper genital tract pathology. PLoS One 9:e95076
Cheng W, Shivshankar P, Li Z, Chen L, Yeh IT, Zhong G (2008) Caspase-1 contributes to *Chlamydia trachomatis*-induced upper urogenital tract inflammatory pathologies without affecting the course of infection. Infect Immun 76:515–522
Choroszy-Krol I, Frej-Madrzak M, Hober M, Sarowska J, Jama-Kmiecik A (2014) Infections caused by *Chlamydophila pneumoniae*. Adv Clin Exp Med 23:123–126
Conway DJ, Holland MJ, Campbell AE, Bailey RL, Krausa P, Peeling RW, Whittle HC, Mabey DC (1996) HLA class I and II polymorphisms and trachomatous scarring in a *Chlamydia trachomatis*-endemic population. J Infect Dis 174:643–646
Darville T, Hiltke TJ (2010) Pathogenesis of genital tract disease due to *Chlamydia trachomatis*. J Infect Dis 201(Suppl 2):S114–S125

Darville T, O'Neill JM, Andrews CW Jr, Nagarajan UM, Stahl L, Ojcius DM (2003) Toll-like receptor-2, but not toll-like receptor-4, is essential for development of oviduct pathology in chlamydial genital tract infection. J Immunol 171:6187–6197

De CE, Kalmar I, Vanrompay D (2013) Animal models for studying female genital tract infection with *Chlamydia trachomatis*. Infect Immun 81:3060–3067

Deniset JF, Cheung PK, Dibrov E, Lee K, Steigerwald S, Pierce GN (2010) *Chlamydophila pneumoniae* infection leads to smooth muscle cell proliferation and thickening in the coronary artery without contributions from a host immune response. Am J Pathol 176:1028–1037

Derrick T, Roberts C, Last AR, Burr SE, Holland MJ (2015) Trachoma and ocular chlamydial infection in the Era of genomics. Mediators Inflamm 2015:791847

Domeika M, Domeika K, Paavonen J, Mardh PA, Witkin SS (1998) Humoral immune response to conserved epitopes of *Chlamydia trachomatis* and human 60-kDa heat-shock protein in women with pelvic inflammatory disease. J Infect Dis 177:714–719

Dong X, Liu Y, Chang X, Lei L, Zhong G (2014) Signaling via tumor necrosis factor receptor 1 but not Toll-like receptor 2 contributes significantly to hydrosalpinx development following *Chlamydia muridarum* infection. Infect Immun 82:1833–1839

Erkkila L, Laitinen K, Laurila A, Saikku P, Leinonen M (2002) Experimental *Chlamydia pneumoniae* infection in NIH/S mice: effect of reinoculation with chlamydial or cell preparation on culture, PCR and histological findings of lung tissue. Vaccine 20:2318–2324

Faal N, Bailey RL, Jeffries D, Joof H, Sarr I, Laye M, Mabey DC, Holland MJ (2006) Conjunctival FOXP3 expression in trachoma: do regulatory T cells have a role in human ocular *Chlamydia trachomatis* infection? PLoS Med 3:e266

Fankhauser SC, Starnbach MN (2014) PD-L1 limits the mucosal $CD8^+$ T cell response to *Chlamydia trachomatis*. J Immunol 192:1079–1090

Farris CM, Morrison SG, Morrison RP (2010) $CD4^+$ T cells and antibody are required for optimal major outer membrane protein vaccine-induced immunity to *Chlamydia muridarum* genital infection. Infect Immun 78:4374–4383

Fling SP, Sutherland RA, Steele LN, Hess B, D'Orazio SE, Maisonneuve J, Lampe MF, Probst P, Starnbach MN (2001) $CD8^+$ T cells recognize an inclusion membrane-associated protein from the vacuolar pathogen *Chlamydia trachomatis*. Proc Natl Acad Sci USA 98:1160–1165

Frazer LC, O'Connell CM, Andrews CW Jr, Zurenski MA, Darville T (2011) Enhanced neutrophil longevity and recruitment contribute to the severity of oviduct pathology during *Chlamydia muridarum* infection. Infect Immun 79:4029–4041

Frazer LC, Scurlock AM, Zurenski MA, Riley MM, Mintus M, Pociask DA, Sullivan JE, Andrews CW Jr, Darville T (2013) IL-23 induces IL-22 and IL-17 production in response to *Chlamydia muridarum* genital tract infection, but the absence of these cytokines does not influence disease pathogenesis. Am J Reprod Immunol 70:472–484

Geisler WM (2010) Duration of untreated, uncomplicated *Chlamydia trachomatis* genital infection and factors associated with *Chlamydia* resolution: a review of human studies. J Infect Dis 201 (Suppl 2):S104–S113

Grayston JT, Wang SP, Yeh LJ, Kuo CC (1985) Importance of reinfection in the pathogenesis of trachoma. Rev Infect Dis 7:717–725

Grayston JT, Kuo CC, Wang SP, Altman J (1986) A new *Chlamydia psittaci* strain, TWAR, isolated in acute respiratory tract infections. N Engl J Med 315:161–168

Grayston JT, Aldous MB, Easton A, Wang SP, Kuo CC, Campbell LA, Altman J (1993) Evidence that *Chlamydia pneumoniae* causes pneumonia and bronchitis. J Infect Dis 168:1231–1235

Grayston JT, Belland RJ, Byrne GI, Kuo CC, Schachter J, Stamm WE, Zhong G (2015) Infection with *Chlamydia pneumoniae* as a cause of coronary heart disease: the hypothesis is still untested. Pathog Dis 73:1–9

Hahn DL, Dodge RW, Golubjatnikov R (1991) Association of *Chlamydia pneumoniae* (strain TWAR) infection with wheezing, asthmatic bronchitis, and adult-onset asthma. JAMA 266:225–230

Hansbro PM, Beagley KW, Horvat JC, Gibson PG (2004) Role of atypical bacterial infection of the lung in predisposition/protection of asthma. Pharmacol Ther 101:193–210

Harkinezhad T, Schautteet K, Vanrompay D (2009) Protection of budgerigars (*Melopsittacus undulatus*) against *Chlamydophila psittaci* challenge by DNA vaccination. Vet Res 40:61

Honarmand H (2013) Atherosclerosis induced by *Chlamydophila pneumoniae*: a controversial theory. Interdiscip Perspect Infect Dis 2013:941392

Howard LV, O'Leary MP, Nichols RL (1976) Animal model studies of genital chlamydial infections. Immunity to re-infection with guinea-pig inclusion conjunctivitis agent in the urethra and eye of male guinea-pigs. Br J Vener Dis 52:261–265

Ibana JA, Schust DJ, Sugimoto J, Nagamatsu T, Greene SJ, Quayle AJ (2011) *Chlamydia trachomatis* immune evasion via downregulation of MHC class I surface expression involves direct and indirect mechanisms. Infect Dis Obstet Gynecol 2011:420905

Igietseme JU, Magee DM, Williams DM, Rank RG (1994) Role for CD8 + T cells in antichlamydial immunity defined by *Chlamydia*-specific T-lymphocyte clones. Infect Immun 62:5195–5197

Igietseme JU, He Q, Joseph K, Eko FO, Lyn D, Ananaba G, Campbell A, Bandea C, Black CM (2009) Role of T lymphocytes in the pathogenesis of *Chlamydia* disease. J Infect Dis 200:926–934

Igietseme JU, Omosun Y, Partin J, Goldstein J, He Q, Joseph K, Ellerson D, Ansari U, Eko FO, Bandea C, Zhong G, Black CM (2013) Prevention of *Chlamydia*-induced infertility by inhibition of local caspase activity. J Infect Dis 207:1095–1104

Igietseme JU, Omosun Y, Stuchlik O, Reed MS, Partin J, He Q, Joseph K, Ellerson D, Bollweg B, George Z, Eko FO, Bandea C, Liu H, Yang G, Shieh WJ, Pohl J, Karem K, Black CM (2015a) Role of epithelial-mesenchyme transition in *Chlamydia* pathogenesis. PLoS One 10:e0145198

Igietseme JU, Omosun Y, Stuchlik O, Reed MS, Partin J, He Q, Joseph K, Ellerson D, Bollweg B, George Z, Eko FO, Bandea C, Liu H, Yang G, Shieh WJ, Pohl J, Karem K, Black CM (2015) Role of epithelial-mesenchyme transition in *Chlamydia* Pathogenesis. PLoS One 10:e0145198

Imtiaz MT, Distelhorst JT, Schripsema JH, Sigar IM, Kasimos JN, Lacy SR, Ramsey KH (2007) A role for matrix metalloproteinase-9 in pathogenesis of urogenital *Chlamydia muridarum* infection in mice. Microbes Infect 9:1561–1566

Jiang J, Champion CI, Wei B, Liu G, Kelly KA (2013) CD8(+)CXCR5(+) T cells regulate pathology in the genital tract. Infect Dis Obstet Gynecol 2013:813238

Johnson RM, Brunham RC (2016) Tissue resident T cells as the central paradigm of *Chlamydia* immunity. Infect Immun 84:868–873

Johnson RM, Yu H, Kerr MS, Slaven JE, Karunakaran KP, Brunham RC (2012) PmpG303-311, a protective vaccine epitope that elicits persistent cellular immune responses in *Chlamydia muridarum*-immune mice. Infect Immun 80:2204–2211

Johnson RM, Kerr MS, Slaven JE (2014) An atypical CD8 T-cell response to *Chlamydia muridarum* genital tract infections includes T cells that produce interleukin-13. Immunology 142:248–257

Kavathas PB, Boeras CM, Mulla MJ, Abrahams VM (2013) Nod1, but not the ASC inflammasome, contributes to induction of IL-1beta secretion in human trophoblasts after sensing of *Chlamydia trachomatis*. Mucosal Immunol 6:235–243

Khader SA, Gaffen SL, Kolls JK (2009) Th17 cells at the crossroads of innate and adaptive immunity against infectious diseases at the mucosa. Mucosal Immunol 2:403–411

Kimani J, Maclean IW, Bwayo JJ, MacDonald K, Oyugi J, Maitha GM, Peeling RW, Cheang M, Nagelkerke NJ, Plummer FA, Brunham RC (1996) Risk factors for *Chlamydia trachomatis* pelvic inflammatory disease among sex workers in Nairobi, Kenya. J Infect Dis 173:1437–1444

Kinnunen A, Molander P, Morrison R, Lehtinen M, Karttunen R, Tiitinen A, Paavonen J, Surcel HM (2002) Chlamydial heat shock protein 60–specific T cells in inflamed salpingeal tissue. Fertil Steril 77:162–166

Lee HY, Schripsema JH, Sigar IM, Lacy SR, Kasimos JN, Murray CM, Ramsey KH (2010a) A role for CXC chemokine receptor-2 in the pathogenesis of urogenital *Chlamydia muridarum* infection in mice. FEMS Immunol Med Microbiol 60:49–56

Lee HY, Schripsema JH, Sigar IM, Murray CM, Lacy SR, Ramsey KH (2010b) A link between neutrophils and chronic disease manifestations of *Chlamydia muridarum* urogenital infection of mice. FEMS Immunol Med Microbiol 59:108–116

Leslie M (2016) Immunity goes local. Science 352:21–23

Li LX, McSorley SJ (2013) B cells enhance antigen-specific CD4 T cell priming and prevent bacteria dissemination following *Chlamydia muridarum* genital tract infection. PLoS Pathog 9: e1003707

Lu C, Holland MJ, Gong S, Peng B, Bailey RL, Mabey DW, Wu Y, Zhong G (2012a) Genome-wide identification of *Chlamydia trachomatis* antigens associated with trachomatous trichiasis. Invest Ophthalmol Vis Sci 53:2551–2559

Lu C, Zeng H, Li Z, Lei L, Yeh IT, Wu Y, Zhong G (2012b) Protective immunity against mouse upper genital tract pathology correlates with high IFNgamma but low IL-17 T cell and anti-secretion protein antibody responses induced by replicating chlamydial organisms in the airway. Vaccine 30:475–485

Luense LJ, Carletti MZ, Christenson LK (2009) Role of dicer in female fertility. Trends Endocrinol Metab 20:265–272

Mabey DC, Hu V, Bailey RL, Burton MJ, Holland MJ (2014) Towards a safe and effective chlamydial vaccine: lessons from the eye. Vaccine 32:1572–1578

Manam S, Nicholson BJ, Murthy AK (2013) OT-1 mice display minimal upper genital tract pathology following primary intravaginal *Chlamydia muridarum* infection. Pathog Dis 67:221–224

Manam S, Thomas JD, Li W, Maladore A, Schripsema JH, Ramsey KH, Murthy AK (2015) Tumor Necrosis Factor (TNF) receptor superfamily member 1b on $CD8^+$ T cells and TNF receptor superfamily member 1a on Non-$CD8^+$ T cells contribute significantly to upper genital tract pathology following chlamydial infection. J Infect Dis 211:2014–2022

Marks E, Verolin M, Stensson A, Lycke N (2007) Differential CD28 and inducible costimulatory molecule signaling requirements for protective $CD4^+$ T-cell-mediated immunity against genital tract *Chlamydia trachomatis* infection. Infect Immun 75:4638–4647

Marks E, Tam MA, Lycke NY (2010) The female lower genital tract is a privileged compartment with IL-10 producing dendritic cells and poor Th1 immunity following *Chlamydia trachomatis* infection. PLoS Pathog 6:e1001179

Masson L, Salkinder AL, Olivier AJ, McKinnon LR, Gamieldien H, Mlisana K, Scriba TJ, Lewis DA, Little F, Jaspan HB, Ronacher K, Denny L, Abdool Karim SS, Passmore JA (2015) Relationship between female genital tract infections, mucosal interleukin-17 production and local T helper type 17 cells. Immunology 146:557–567

Menon S, Timms P, Allan JA, Alexander K, Rombauts L, Horner P, Keltz M, Hocking J, Huston WM (2015) Human and pathogen factors associated with *Chlamydia trachomatis*-related infertility in women. Clin Microbiol Rev 28:969–985

Moniz RJ, Chan AM, Gordon LK, Braun J, Arditi M, Kelly KA (2010) Plasmacytoid dendritic cells modulate nonprotective T-cell responses to genital infection by *Chlamydia muridarum*. FEMS Immunol Med Microbiol 58:397–404

Moore DE, Cates W (1990) Sexually transmitted diseases and infertility. In: Holmes KK, Mardh PA, Sparling PF, Weisner PJ (eds) Sexually transmitted diseases. NY, McGraw-Hill, New York, pp 763–771

Moore T, Ananaba GA, Bolier J, Bowers S, Belay T, Eko FO, Igietseme JU (2002) Fc receptor regulation of protective immunity against *Chlamydia trachomatis*. Immunology 105:213–221

Moore-Connors JM, Fraser R, Halperin SA, Wang J (2013) CD4(+)CD25(+)Foxp3(+) regulatory T cells promote Th17 responses and genital tract inflammation upon intracellular *Chlamydia muridarum* infection. J Immunol 191:3430–3439

Morrison RP, Caldwell HD (2002) Immunity to murine chlamydial genital infection. Infect Immun 70:2741–2751

Morrison RP, Lyng K, Caldwell HD (1989a) Chlamydial disease pathogenesis. Ocular hypersensitivity elicited by a genus-specific 57-kD protein. J Exp Med 169:663–675

Morrison RP, Belland RJ, Lyng K, Caldwell HD (1989b) Chlamydial disease pathogenesis. The 57-kD chlamydial hypersensitivity antigen is a stress response protein. J Exp Med 170:1271–1283

Mueller SN, Mackay LK (2016) Tissue-resident memory T cells: local specialists in immune defence. Nat Rev Immunol 16:79–89

Muhlestein JB (2000) *Chlamydia pneumoniae*-induced atherosclerosis in a rabbit model. J Infect Dis 181(Suppl 3):S505–S507

Murthy AK, Chambers JP, Meier PA, Zhong G, Arulanandam BP (2007) Intranasal vaccination with a secreted chlamydial protein enhances resolution of genital *Chlamydia muridarum* infection, protects against oviduct pathology, and is highly dependent upon endogenous gamma interferon production. Infect Immun 75:666–676

Murthy AK, Chaganty BK, Li W, Guentzel MN, Chambers JP, Seshu J, Zhong G, Arulanandam BP (2009) A limited role for antibody in protective immunity induced by rCPAF and CpG vaccination against primary genital *Chlamydia muridarum* challenge. FEMS Immunol Med Microbiol 55:271–279

Murthy AK, Li W, Guentzel MN, Zhong G, Arulanandam BP (2011a) Vaccination with the defined chlamydial secreted protein CPAF induces robust protection against female infertility following repeated genital chlamydial challenge. Vaccine 29:2519–2522

Murthy AK, Li W, Chaganty BK, Kamalakaran S, Guentzel MN, Seshu J, Forsthuber TG, Zhong G, Arulanandam BP (2011b) Tumor necrosis factor alpha production from CD8 + T cells mediates oviduct pathological sequelae following primary genital *Chlamydia muridarum* infection. Infect Immun 79:2928–2935

Nagarajan UM, Ojcius DM, Stahl L, Rank RG, Darville T (2005) *Chlamydia trachomatis* induces expression of IFN-gamma-inducible protein 10 and IFN-beta independent of TLR2 and TLR4, but largely dependent on MyD88. J Immunol 175:450–460

Nagarajan UM, Prantner D, Sikes JD, Andrews CW Jr, Goodwin AM, Nagarajan S, Darville T (2008) Type I interferon signaling exacerbates *Chlamydia muridarum* genital infection in a murine model. Infect Immun 76:4642–4648

Nagarajan UM, Sikes JD, Yeruva L, Prantner D (2012) Significant role of IL-1 signaling, but limited role of inflammasome activation, in oviduct pathology during *Chlamydia muridarum* genital infection. J Immunol 188:2866–2875

Nelson DE, Virok DP, Wood H, Roshick C, Johnson RM, Whitmire WM, Crane DD, Steele-Mortimer O, Kari L, McClarty G, Caldwell HD (2005) Chlamydial IFN-gamma immune evasion is linked to host infection tropism. Proc Natl Acad Sci USA 102:10658–10663

Ness RB, Soper DE, Richter HE, Randall H, Peipert JF, Nelson DB, Schubeck D, McNeeley SG, Trout W, Bass DC, Hutchison K, Kip K, Brunham RC (2008) *Chlamydia* antibodies, chlamydia heat shock protein, and adverse sequelae after pelvic inflammatory disease: the PID Evaluation and Clinical Health (PEACH) study. Sex Transm Dis 35:129–135

O'Meara CP, Armitage CW, Harvie MC, Andrew DW, Timms P, Lycke NY, Beagley KW (2014a) Immunity against a *Chlamydia* infection and disease may be determined by a balance of IL-17 signaling. Immunol Cell Biol 92:287–297

O'Meara CP, Andrew DW, Beagley KW (2014b) The mouse model of *Chlamydia* genital tract infection: a review of infection, disease, immunity and vaccine development. Curr Mol Med 14:396–421

Oakeshott P, Kerry S, Aghaizu A, Atherton H, Hay S, Taylor-Robinson D, Simms I, Hay P (2010) Randomised controlled trial of screening for *Chlamydia trachomatis* to prevent pelvic inflammatory disease: the POPI (prevention of pelvic infection) trial. BMJ 340:c1642

Olivares-Zavaleta N, Whitmire WM, Kari L, Sturdevant GL, Caldwell HD (2014) $CD8^+$ T cells define an unexpected role in live-attenuated vaccine protective immunity against *Chlamydia trachomatis* infection in macaques. J Immunol 192:4648–4654

Paavonen J, Westrom L, Eschenbach D (2008) Pelvic inflammatory disease. In: Holmes KK, Sparling PF, Stamm WE, Piot P, Wasserheit JN, Corey L, Cohen MS, Watts DH (eds) Sexually transmitted diseases, 4th edn. NY, McGraw Hill, New York, pp 1017–1050

Penttila T, Haveri A, Tammiruusu A, Vuola JM, Lahesmaa R, Puolakkainen M (2008) *Chlamydia pneumoniae* infection in IL-10 knock out mice: accelerated clearance but severe pulmonary inflammatory response. Microb Pathog 45:25–29

Player MS, Mainous AG III, Everett CJ, Diaz VA, Knoll ME, Wright RU (2014) *Chlamydia pneumoniae* and progression of subclinical atherosclerosis. Eur J Prev Cardiol 21:559–565

Porcella SF, Carlson JH, Sturdevant DE, Sturdevant GL, Kanakabandi K, Virtaneva K, Wilder H, Whitmire WM, Song L, Caldwell HD (2015) Transcriptional profiling of human epithelial cells infected with plasmid-bearing and plasmid-deficient *Chlamydia trachomatis*. Infect Immun 83:534–543

Prantner D, Darville T, Sikes JD, Andrews CW Jr, Brade H, Rank RG, Nagarajan UM (2009) Critical role for interleukin-1beta (IL-1beta) during *Chlamydia muridarum* genital infection and bacterial replication-independent secretion of IL-1beta in mouse macrophages. Infect Immun 77:5334–5346

Ramsey KH, Sigar IM, Rana SV, Gupta J, Holland SM, Byrne GI (2001) Role for inducible nitric oxide synthase in protection from chronic *Chlamydia trachomatis* urogenital disease in mice and its regulation by oxygen free radicals. Infect Immun 69:7374–7379

Ramsey KH, Sigar IM, Schripsema JH, Townsend KE, Barry RJ, Peters J, Platt KB (2016) Detection of *Chlamydia* infection in *Peromyscus* species rodents from sylvatic and laboratory sources. Pathog Dis 74

Rank RG (1994) Animal models for urogenital infections. Methods Enzymol 235:83–93

Rank RG, Barron AL (1987) Specific effect of estradiol on the genital mucosal antibody response in chlamydial ocular and genital infections. Infect Immun 55:2317–2319

Rank RG, Whittum-Hudson JA (1994) Animal models for ocular infections. Methods Enzymol 235:69–83

Rank RG, White HJ, Hough AJ Jr, Pasley JN, Barron AL (1982) Effect of estradiol on chlamydial genital infection of female guinea pigs. Infect Immun 38:699–705

Rank RG, Dascher C, Bowlin AK, Bavoil PM (1995) Systemic immunization with Hsp60 alters the development of chlamydial ocular disease. Invest Ophthalmol Vis Sci 36:1344–1351

Rank RG, Bowlin AK, Reed RL, Darville T (2003) Characterization of chlamydial genital infection resulting from sexual transmission from male to female guinea pigs and determination of infectious dose. Infect Immun 71:6148–6154

Rasmussen SJ, Eckmann L, Quayle AJ, Shen L, Zhang YX, Anderson DJ, Fierer J, Stephens RS, Kagnoff MF (1997) Secretion of proinflammatory cytokines by epithelial cells in response to *Chlamydia* infection suggests a central role for epithelial cells in chlamydial pathogenesis. J Clin Invest 99:77–87

Ripa KT, Moller BR, Mardh PA, Freundt EA, Melsen F (1979) Experimental acute salpingitis in grivet monkeys provoked by *Chlamydia trachomatis*. Acta Pathol Microbiol Scand B 87B:65–70

Roberts CH, Molina S, Makalo P, Joof H, Harding-Esch EM, Burr SE, Mabey DC, Bailey RL, Burton MJ, Holland MJ (2014) Conjunctival scarring in trachoma is associated with the HLA-C ligand of KIR and is exacerbated by heterozygosity at KIR2DL2/KIR2DL3. PLoS Negl Trop Dis 8:e2744

Roulis E, Polkinghorne A, Timms P (2013) *Chlamydia pneumoniae*: modern insights into an ancient pathogen. Trends Microbiol 21:120–128

Saikku P, Laitinen K, Leinonen M (1998) Animal models for *Chlamydia pneumoniae* infection. Atherosclerosis 140(Suppl 1):S17–S19

Sakaguchi S, Miyara M, Costantino CM, Hafler DA (2010) FOXP3 + regulatory T cells in the human immune system. Nat Rev Immunol 10:490–500

Sakurai-Komada N, Iso H, Koike KA, Ikeda A, Umesawa M, Ikehara S, Inoue M, Tsugane S (2014) Association between *Chlamydophila pneumoniae* infection and risk of coronary heart disease for Japanese: the JPHC study. Atherosclerosis 233:338–342

Schautteet K, De CE, Jonsson Y, Lagae S, Chiers K, Cox E, Vanrompay D (2012) Protection of pigs against genital *Chlamydia trachomatis* challenge by parenteral or mucosal DNA immunization. Vaccine 30:2869–2881

Scurlock AM, Frazer LC, Andrews CW Jr, O'Connell CM, Foote IP, Bailey SL, Chandra-Kuntal K, Kolls JK, Darville T (2011) Interleukin-17 contributes to generation of Th1 immunity and neutrophil recruitment during *Chlamydia muridarum* genital tract infection but is not required for macrophage influx or normal resolution of infection. Infect Immun 79:1349–1362

Sessa R, Pietro MD, Filardo S, Turriziani O (2014) Infectious burden and atherosclerosis: a clinical issue. World J Clin Cases 2:240–249

Shah AA, Schripsema JH, Imtiaz MT, Sigar IM, Kasimos J, Matos PG, Inouye S, Ramsey KH (2005) Histopathologic changes related to fibrotic oviduct occlusion after genital tract infection of mice with *Chlamydia muridarum*. Sex Transm Dis 32:49–56

Sobottka B, Harrer MD, Ziegler U, Fischer K, Wiendl H, Hunig T, Becher B, Goebels N (2009) Collateral bystander damage by myelin-directed $CD8^+$ T cells causes axonal loss. Am J Pathol 175:1160–1166

Stamm WE, Batteiger BE (2010) *Chlamydia trachomatis* (trachoma, perinatal infections, lymphogranuloma venereum, and other genital infections). In: Mandell GLBJEDRe (ed) Principles and practice of infectious diseases, 7th edn, vol 2. pp 2443–2461

Stamm WE, Holmes KK (1990) Chlamydia trachomatis infections of the adult. In: Holmes KK, Sparling PF, Stamm WE, Piot P, Wasserhiet JN, Corey Le (eds) 2nd Ed. New York, NY, McGraw-Hill

Starnbach MN, Bevan MJ, Lampe MF (1994) Protective cytotoxic T lymphocytes are induced during murine infection with *Chlamydia trachomatis*. J Immunol 153:5183–5189

Starnbach MN, Loomis WP, Ovendale P, Regan D, Hess B, Alderson MR, Fling SP (2003) An inclusion membrane protein from *Chlamydia trachomatis* enters the MHC class I pathway and stimulates a $CD8^+$ T cell response. J Immunol 171:4742–4749

Stary G, Olive A, Radovic-Moreno AF, Gondek D, Alvarez D, Basto PA, Perro M, Vrbanac VD, Tager AM, Shi J, Yethon JA, Farokhzad OC, Langer R, Starnbach MN, von Andrian UH (2015) VACCINES. A mucosal vaccine against *Chlamydia trachomatis* generates two waves of protective memory T cells. Science 348:aaa8205

Stephens RS (2003) The cellular paradigm of chlamydial pathogenesis. Trends Microbiol 11:44–51

Stoner BP, Cohen SE (2015) Lymphogranuloma venereum 2015: clinical presentation, diagnosis, and treatment. Clin Infect Dis 61(Suppl 8):S865–S873

Sturdevant GL, Kari L, Gardner DJ, Olivares-Zavaleta N, Randall LB, Whitmire WM, Carlson JH, Goheen MM, Selleck EM, Martens C, Caldwell HD (2010) Frameshift mutations in a single novel virulence factor alter the in vivo pathogenicity of *Chlamydia trachomatis* for the female murine genital tract. Infect Immun 78:3660–3668

Su H, Feilzer K, Caldwell HD, Morrison RP (1997) *Chlamydia trachomatis* genital tract infection of antibody-deficient gene knockout mice. Infect Immun 65:1993–1999

Taylor HR (1985) Ocular models of chlamydial infection. Rev Infect Dis 7:737–740

Taylor HR, Prendergast RA, Dawson CR, Schachter J, Silverstein AM (1981) An animal model for cicatrizing trachoma. Invest Ophthalmol Vis Sci 21:422–433

Taylor HR, Johnson SL, Prendergast RA, Schachter J, Dawson CR, Silverstein AM (1982) An animal model of trachoma II. The importance of repeated reinfection. Invest Ophthalmol Vis Sci 23:507–515

Taylor HR, Kolarczyk RA, Johnson SL, Schachter J, Prendergast RA (1984) Effect of bacterial secondary infection in an animal model of trachoma. Infect Immun 44:614–616

Taylor HR, Johnson SL, Schachter J, Caldwell HD, Prendergast RA (1987) Pathogenesis of trachoma: the stimulus for inflammation. J Immunol 138:3023–3027

Taylor HR, Burton MJ, Haddad D, West S, Wright H (2014) Trachoma. Lancet 384:2142–2152

Tiszlavicz Z, Somogyvari F, Kocsis AK, Szolnoki Z, Sztriha LK, Kis Z, Vecsei L, Mandi Y (2009) Relevance of the genetic polymorphism of NOD1 in *Chlamydia pneumoniae* seropositive stroke patients. Eur J Neurol 16:1224–1229

Tuffrey M, Falder P, Gale J, Taylor-Robinson D (1986) Salpingitis in mice induced by human strains of *Chlamydia trachomatis*. Br J Exp Pathol 67:605–616

Van Voorhis WC, Barrett LK, Sweeney YT, Kuo CC, Patton DL (1996) Analysis of lymphocyte phenotype and cytokine activity in the inflammatory infiltrates of the upper genital tract of female macaques infected with *Chlamydia trachomatis*. J Infect Dis 174:647–650

Van Voorhis WC, Barrett LK, Sweeney YT, Kuo CC, Patton DL (1997) Repeated *Chlamydia trachomatis* infection of Macaca nemestrina fallopian tubes produces a Th1-like cytokine response associated with fibrosis and scarring. Infect Immun 65:2175–2182

Vasilevsky S, Greub G, Nardelli-Haefliger D, Baud D (2014) Genital *Chlamydia trachomatis*: understanding the roles of innate and adaptive immunity in vaccine research. Clin Microbiol Rev 27:346–370

Vlcek KR, Li W, Manam S, Zanotti B, Nicholson BJ, Ramsey KH, Murthy AK (2016) The contribution of *Chlamydia*-specific CD8(+) T cells to upper genital tract pathology. Immunol Cell Biol 94:208–212

von Hertzen L, Alakarppa H, Koskinen R, Liippo K, Surcel HM, Leinonen M, Saikku P (1997) *Chlamydia pneumoniae* infection in patients with chronic obstructive pulmonary disease. Epidemiol Infect 118:155–164

Watkins NG, Hadlow WJ, Moos AB, Caldwell HD (1986) Ocular delayed hypersensitivity: a pathogenetic mechanism of chlamydial-conjunctivitis in guinea pigs. Proc Natl Acad Sci USA 83:7480–7484

Waugh CA, Timms P, Andrew D, Rawlinson G, Brumm J, Nilsson K, Beagley KW (2015) Comparison of subcutaneous versus intranasal immunization of male koalas (*Phascolarctos cinereus*) for induction of mucosal and systemic immunity against *Chlamydia pecorum*. Vaccine 33:855–860

Welter-Stahl L, Ojcius DM, Viala J, Girardin S, Liu W, Delarbre C, Philpott D, Kelly KA, Darville T (2006) Stimulation of the cytosolic receptor for peptidoglycan, Nod1, by infection with *Chlamydia trachomatis* or *Chlamydia muridarum*. Cell Microbiol 8:1047–1057

Westrom L, Mardh PA (1990) Acute pelvic inflammatory disease. In: Holmes KK, Mardh PA, Sparling PF, Weisner PJ (eds) Sexually transmitted diseases. NY, McGraw-Hill, New York, pp 593–615

WHO (2016) Global strategy for the prevention and control of sexually transmitted infection: 2006–2015

Witkin SS, Jeremias J, Toth M, Ledger WJ (1994) Proliferative response to conserved epitopes of the *Chlamydia trachomatis* and human 60-kilodalton heat-shock proteins by lymphocytes from women with salpingitis. Am J Obstet Gynecol 171:455–460

Wolner-Hanssen P, Kiviat NB, Holmes KK (1990) Atypical pelvic inflammatory disease: subacute, chronic, or subclinical upper genital tract infection in women. In: Holmes KK, Mardh PA, Sparling PF, Weisner PJ (eds) Sexually transmitted diseases. NY, McGraw-Hill, New York, pp 763–771

Yang X, Brunham RC (1998) Gene knockout B cell-deficient mice demonstrate that B cells play an important role in the initiation of T cell responses to *Chlamydia trachomatis* (mouse pneumonitis) lung infection. J Immunol 161:1439–1446

Yang X, Gartner J, Zhu L, Wang S, Brunham RC (1999) IL-10 gene knockout mice show enhanced Th1-like protective immunity and absent granuloma formation following *Chlamydia trachomatis* lung infection. J Immunol 162:1010–1017

Yi Y, Zhong G, Brunham RC (1993) Continuous B-cell epitopes in *Chlamydia trachomatis* heat shock protein 60. Infect Immun 61:1117–1120

Zafiratos MT, Manam S, Henderson KK, Ramsey KH, Murthy AK (2015) $CD8^+$ T cells mediate *Chlamydia pneumoniae*-induced atherosclerosis in mice. Pathog Dis 73

Zhang YX, Fox JG, Ho Y, Zhang L, Stills HF Jr, Smith TF (1993) Comparison of the major outer-membrane protein (MOMP) gene of mouse pneumonitis (MoPn) and hamster SFPD strains of *Chlamydia trachomatis* with other *Chlamydia* strains. Mol Biol Evol 10:1327–1342

Zhong G, Liu L, Fan T, Fan P, Ji H (2000) Degradation of transcription factor RFX5 during the inhibition of both constitutive and interferon gamma-inducible major histocompatibility complex class I expression in *Chlamydia*-infected cells. J Exp Med 191:1525–1534

Zhou X, Chen Q, Moore J, Kolls JK, Halperin S, Wang J (2009) Critical role of the interleukin-17/interleukin-17 receptor axis in regulating host susceptibility to respiratory infection with *Chlamydia* species. Infect Immun 77:5059–5070

Chlamydia trachomatis: Protective Adaptive Responses and Prospects for a Vaccine

Taylor B. Poston and Toni Darville

Abstract *Chlamydia trachomatis* is the most common cause of sexually transmitted bacterial infection globally. These infections translate to a significant public health burden, particularly women's healthcare costs due to serious disease sequelae such as pelvic inflammatory disease (PID), tubal factor infertility, chronic pelvic pain, and ectopic pregnancy. There is no evidence that natural immunity can provide complete, long-term protection necessary to prevent chronic pathology, making human vaccine development critical. Vaccine design will require careful consideration of protective versus pathological host-response mechanisms in concert with elucidation of optimal antigens and adjuvants. Evidence suggests that a Th1 response, facilitated by IFN-γ-producing CD4 T cells, will be instrumental in generating long-term, sterilizing immunity. Although the role of antibodies is not completely understood, they have exhibited a protective effect by enhancing chlamydial clearance. Future work will require investigation of broadly neutralizing antibodies and antibody-augmented cellular immunity to successfully design a vaccine that potently elicits both arms of the immune response. Sterilizing immunity is the ultimate goal. However, vaccine-induced partial immunity that prevents upper genital tract infection and inflammation would be cost-effective compared to current screening and treatment strategies. In this chapter, we examine evidence from animal and human studies demonstrating protective adaptive immune responses to *Chlamydia* and discuss future challenges and prospects for vaccine development.

T.B. Poston · T. Darville (✉)
Department of Pediatrics, University of North Carolina, Chapel Hill, NC, USA
e-mail: lad@email.unc.edu

Current Topics in Microbiology and Immunology (2018) 412:217–238
DOI 10.1007/82_2016_6

Published Online: 01 April 2016

Contents

1 Overview

Chlamydia trachomatis is a Gram-negative, obligate intracellular bacterium that can infect human ocular, genital tract, and respiratory epithelium. Globally, trachoma (serovars A, B, C) is the leading cause of infectious blindness. Repeated infections within endemic areas result in chronic inflammation and damaged conjunctiva that leads to trichiasis, scarring, and blindness. Genital infection can cause urethritis and proctitis in men, and urethritis, cervicitis, endometritis, and salpingitis in women with serious sequelae including pelvic inflammatory disease (PID), tubal factor infertility, ectopic pregnancy, and chronic pelvic pain. Furthermore, *Chlamydia* leads to increased transmission and acquisition of human immunodeficiency virus (HIV) (Schust et al. 2012). Recent estimates suggest that there are approximately 3.0 million sexually transmitted chlamydial infections in the USA (Satterwhite et al. 2013) and 90 million new infections globally each year (Gonzales et al. 2004). Genital infection is most prevalent among adolescents and young adults, affecting approximately 4 % of 18–26-year-olds in the USA (Miller et al. 2004). Screening programs can identify and treat at-risk populations; however, these programs are costly and may prevent natural immunity from developing—a concept referred to as the "arrested immunity hypothesis" (Brunham and Rekart 2008). Animal models demonstrate that partial and even sterilizing immunity can develop after infection, but this protection is short-lived. There is no evidence that natural immunity can provide complete, long-term protection necessary to prevent pathologic sequelae. Although partial immunity results in reduced bacterial burden and duration of infection upon challenge, individuals are not necessarily protected from upper genital tract disease. Nevertheless, the ability of natural infection to induce at least partial protection from reinfection is promising evidence for the feasibility of a protective vaccine, whether sterilizing or preventive of pathology (Murthy et al.

2007). Evidence for immune protection in humans includes decreased prevalence of ocular and genital infections with increasing age despite ongoing exposure, decreased genital bacterial load in older individuals, decreased infection concordance with increased age of sexual partnerships, and increased infection rates in individuals with no prior history of infection (Arno et al. 1994; Batteiger et al. 2010). A prospective longitudinal study of young females revealed that those who spontaneously cleared infection were able to resist reinfection (Geisler et al. 2013), providing further evidence of the potential for protective immunity to be achieved. Nonetheless, chronic (Molano et al. 2005) and repeated infections are common, demonstrating the ability of *C. trachomatis* to evade the host immune response and illustrating the necessity for an efficacious vaccine to overcome these evasion strategies by providing robust immunity that is accelerated beyond that induced by natural infection.

2 Obstacles to Vaccine Development

Chlamydiales have adapted numerous mechanisms to infect the host cell, evade the host immune response, and replicate in a protective, intracellular inclusion. The infectious elementary body (EB) form contains cross-linked protein complexes that render the EB metabolically inactive and resistant to extracellular osmotic stress. The polymorphic, major out member protein (MOMP) is the most abundant component of the bacterium's envelope. MOMP acts as a cytoadhesin and binds to heparin sulfate proteoglycan receptors on the host cells to invade (Su et al. 1996). Additional proteins on the chlamydial outer membrane complex have been shown to be important for cellular invasion. The outer membrane complex B (OmcB) functions as an adhesin with specificity for glycosaminoglycan receptors on host cells (Fadel and Eley 2007), and the bacterium has also been shown to utilize the cystic fibrosis transmembrane conductance regulator (CFTCR) apical anion channel for internalization (Ajonuma et al. 2010). Multiple studies have demonstrated that *Chlamydia* can utilize estrogen receptors, particularly the protein disulfide isomerase component, for entry into host cells (Abromaitis and Stephens 2009; Conant and Stephens 2007; Davis et al. 2002; Hall et al. 2011). The EphrinA2 receptor has most recently been shown to be an adherence and invasion receptor for infection (Subbarayal et al. 2015). It is evident that the bacterium has evolved numerous mechanisms to invade the host cell. Additional research is required to identify broadly neutralizing antibodies due to the polymorphic nature of chlamydial-binding proteins.

The biphasic developmental cycle of *Chlamydia* creates another obstacle to vaccine development. After host cell entry, the EB avoids the host lysosomal pathway, disulfide bonds are reduced, and the bacterium enters a reticulate body (RB) form (Scidmore et al. 2003; Dautry-Varsat et al. 2005). The RB is metabolically active and capable of generating its own stores of energy and essential compounds, but is also capable of hijacking host cell nutrients for growth and replication from the inside of a protective intracellular vacuole called an inclusion. During stress and in response to host cytokines, *Chlamydia* can enter a delayed growth state characterized by large aberrant bodies that may allow for chronic infections less susceptible to antimicrobial killing (Schoborg 2011). The multiple mechanisms utilized by *Chlamydia* to escape the immune system have been well summarized (Bastidas et al. 2013). Thus, a vaccine inducing strong cellular immunity is essential to prevent chlamydial infection and disease.

3 Immune Responses and Pathogenesis

Inflammatory mediators are capable of inducing tissue destruction and pathogenic immune responses during chlamydial infection (Brunham and Rey-Ladino 2005). Animal models of trachoma and of female genital infection reveal a direct correlation between neutrophil influx and activation and development of tissue damage (Imtiaz et al. 2007; Darville et al. 1997; Lacy et al. 2011; Prantner et al. 2009; Ramsey et al. 2001; Shah et al. 2005). In addition, human transcriptional profiling and genetic studies have determined an association of enhanced innate proinflammatory responses with trachomatous scarring (Burton et al. 2004; Hu et al. 2012; Shah et al. 2005). Finally, there is in vitro evidence for IL-1, a prominent cytokine released by neutrophils and monocytes, to cause direct oviduct cell damage (Hvid et al. 2007). Since the innate inflammatory response is induced by the interaction of pathogen-associated molecular patterns (PAMPs) with pathogen recognition receptors (PRRs) on innate inflammatory cells and host epithelial cells, it should not be surprising that increased bacterial burden leads to enhanced innate inflammation and disease (Zhang et al. 2014; Darville et al. 1997; Qu et al. 2015). Using the mouse model of genital infection, we demonstrated that repeated abbreviated infections with *Chlamydia muridarum* led to the protection from oviduct disease that was associated with a significant reduction in the frequency of neutrophils and an increase in the frequency of T cells infiltrating the genital tract upon challenge (Riley et al. 2012). Furthermore, a single infection with a plasmid-deficient strain of *C. muridarum* protects mice from oviduct disease upon challenge with the fully virulent parental strain (O'Connell et al. 2007). This protection is again associated with reduced neutrophil influx and an anamnestic T cell response (Riley et al. 2012). Thus, avoidance of chlamydial-induced neutrophil influx and neutrophil activation appears essential for disease prevention. A vaccine that promotes adaptive T cell responses that are innocuous for the tissue but potently chlamydiacidal should protect from disease by the avoidance of PAMP-induced tissue-damaging responses from neutrophils. This is further supported by murine vaccine studies using a variety of antigens and adjuvants that reveal a direct correlation between protection and the strength of the adaptive IFN-γ-producing CD4 T cell response induced by vaccination (Eko et al. 2003; Ifere et al. 2007; Farris et al. 2010; Murthy et al. 2007; Stary et al. 2015; Yu et al. 2010).

Human epidemiological studies demonstrate an increased risk of disease with recurrent infections (Kimani et al. 1996; Bakken et al. 2007). However, the contribution of pathological effects of the primary infection versus subsequent infections is unknown, and each successful infection would induce an element of tissue-damaging innate responses. Cytokines that have been proposed to play an important role in disease include interleukin-1 (IL-1) (Hvid et al. 2007; Nagarajan et al. 2012) and tumor necrosis factor alpha (TNF-α) (Manam et al. 2015). Interferon-γ and IL-12 mediate protective T helper 1 (Th1) responses (Perry et al. 1997), while T helper 2 (Th2) responses have been shown to be non-protective and pathogenic (Holland et al. 1996). The T helper 17 (Th17) response contributes to the generation of Th1 immunity, but is dispensable for both protection and pathogenesis in the mouse model (Frazer et al. 2013; Scurlock et al. 2011). Further experimentation is needed to discern the role of Th17 cells in human chlamydial infection. CD8 T cells have been shown to play a role in pathogenesis in the macaque and mouse models of genital tract infection, possibly through the production of TNF-α (Murthy et al. 2011a; Van Voorhis et al. 1997). Currently, there is no evidence for the role of B cells in tissue pathology during chlamydial infection. Recent technological advances in immune profiling using animal models and human clinical samples provide an opportunity to discern specific components of the immune response that contribute to pathology and provide insight for safe vaccination strategies.

4 Protective Adaptive Responses

4.1 CD4 T Cells

The critical role of T cells in chlamydial immunity was first demonstrated 30 years ago with the observation that athymic *nude* mice developed a chronic *C. muridarum* infection (Rank et al. 1985). T cells are detected at the site of infection in mice and humans; antigen-presenting cells can prime T cells in the lymph nodes, where they migrate to inductive sites within the genital tract to clonally expand in response to chlamydial infection. These inductive sites mainly contain CD4 T cells that form perivascular lymphoid clusters (Morrison and Morrison 2000; Kiviat et al. 1990). CD4 T cells that produce IFN-γ likely mediate protection from *C. muridarum* and *C. trachomatis*. Mice deficient in MHC class II (Morrison et al. 1995), CD4 (Morrison et al. 2000), IL-12 (Perry et al. 1997), IFN-γ (Wang et al. 1999), or the IFN-γ receptor (Johansson et al. 1997) have an enhanced susceptibility to infection. Th2 responses correlate with disease progression and pathology during human ocular infection (Holland et al. 1996). Transfer of chlamydial-specific Th2 clones fails to protect mice from genital infection (Hawkins et al. 2002). IFN-γ-mediated control of in vivo infection is not fully understood, but IFN-γ controls in vitro growth of *C. trachomatis* in human cells by inducing the production of indoleamine-2,3-dioxygenase (IDO) (Beatty et al. 1994). IDO leads to tryptophan degradation and lethality to *C. trachomatis* by starvation of the essential amino acid, but the bacterium can be rescued through the addition of indole (Nelson et al. 2005). IFN-γ-producing Th1 cells are essential and sufficient for the resolution of infection, but some evidence suggests that a polyfunctional response that includes TNF-α may enhance immunity (Li et al. 2008; Yu et al. 2011). Additional effector mechanisms include the activation of phagocytic macrophages (Bancroft et al. 1987) and CD4 T cell cytotoxicity (Cheroutre and Husain 2013; Johnson et al. 2012). CD4 T cell recruitment into the female genital tract following infection is dependent on CXCR3 and CCR5, coincident with expression of CCL3, CCL5, and CXCL10 in mucosal tissues (Belay et al. 2002; Olive et al. 2011). T cell recruitment is dependent on the α4β1 integrin–VCAM1 and α4β7–MAdCAM leukocyte adhesion pathways that are upregulated in human genital tract mucosa (Davila et al. 2014; Kelly and Rank 1997; Perry et al. 1998; Kelly et al. 2009). Evidence suggests that a Th1 CD4 response that generates long-term, sterilizing mucosal immunity will be the optimal goal of immunization.

4.2 Resident Memory CD4 T Cells

Tissue-resident memory T (TRM) cells have emerged as an important subset of memory T cells in tissue-specific immune responses. These cells reside in epithelial barrier tissues that interface with the environment, such as the gut, lungs, skin, and reproductive tract, and can provide rapid, effective immunity against previously encountered pathogens. TRM cells are able to respond to a pathogen challenge independent of recruited, circulating systemic T cells (Clark 2015). The female genital tract mucosa is an important barrier to pathogenic microorganisms. Mouse studies illustrate that HSV infection and vaccination generate accumulation of CD4 TRM cells in the vaginal mucosa that are maintained by a local chemokine gradient and mount a rapid, anamnestic response upon antigenic challenge (Iijima and Iwasaki 2014; Shin and Iwasaki 2012). Mucosal immunization with ultraviolet light (UV)-inactivated *C. trachomatis* complexed with charge-switching synthetic adjuvant particles (cSAPs) incorporating the TLR7 agonist resiquimod elicited long-lived protection against chlamydial infection in conventional and humanized mice (Stary et al. 2015). Vaccination generated mucosal and systemic T cell responses, but optimal clearance required TRM induction in the uterine mucosa. Mucosal CD4 Th1 cells will likely be instrumental to *Chlamydia* vaccine success, as the intensity of mucosal CD4 Th1 cellular responses is an important correlate of immunity (Igietseme and Rank 1991).

4.3 CD8 T Cells

Ample evidence from mice and humans supports the role of CD4 T cells in the resolution of *Chlamydia* infection, but the role of CD8 T cells remains less clear. Mouse models demonstrate that CD8 T cells are not needed for infection clearance; however, antigen-specific CD8 T cell clones can home to the genital tract and enhance clearance through their production of IFN-γ (Igietseme et al. 1994; Wizel et al. 2008). Evidence suggests that upregulation of PD-L1 in the genital tract following infection may impair CD8 T cell expansion via PD-1 ligation, hampering the development of CD8 memory responses (Fankhauser and Starnbach 2014). This could be a mechanism to avoid cell-mediated uterine pathology, as CD8 T cells can play a role in tissue damage via production of TNF-α (Murthy et al. 2011a). Current data suggest that despite the ability of CD8 T cells to contribute to host defense against *Chlamydia*, immunization should seek the induction of Th1 CD4 T cells with the ability to produce high levels of IFN-γ at the site of infection.

4.4 B Cells and Antibodies

The role of B cells and antibody in the context of antichlamydial immunity is not completely understood (Li and McSorley 2015). Mice lacking B cells do not demonstrate an altered course of primary genital infection with *C. muridarum* (Ramsey et al. 1988), but are more susceptible to reinfection (Su et al. 1997). Immune wild-type mice depleted of CD4 or CD8 T cells clear a secondary challenge; however, B cell-deficient mice are unable to resolve secondary infection after CD4 T cell depletion (Morrison and Morrison 2001; Morrison et al. 2000). Passive transfer of immune serum to naïve mice does not provide protection, but antigen-experienced mice with primed CD4 T cells and immune serum are afforded optimal protection (Morrison and Morrison 2005). Additionally, B cell-deficient mice have a reduced capacity to prime CD4 T cells leading to bacterial dissemination (Li and McSorley 2013). Studies utilizing B cell-deficient mice are an attractive model, but are limited due to the inherent reduction of a significant antigen-presenting cell (APC) population and cytokine source, less efficient memory CD4 T cell initiation, possible disruption of lymphoid architecture and subcapsular sinus macrophages, and enhanced chlamydial dissemination (Li and McSorley 2015).

Antibodies play a role in chlamydial immunity, but their protective effects are likely due to their ability to enhance Th1 activation and cellular effector responses (Brady 2005). Although early human studies suggested that *Chlamydia*-specific antibodies might play a role in *C. trachomatis* immunity based on in vitro neutralization assays (Barenfanger and MacDonald 1974; Jawetz et al. 1965; Byrne et al. 1993), epidemiological studies indicate that high antibody titers are associated with infertility and do not correlate with infection resolution or control of ascending infection (Punnonen et al. 1979; Russell et al. 2015). Murine studies indicate that antibody can contribute to pathogen clearance during a secondary infection, but the protective response occurs only if CD4 T cells are present during primary infection (Morrison and Morrison 2001; Morrison et al. 2000). The difficulty in developing protective antibodies relates to identifying epitopes needed for recognition and neutralization. Antibodies specific for chlamydial outer membrane proteins have shown efficacy in animal models and correlate with protection (Zhang et al. 1987; Zhong et al. 1994). However, data identifying antigen-specific protective or pathogenic antibodies are limited. Although evidence supports a role for antibody in chlamydial immunity, the protective mechanism seems to be primarily mediated through antibody-augmented cellular immunity.

5 Vaccinology

5.1 Antigens

Induction of sterilizing immunity against *C. trachomatis* by immunization will require protective antigens targeted to CD4 T cells. Novartis assessed 120 *Chlamydia* proteins for immunogenicity using two parallel high-throughput approaches and identified 16 MHC class II-specific IFN-γ-inducing antigens in mice and five that induced both humoral and cellular responses. Their assessment in the mouse model identified seven novel antigens conferring partial protection to lung infection (Finco et al. 2011). A second large-scale antigen discovery approach utilized genomewide screening of human antibodies to over 80 % of the expressed *C. trachomatis* proteome (Wang et al. 2010). Of the 99 infected women studied, only 27 proteins were recognized by at least half of the subjects. The ability of these antigens to induce T cell responses was not analyzed. Another proteomic approach to identify T cell epitopes utilized pulsing of dendritic cells with live *Chlamydia* to identify peptides loaded onto MHC class II molecules (Karunakaran et al. 2008). Five proteins with MHC class II epitopes elicited partial protection in the murine model of genital infection. Most recently, the use of ATLAS technology has allowed for the profiling of T cell responses in human subjects in response to *C. trachomatis* infection (Picard et al. 2015). ATLAS uses a proteomic library with *E. coli* expressing proteins of interest that are fed to APCs, which present the respective antigens to human T cells for high-throughput cytokine detection (Grubaugh et al. 2013). Examination of CD4 and CD8 IFN-γ responses after in vitro exposure to CT antigens in a cohort of 141 subjects led to the identification of 8 CD4 and 18 CD8 antigens associated with spontaneous clearance or resistance to infection. The proteins were varied and included those involved in membrane transport, central metabolism, and secretion pathways. Proteins that were immunodominant were not associated with effective immune responses. Antigens that have been found to induce protection in the mouse model (e.g., MOMP, PmpG,

CPAF) were not highly recognized by subjects identified in this cohort as having effective immune responses. However, recent data in the mouse model using a novel vaccine formulation with a multivalent major outer membrane protein (MOMP) VD4 construct containing a conserved *C. trachomatis* epitope induced robust Th1 responses, broadly neutralizing antibodies, and reduced bacterial burden upon challenge (Olsen et al. 2015). These data illustrate the importance of selecting protective immunogenic epitopes and the appropriate configuration for optimal vaccine-induced immunity. Future work is needed to identify protective antigens and optimally construct them to induce protective cellular and humoral responses in humans.

5.2 Types of Vaccines

5.2.1 Live Vaccines

A human vaccine capable of activating the cellular and humoral arms of the adaptive response to *Chlamydia* is lacking. The complex physiology of the female genital tract, a paucity of effective mucosal adjuvants, and limited knowledge of protective antigens further complicate vaccine development. An effective vaccine should induce mucosal and systemic immune responses devoid of cross-reactive autoantibodies and pathology. The first *C. trachomatis* vaccines were live vaccines (Grayston and Wang 1978). Initial studies focused on ocular, rather than genital infection. Results varied from limited, short-lived protection to substantial protection against infection and pathology. Notably, vaccination of Taiwanese children with formalin-fixed *Chlamydia* exhibited partial protection during three years of follow-up (Grayston et al. 1963). A similar study using two preparations of live *C. trachomatis* in Gambian children also elicited partial protection, similar to the Taiwan study (Sowa et al. 1969). The original interpretation of the Gambian trials indicated vaccine-induced hypersensitivity occurred in some vaccinated children, but at the time, scarring was scored as a positive indicator of protection. A reanalysis of the original Gambian trials in the context of current knowledge about disease pathogenesis found that vaccine-induced hypersensitivity did not occur (Derrick et al. 2015). Live vaccines are advantageous since they contain all antigens in correct conformation; however, large-scale propagation of *Chlamydia* is challenging and requires cold storage, and avirulent strains could potentially revert to infectious wild-type strains (Detmer and Glenting 2006). These safety concerns resulted in a switch to vaccine studies of inactivated bacteria, but killed organisms led to a suboptimal immune response. The use of attenuated plasmid-deficient *C. muridarum* and *C. trachomatis* strains has been explored as vaccination strategies; however, success in the genital tract mouse model did not translate to NHP (O'Connell et al. 2007; Olivares-Zavaleta et al. 2010; Qu et al. 2015). Yet, ocular inoculation of NHP with a plasmid-deficient strain of *C. trachomatis* elicited partial protection against ocular infection in a subset of macaques (Kari et al. 2011).

This illustrates the potential need for differences in the future formulation of a protective vaccine for ocular or genital *Chlamydia* infection.

5.2.2 Subunits

Purified antigenic determinants known to elicit immune responses have been explored as a vaccination strategy. These vaccines are safer since they are unable to cause infection and lack virulent components. MOMP is the most well-studied vaccine candidate from *C. trachomatis*. Murine immunization with purified refolded MOMP reconstituted with Freund's adjuvant significantly reduced bacterial burden after genital challenge (Pal et al. 2001). MOMP immunization combined with saponin-based ISCOM (immune-stimulating complex) elicited Th1 antigen-specific responses, and mice cleared vaginal infection within one week (Igietseme and Murdin 2000). Similar results have been achieved with subunit B cholera toxin (CTB-CpG), CPG-2395, and Montanide ISA 720 as adjuvants for MOMP vaccination in mice (Cheng et al. 2009), and CPG-2395- and Montanide ISA 720-formulated vaccines induced robust antibody and T cell responses in non-human primates (Cheng et al. 2009, 2011). However, MOMP subunit vaccines present the challenge of extracting, refolding, and purifying protein complexes at a high cost that are not standardized.

5.2.3 Recombinant Protein

Molecular cloning has afforded the ability to express an abundance of bacterial proteins. Protein configuration remains challenging in this system. However, the use of plant biotechnology may be useful for the large-scale production of antigenic proteins like recombinant MOMP (Kalbina et al. 2011). Additional vaccine candidates such as recombinant CPAF and an OmcB-CT521 fusion protein have elicited Th1 responses and markedly reduced bacterial burdens in mice (Murthy et al. 2007, 2011b).

5.2.4 DNA Plasmid

DNA vaccines that inject plasmids carrying the protein(s) of interest confer many advantages. DNA plasmids can be constructed quickly and purified and can encode multiple epitopes in native three-dimensional structures. A DNA vaccine overcomes the concerns of reversion to virulent forms. While anti-DNA antibodies could be induced, clinical trials have not demonstrated changes in clinical markers of autoimmunity (Ferraro et al. 2011). Despite minimal work in this field, some interesting findings have been generated. DNA vaccine delivery encoding MOMP coadministered with the adjuvants GM-CSF and *E. Coli* enterotoxin subunits A and B generated robust protection against *C. trachomatis* genital challenge in pigs

(Schautteet et al. 2012). A plasmid encoding MOMP epitopes inserted into human papilloma virus (HPV) was protective against vaginal infection and elicited a Th1 response in mice (Xu et al. 2011). Other studies have shown DNA vaccination to be immunogenic with only modest protection in mice (Dong-Ji et al. 2000; Pal et al. 1999). These studies demonstrate the feasibility of a DNA-based vaccine, and additional studies may be warranted for the development of protective animal vaccines. However, DNA vaccine studies have largely been abandoned in humans due to the inability to transfer adequate DNA concentrations. The low immunogenicity due to poor uptake has led to efforts to optimize delivery and immune responses (Grunwald and Ulbert 2015).

5.3 Adjuvants

Due to safety concerns of attenuated or whole-organism killed vaccines, a subunit vaccine is an attractive approach to the vaccine development. Administration of innocuous protein subunits is subimmunogenic and requires adjuvants. Natural or artificial adjuvants aim to replicate host induction of an immunologic response during a live infection. Identifying protective antigens, in combination with an optimal adjuvant, is a crucial goal in vaccine development. An effective vaccine requires an adjuvant that can activate innate effector cells, induce type-1 cytokines, enhance antigen presentation, and induce protective effector cellular and humoral responses. Despite the use of adjuvants in research for many years, there are a limited number of effective adjuvants approved for vaccine usage. Alum hydroxide (Alum), AS04 (monophosphoryl lipid A with alum), AS03 and MF59 (squalene-based), and liposomes are included in adjuvants currently utilized (Mbow et al. 2010). Binding of the adjuvant and antigen allows for costimulation of immune cells, particularly maturation and antigen presentation by dendritic cells and macrophage polarization. Antigen delivery systems with adjuvants can include immune-stimulating complexes (ISCOMs), virus-like particles, nanoparticles, emulsions, liposomes, calcium phosphate, tyrosine, and alum (O'Hagan and Fox 2015). When Th1 immunity is required, as in chlamydial protection, there is a dearth of adjuvants. Recently, development of adjuvants derived from plant carbohydrates (e.g., inulin, saponin) has shown the ability to induce protective type-1 responses (Buchmann et al. 2013; Picard et al. 2012). Other immune potentiators have been explored, usually comprised of purified bacterial or viral components or synthetic mimics. Monophosphoryl lipid A (MPL), muramyl dipeptide, CpG, lipopeptides, dsRNA, and bacterial or viral components have been explored as vaccine adjuvants. MPL is a less toxic form of LPS and is licensed for vaccines against HPV and hepatitis B. The cationic liposome formulation of dimethyldioctadecylammonium (DDA) and trehalose 6,6′-dibehenate (TDB) is currently in human clinical trials for vaccines against tuberculosis and HIV. LTK63, a non-toxic mutant of heat-labile toxin, is the only mucosal adjuvant shown to be safe in human trials (Stephenson et al. 2006), and a LTK/CpG formulation generated strong Th1 immune responses against *C. muridarum* in the mouse model (Finco et al. 2011). There is an unquestioned need to investigate the efficacy of these adjuvants and develop optimal epitope-based vaccines.

5.4 Vaccination Routes

An efficacious chlamydial vaccine may need to target and induce protective mucosal immunity. The route of vaccination reflects this necessity, and an approach targeting relevant mucosal immune responses at inductive sites of the genital mucosa could be necessary. Mucosal immunization has been shown to be more effective than systemic immunization against mucosal tissue-tropic pathogens (De Magistris 2006). *Chlamydia* vaccines should be optimized with appropriate delivery vehicles and adjuvants to induce mucosal immunity, and selection of the appropriate route of vaccination is imperative to generate the most robust mucosal Th1 effector response. Nasal immunization can result in partial genital immunity (Pal et al. 2001; Stary et al. 2015), but recent evidence demonstrates the ability of vaginal immunization to induce robust genital tract and systemic T cell responses (Stary et al. 2015).

6 Future Challenges and Conclusions

Critical advances have been made in the field of chlamydial immunology that includes identification of the basic correlates of protective immunity and capacity of vaccination to induce resident memory T cells. However, there are many challenges and questions that need to be addressed regarding the adaptive response to infection, in order to develop an efficacious chlamydial vaccine. The use of the mouse model is limited because T cell-mediated clearance operates through different mechanisms compared to humans. Additionally, the role of antibody and capacity to induce broadly neutralizing antibodies to multiple serovars remain unresolved; however, the recent ability to induce broadly neutralizing antibodies to the MOMP VD4 region shows promise. The mechanism by which *C. trachomatis* induces genital tract pathology in humans is also unclear, and we lack understanding of why some patients remain asymptomatic with no pathology and others develop PID. Additionally, there is a basic requirement to characterize the correlates of immunity that allow for chronic infection versus spontaneous clearance. Exacerbating this problem is the paucity of data reflecting protective responses in humans, and the NHP model for vaccine testing has demonstrated more success for trachoma than genital infection. There is a need for more basic testing of the NHP response to infection and vaccination and exploration of human responses to infection.

Furthermore, identification of protective human antigens is in its infancy (Finco et al. 2011; Picard et al. 2015). Current research is focused on delineating protective versus pathogenic antigen-specific responses.

A better understanding of mucosal immunity is necessary to address proper adjuvants and vaccine delivery methods. To enhance and guide the proper immune response to vaccination, current mucosal adjuvants will require further testing and new adjuvants may need to be developed. Additionally, a vaccine may require reformulation to protect against ocular or genital tract infection, if a single vaccine does not prove efficacious against both routes of transmission. A mucosal vaccine may not be necessary if systemic immunity is capable of preventing upper genital tract infection and pathology. Sterilizing immunity is the ultimate goal; however, a partially protective vaccine that could be boosted by a live infection may be more pragmatic, particularly if it is able to prevent disease and transmission and seed the genital mucosa with TRM. Ideally, a chlamydial vaccine would be combined with other vaccinations delivered during childhood or adolescence to enhance vaccine uptake, improve marketability, and avoid multiple immunizations. Economic analysis suggests that a vaccine that provides partial immunity would be cost-effective compared to current screening and treatment strategies (Owusu-Edusei et al. 2015). A partially protective vaccine would reduce the prevalence of genital infection (Gray et al. 2009), and vaccination of both sexes could synergize to impart sterilizing immunity against sexual transmission (O'Meara et al. 2015). Current research must continue to focus on identifying correlates of protective immunity versus pathogenic responses and delineate adjuvants and antigens that can enhance protective T cell responses.

References

Abromaitis S, Stephens RS (2009) Attachment and entry of Chlamydia have distinct requirements for host protein disulfide isomerase. PLoS Pathog 5(4):e1000357. doi:10.1371/journal.ppat.1000357

Ajonuma LC, Fok KL, Ho LS, Chan PK, Chow PH, Tsang LL, Wong CH, Chen J, Li S, Rowlands DK, Chung YW, Chan HC (2010) CFTR is required for cellular entry and internalization of *Chlamydia trachomatis*. Cell Biol Int 34(6):593–600. doi:10.1042/CBI20090227

Arno JN, Katz BP, McBride R, Carty GA, Batteiger BE, Caine VA, Jones RB (1994) Age and clinical immunity to infections with *Chlamydia trachomatis*. Sex Transm Dis 21(1):47–52

Bakken IJ, Skjeldestad FE, Nordbo SA (2007) *Chlamydia trachomatis* infections increase the risk for ectopic pregnancy: a population-based, nested case-control study. Sex Transm Dis 34 (3):166–169. doi:10.1097/01.olq.0000230428.06837.f7

Bancroft GJ, Schreiber RD, Bosma GC, Bosma MJ, Unanue ER (1987) A T cell-independent mechanism of macrophage activation by interferon-gamma. J Immunol 139(4):1104–1107

Barenfanger J, MacDonald AB (1974) The role of immunoglobulin in the neutralization of trachoma infectivity. J Immunol 113(5):1607–1617

Bastidas RJ, Elwell CA, Engel JN, Valdivia RH (2013) Chlamydial intracellular survival strategies. Cold Spring Harbor Perspect Med 3(5):a010256. doi:10.1101/cshperspect.a010256

Batteiger BE, Xu F, Johnson RE, Rekart ML (2010) Protective immunity to *Chlamydia trachomatis* genital infection: evidence from human studies. J Infect Dis 201(Suppl 2):S178–189

Beatty WL, Belanger TA, Desai AA, Morrison RP, Byrne GI (1994) Tryptophan depletion as a mechanism of gamma interferon-mediated chlamydial persistence. Infect Immun 62(9):3705–3711

Belay T, Eko FO, Ananaba GA, Bowers S, Moore T, Lyn D, Igietseme JU (2002) Chemokine and chemokine receptor dynamics during genital chlamydial infection. Infect Immun 70(2):844–850

Brady LJ (2005) Antibody-mediated immunomodulation: a strategy to improve host responses against microbial antigens. Infect Immun 73(2):671–678. doi:10.1128/IAI.73.2.671-678.2005

Brunham RC, Rekart ML (2008) The arrested immunity hypothesis and the epidemiology of chlamydia control. Sex Transm Dis 35(1):53–54. doi:10.1097/OLQ.0b013e31815e41a3

Brunham RC, Rey-Ladino J (2005) Immunology of Chlamydia infection: implications for a *Chlamydia trachomatis* vaccine. Nat Rev Immunol 5(2):149–161. doi:10.1038/nri1551

Buchmann P, Dembek C, Kuklick L, Jager C, Tedjokusumo R, von Freyend MJ, Drebber U, Janowicz Z, Melber K, Protzer U (2013) A novel therapeutic hepatitis B vaccine induces cellular and humoral immune responses and breaks tolerance in hepatitis B virus (HBV) transgenic mice. Vaccine 31(8):1197–1203. doi:10.1016/j.vaccine.2012.12.074

Burton MJ, Bailey RL, Jeffries D, Mabey DC, Holland MJ (2004) Cytokine and fibrogenic gene expression in the conjunctivas of subjects from a Gambian community where trachoma is endemic. Infect Immun 72(12):7352–7356. doi:10.1128/IAI.72.12.7352-7356.2004

Byrne GI, Stephens RS, Ada G, Caldwell HD, Su H, Morrison RP, Van der Pol B, Bavoil P, Bobo L, Everson S et al (1993) Workshop on in vitro neutralization of *Chlamydia trachomatis*: summary of proceedings. J Infect Dis 168(2):415–420

Cheng C, Bettahi I, Cruz-Fisher MI, Pal S, Jain P, Jia Z, Holmgren J, Harandi AM, de la Maza LM (2009) Induction of protective immunity by vaccination against *Chlamydia trachomatis* using the major outer membrane protein adjuvanted with CpG oligodeoxynucleotide coupled to the nontoxic B subunit of cholera toxin. Vaccine 27(44):6239–6246. doi:10.1016/j.vaccine.2009.07.108

Cheng C, Pal S, Bettahi I, Oxford KL, Barry PA, de la Maza LM (2011) Immunogenicity of a vaccine formulated with the *Chlamydia trachomatis* serovar F, native major outer membrane protein in a nonhuman primate model. Vaccine 29(18):3456–3464. doi:10.1016/j.vaccine.2011.02.057

Cheroutre H, Husain MM (2013) CD4 CTL: living up to the challenge. Semin Immunol 25 (4):273–281. doi:10.1016/j.smim.2013.10.022

Clark RA (2015) Resident memory T cells in human health and disease. Sci Transl Med 7 (269):269rv261. doi:10.1126/scitranslmed.3010641

Conant CG, Stephens RS (2007) Chlamydia attachment to mammalian cells requires protein disulfide isomerase. Cell Microbiol 9(1):222–232. doi:10.1111/j.1462-5822.2006.00783.x

Darville T, Andrews CW Jr, Laffoon KK, Shymasani W, Kishen LR, Rank RG (1997) Mouse strain-dependent variation in the course and outcome of chlamydial genital tract infection is associated with differences in host response. Infect Immun 65(8):3065–3073

Dautry-Varsat A, Subtil A, Hackstadt T (2005) Recent insights into the mechanisms of Chlamydia entry. Cell Microbiol 7(12):1714–1722. doi:10.1111/j.1462-5822.2005.00627.x

Davila SJ, Olive AJ, Starnbach MN (2014) Integrin alpha4beta1 is necessary for CD4+ T cell-mediated protection against genital *Chlamydia trachomatis* infection. J Immunol 192 (9):4284–4293. doi:10.4049/jimmunol.1303238

Davis CH, Raulston JE, Wyrick PB (2002) Protein disulfide isomerase, a component of the estrogen receptor complex, is associated with *Chlamydia trachomatis* serovar E attached to human endometrial epithelial cells. Infect Immun 70(7):3413–3418

De Magistris MT (2006) Mucosal delivery of vaccine antigens and its advantages in pediatrics. Adv Drug Deliv Rev 58(1):52–67. doi:10.1016/j.addr.2006.01.002

Derrick T, Roberts C, Last AR, Burr SE, Holland MJ (2015) Trachoma and ocular chlamydial infection in the era of genomics. Mediat Inflamm 2015:791847. doi:10.1155/2015/791847
Detmer A, Glenting J (2006) Live bacterial vaccines–a review and identification of potential hazards. Microb Cell Fact 5:23. doi:10.1186/1475-2859-5-23
Dong-Ji Z, Yang X, Shen C, Lu H, Murdin A, Brunham RC (2000) Priming with *Chlamydia trachomatis* major outer membrane protein (MOMP) DNA followed by MOMP ISCOM boosting enhances protection and is associated with increased immunoglobulin A and Th1 cellular immune responses. Infect Immun 68(6):3074–3078
Eko FO, Lubitz W, McMillan L, Ramey K, Moore TT, Ananaba GA, Lyn D, Black CM, Igietseme JU (2003) Recombinant Vibrio cholerae ghosts as a delivery vehicle for vaccinating against *Chlamydia trachomatis*. Vaccine 21(15):1694–1703
Fadel S, Eley A (2007) *Chlamydia trachomatis* OmcB protein is a surface-exposed glycosaminoglycan-dependent adhesin. J Med Microbiol 56(Pt 1):15–22. doi:10.1099/jmm.0.46801-0
Fankhauser SC, Starnbach MN (2014) PD-L1 limits the mucosal CD8+ T cell response to *Chlamydia trachomatis*. J Immunol 192(3):1079–1090. doi:10.4049/jimmunol.1301657
Farris CM, Morrison SG, Morrison RP (2010) CD4+ T cells and antibody are required for optimal major outer membrane protein vaccine-induced immunity to *Chlamydia muridarum* genital infection. Infect Immun 78(10):4374–4383. doi:10.1128/IAI.00622-10
Ferraro B, Morrow MP, Hutnick NA, Shin TH, Lucke CE, Weiner DB (2011) Clinical applications of DNA vaccines: current progress. Clin Infect Dis 53(3):296–302. doi:10.1093/cid/cir334 (an official publication of the Infectious Diseases Society of America)
Finco O, Frigimelica E, Buricchi F, Petracca R, Galli G, Faenzi E, Meoni E, Bonci A, Agnusdei M, Nardelli F, Bartolini E, Scarselli M, Caproni E, Laera D, Zedda L, Skibinski D, Giovinazzi S, Bastone R, Ianni E, Cevenini R, Grandi G, Grifantini R (2011) Approach to discover T- and B-cell antigens of intracellular pathogens applied to the design of *Chlamydia trachomatis* vaccines. Proc Natl Acad Sci USA 108(24):9969–9974. doi:10.1073/pnas.1101756108
Frazer LC, Scurlock AM, Zurenski MA, Riley MM, Mintus M, Pociask DA, Sullivan JE, Andrews CW Jr, Darville T (2013) IL-23 induces IL-22 and IL-17 production in response to *Chlamydia muridarum* genital tract infection, but the absence of these cytokines does not influence disease pathogenesis. Am J Reprod Immunol 70(6):472–484. doi:10.1111/aji.12171
Geisler WM, Lensing SY, Press CG, Hook EW 3rd (2013) Spontaneous resolution of genital *Chlamydia trachomatis* infection in women and protection from reinfection. J Infect Dis 207 (12):1850–1856. doi:10.1093/infdis/jit094
Gonzales GF, Munoz G, Sanchez R, Henkel R, Gallegos-Avila G, Diaz-Gutierrez O, Vigil P, Vasquez F, Kortebani G, Mazzolli A, Bustos-Obregon E (2004) Update on the impact of *Chlamydia trachomatis* infection on male fertility. Andrologia 36(1):1–23
Gray RT, Beagley KW, Timms P, Wilson DP (2009) Modeling the impact of potential vaccines on epidemics of sexually transmitted *Chlamydia trachomatis* infection. J Infect Dis 199(11):1680–1688. doi:10.1086/598983
Grayston JT, Wang SP (1978) The potential for vaccine against infection of the genital tract with *Chlamydia trachomatis*. Sex Transm Dis 5(2):73–77
Grayston JT, Woolridge RL, Wang SP, Yen CH, Yang CY, Cheng KH, Chang IH (1963) Field studies of protection from infection by experimental trachoma virus vaccine in preschool-aged children on Taiwan. Proc Soc Exp Biol Med 112:589–595
Grubaugh D, Flechtner JB, Higgins DE (2013) Proteins as T cell antigens: methods for high-throughput identification. Vaccine 31(37):3805–3810. doi:10.1016/j.vaccine.2013.06.046
Grunwald T, Ulbert S (2015) Improvement of DNA vaccination by adjuvants and sophisticated delivery devices: vaccine-platforms for the battle against infectious diseases. Clin Exp Vaccine Res 4(1):1–10. doi:10.7774/cevr.2015.4.1.1
Hall JV, Schell M, Dessus-Babus S, Moore CG, Whittimore JD, Sal M, Dill BD, Wyrick PB (2011) The multifaceted role of oestrogen in enhancing *Chlamydia trachomatis* infection in

polarized human endometrial epithelial cells. Cell Microbiol 13(8):1183–1199. doi:10.1111/j.1462-5822.2011.01608.x

Hawkins RA, Rank RG, Kelly KA (2002) A *Chlamydia trachomatis*-specific Th2 clone does not provide protection against a genital infection and displays reduced trafficking to the infected genital mucosa. Infect Immun 70(9):5132–5139

Holland MJ, Bailey RL, Conway DJ, Culley F, Miranpuri G, Byrne GI, Whittle HC, Mabey DC (1996) T helper type-1 (Th1)/Th2 profiles of peripheral blood mononuclear cells (PBMC); responses to antigens of *Chlamydia trachomatis* in subjects with severe trachomatous scarring. Clin Exp Immunol 105(3):429–435

Hu VH, Weiss HA, Ramadhani AM, Tolbert SB, Massae P, Mabey DC, Holland MJ, Bailey RL, Burton MJ (2012) Innate immune responses and modified extracellular matrix regulation characterize bacterial infection and cellular/connective tissue changes in scarring trachoma. Infect Immun 80(1):121–130. doi:10.1128/IAI.05965-11

Hvid M, Baczynska A, Deleuran B, Fedder J, Knudsen HJ, Christiansen G, Birkelund S (2007) Interleukin-1 is the initiator of Fallopian tube destruction during *Chlamydia trachomatis* infection. Cell Microbiol 9(12):2795–2803. doi:10.1111/j.1462-5822.2007.00996.x

Ifere GO, He Q, Igietseme JU, Ananaba GA, Lyn D, Lubitz W, Kellar KL, Black CM, Eko FO (2007) Immunogenicity and protection against genital Chlamydia infection and its complications by a multisubunit candidate vaccine. J Microbiol Immunol Infect (Wei mian yu gan ran za zhi) 40(3):188–200

Igietseme JU, Murdin A (2000) Induction of protective immunity against *Chlamydia trachomatis* genital infection by a vaccine based on major outer membrane protein-lipophilic immune response-stimulating complexes. Infect Immun 68(12):6798–6806

Igietseme JU, Rank RG (1991) Susceptibility to reinfection after a primary chlamydial genital infection is associated with a decrease of antigen-specific T cells in the genital tract. Infect Immun 59(4):1346–1351

Igietseme JU, Magee DM, Williams DM, Rank RG (1994) Role for CD8+ T cells in antichlamydial immunity defined by Chlamydia-specific T-lymphocyte clones. Infect Immun 62(11):5195–5197

Iijima N, Iwasaki A (2014) T cell memory. A local macrophage chemokine network sustains protective tissue-resident memory CD4 T cells. Science 346(6205):93–98. doi:10.1126/science.1257530

Imtiaz MT, Distelhorst JT, Schripsema JH, Sigar IM, Kasimos JN, Lacy SR, Ramsey KH (2007) A role for matrix metalloproteinase-9 in pathogenesis of urogenital *Chlamydia muridarum* infection in mice. Microbes Infect 9:1561–1566

Jawetz E, Rose L, Hanna L, Thygeson P (1965) Experimental inclusion conjunctivitis in man: measurements of infectivity and resistance. JAMA 194(6):620–632

Johansson M, Schon K, Ward M, Lycke N (1997) Genital tract infection with *Chlamydia trachomatis* fails to induce protective immunity in gamma interferon receptor-deficient mice despite a strong local immunoglobulin A response. Infect Immun 65(3):1032–1044

Johnson RM, Kerr MS, Slaven JE (2012) Plac8-dependent and inducible NO synthase-dependent mechanisms clear *Chlamydia muridarum* infections from the genital tract. J Immunol 188(4):1896–1904. doi:10.4049/jimmunol.1102764

Kalbina I, Wallin A, Lindh I, Engstrom P, Andersson S, Strid K (2011) A novel chimeric MOMP antigen expressed in *Escherichia coli*, *Arabidopsis thaliana*, and *Daucus carota* as a potential *Chlamydia trachomatis* vaccine candidate. Protein Expr Purif 80(2):194–202. doi:10.1016/j.pep.2011.08.010

Kari L, Whitmire WM, Olivares-Zavaleta N, Goheen MM, Taylor LD, Carlson JH, Sturdevant GL, Lu C, Bakios LE, Randall LB, Parnell MJ, Zhong G, Caldwell HD (2011) A live-attenuated chlamydial vaccine protects against trachoma in nonhuman primates. J Exp Med 208(11):2217–2223. doi:10.1084/jem.20111266

Karunakaran KP, Rey-Ladino J, Stoynov N, Berg K, Shen C, Jiang X, Gabel BR, Yu H, Foster LJ, Brunham RC (2008) Immunoproteomic discovery of novel T cell antigens from the obligate intracellular pathogen Chlamydia. J Immunol 180(4):2459–2465

Kelly KA, Rank RG (1997) Identification of homing receptors that mediate the recruitment of CD4 T cells to the genital tract following intravaginal infection with *Chlamydia trachomatis*. Infect Immun 65(12):5198–5208

Kelly KA, Wiley D, Wiesmeier E, Briskin M, Butch A, Darville T (2009) The combination of the gastrointestinal integrin (alpha4beta7) and selectin ligand enhances T-Cell migration to the reproductive tract during infection with *Chlamydia trachomatis*. Am J Reprod Immunol 61 (6):446–452. doi:10.1111/j.1600-0897.2009.00705.x

Kimani J, Maclean IW, Bwayo JJ, MacDonald K, Oyugi J, Maitha GM, Peeling RW, Cheang M, Nagelkerke NJ, Plummer FA, Brunham RC (1996) Risk factors for *Chlamydia trachomatis* pelvic inflammatory disease among sex workers in Nairobi, Kenya. J Infect Dis 173(6):1437–1444

Kiviat NB, Wolner-Hanssen P, Eschenbach DA, Wasserheit JN, Paavonen JA, Bell TA, Critchlow CW, Stamm WE, Moore DE, Holmes KK (1990) Endometrial histopathology in patients with culture-proved upper genital tract infection and laparoscopically diagnosed acute salpingitis. Am J Surg Pathol 14(2):167–175

Lacy HM, Bowlin AK, Hennings L, Scurlock AM, Nagarajan UM, Rank RG (2011) Essential role for neutrophils in pathogenesis and adaptive immunity in Chlamydia caviae ocular infections. Infect Immun 79(5):1889–1897. doi:10.1128/IAI.01257-10

Li LX, McSorley SJ (2013) B cells enhance antigen-specific CD4 T cell priming and prevent bacteria dissemination following *Chlamydia muridarum* genital tract infection. PLoS Pathog 9 (10):e1003707. doi:10.1371/journal.ppat.1003707

Li LX, McSorley SJ (2015) A re-evaluation of the role of B cells in protective immunity to Chlamydia infection. Immunol Lett 164(2):88–93. doi:10.1016/j.imlet.2015.02.004

Li W, Murthy AK, Guentzel MN, Seshu J, Forsthuber TG, Zhong G, Arulanandam BP (2008) Antigen-specific CD4+ T cells produce sufficient IFN-gamma to mediate robust protective immunity against genital *Chlamydia muridarum* infection. J Immunol 180(5):3375–3382

Manam S, Thomas JD, Li W, Maladore A, Schripsema JH, Ramsey KH, Murthy AK (2015) Tumor necrosis factor (TNF) receptor superfamily member 1b on CD8+ T Cells and TNF receptor superfamily member 1a on Non-CD8+ T Cells contribute significantly to upper genital tract pathology following chlamydial infection. J Infect Dis 211(12):2014–2022. doi:10.1093/infdis/jiu839

Mbow ML, De Gregorio E, Valiante NM, Rappuoli R (2010) New adjuvants for human vaccines. Curr Opin Immunol 22(3):411–416. doi:10.1016/j.coi.2010.04.004

Miller WC, Ford CA, Morris M, Handcock MS, Schmitz JL, Hobbs MM, Cohen MS, Harris KM, Udry JR (2004) Prevalence of chlamydial and gonococcal infections among young adults in the United States. JAMA 291(18):2229–2236. doi:10.1001/jama.291.18.2229

Molano M, Meijer CJ, Weiderpass E, Arslan A, Posso H, Franceschi S, Ronderos M, Munoz N, van den Brule AJ (2005) The natural course of *Chlamydia trachomatis* infection in asymptomatic Colombian women: a 5-year follow-up study. J Infect Dis 191(6):907–916. doi:10.1086/428287

Morrison SG, Morrison RP (2000) In situ analysis of the evolution of the primary immune response in murine *Chlamydia trachomatis* genital tract infection. Infect Immun 68(5):2870–2879

Morrison SG, Morrison RP (2001) Resolution of secondary *Chlamydia trachomatis* genital tract infection in immune mice with depletion of both CD4+ and CD8+ T cells. Infect Immun 69 (4):2643–2649. doi:10.1128/IAI.69.4.2643-2649.2001

Morrison SG, Morrison RP (2005) A predominant role for antibody in acquired immunity to chlamydial genital tract reinfection. J Immunol 175(11):7536–7542

Morrison RP, Feilzer K, Tumas DB (1995) Gene knockout mice establish a primary protective role for major histocompatibility complex class II-restricted responses in *Chlamydia trachomatis* genital tract infection. Infect Immun 63(12):4661–4668

Morrison SG, Su H, Caldwell HD, Morrison RP (2000) Immunity to murine *Chlamydia trachomatis* genital tract reinfection involves B cells and CD4(+) T cells but not CD8(+) T cells. Infect Immun 68(12):6979–6987

Murthy AK, Chambers JP, Meier PA, Zhong G, Arulanandam BP (2007) Intranasal vaccination with a secreted chlamydial protein enhances resolution of genital *Chlamydia muridarum* infection, protects against oviduct pathology, and is highly dependent upon endogenous gamma interferon production. Infect Immun 75(2):666–676. doi:10.1128/IAI.01280-06

Murthy AK, Li W, Chaganty BK, Kamalakaran S, Guentzel MN, Seshu J, Forsthuber TG, Zhong G, Arulanandam BP (2011a) Tumor necrosis factor alpha production from CD8+ T cells mediates oviduct pathological sequelae following primary genital *Chlamydia muridarum* infection. Infect Immun 79(7):2928–2935. doi:10.1128/IAI.05022-11

Murthy AK, Li W, Guentzel MN, Zhong G, Arulanandam BP (2011b) Vaccination with the defined chlamydial secreted protein CPAF induces robust protection against female infertility following repeated genital chlamydial challenge. Vaccine 29(14):2519–2522. doi:10.1016/j.vaccine.2011.01.074

Nagarajan UM, Sikes JD, Yeruva L, Prantner D (2012) Significant role of IL-1 signaling, but limited role of inflammasome activation, in oviduct pathology during *Chlamydia muridarum* genital infection. J Immunol 188(6):2866–2875. doi:10.4049/jimmunol.1103461

Nelson DE, Virok DP, Wood H, Roshick C, Johnson RM, Whitmire WM, Crane DD, Steele-Mortimer O, Kari L, McClarty G, Caldwell HD (2005) Chlamydial IFN-gamma immune evasion is linked to host infection tropism. Proc Natl Acad Sci USA 102(30):10658–10663. doi:10.1073/pnas.0504198102

O'Connell CM, Ingalls RR, Andrews CW Jr, Scurlock AM, Darville T (2007) Plasmid-deficient *Chlamydia muridarum* fail to induce immune pathology and protect against oviduct disease. J Immunol 179(6):4027–4034

O'Hagan DT, Fox CB (2015) New generation adjuvants–from empiricism to rational design. Vaccine 33(Suppl 2):B14–B20. doi:10.1016/j.vaccine.2015.01.088

Olivares-Zavaleta N, Whitmire W, Gardner D, Caldwell HD (2010) Immunization with the attenuated plasmidless *Chlamydia trachomatis* L2(25667R) strain provides partial protection in a murine model of female genitourinary tract infection. Vaccine 28(6):1454–1462. doi:10.1016/j.vaccine.2009.11.073

Olive AJ, Gondek DC, Starnbach MN (2011) CXCR3 and CCR5 are both required for T cell-mediated protection against *C. trachomatis* infection in the murine genital mucosa. Mucosal Immunol 4(2):208–216. doi:10.1038/mi.2010.58

Olsen AW, Follmann F, Erneholm K, Rosenkrands I, Andersen P (2015) Protection against *Chlamydia trachomatis* infection and upper genital tract pathological changes by vaccine-promoted neutralizing antibodies directed to the VD4 of the major outer membrane protein. J Infect Dis 212(6):978–989. doi:10.1093/infdis/jiv137

O'Meara CP, Armitage CW, Kollipara A, Andrew DW, Trim L, Plenderleith MB, Beagley KW (2015) Induction of partial immunity in both males and females is sufficient to protect females against sexual transmission of Chlamydia. Mucosal Immunol. doi:10.1038/mi.2015.125

Owusu-Edusei K Jr, Chesson HW, Gift TL, Brunham RC, Bolan G (2015) Cost-effectiveness of chlamydia vaccination programs for young women. Emerg Infect Dis 21(6):960–968. doi:10.3201/eid2106.141270

Pal S, Barnhart KM, Wei Q, Abai AM, Peterson EM, de la Maza LM (1999) Vaccination of mice with DNA plasmids coding for the *Chlamydia trachomatis* major outer membrane protein elicits an immune response but fails to protect against a genital challenge. Vaccine 17(5):459–465

Pal S, Theodor I, Peterson EM, de la Maza LM (2001) Immunization with the *Chlamydia trachomatis* mouse pneumonitis major outer membrane protein can elicit a protective immune response against a genital challenge. Infect Immun 69(10):6240–6247. doi:10.1128/IAI.69.10.6240-6247.2001

Perry LL, Feilzer K, Caldwell HD (1997) Immunity to *Chlamydia trachomatis* is mediated by T helper 1 cells through IFN-gamma-dependent and -independent pathways. J Immunol 158(7):3344–3352

Perry LL, Feilzer K, Portis JL, Caldwell HD (1998) Distinct homing pathways direct T lymphocytes to the genital and intestinal mucosae in Chlamydia-infected mice. J Immunol 160 (6):2905–2914

Picard MD, Cohane KP, Gierahn TM, Higgins DE, Flechtner JB (2012) High-throughput proteomic screening identifies *Chlamydia trachomatis* antigens that are capable of eliciting T cell and antibody responses that provide protection against vaginal challenge. Vaccine 30 (29):4387–4393. doi:10.1016/j.vaccine.2012.01.017

Picard MD, Bodmer JL, Gierahn TM, Lee A, Price J, Cohane K, Clemens V, DeVault VL, Gurok G, Kohberger R, Higgins DE, Siber GR, Flechtner JB, Geisler WM (2015) Resolution of *Chlamydia trachomatis* Infection Is Associated with a Distinct T Cell Response Profile. Clin Vaccine Immunol: CVI 22(11):1206–1218. doi:10.1128/CVI.00247-15

Prantner D, Darville T, Sikes JD, Andrews CW Jr, Brade H, Rank RG, Nagarajan UM (2009) Critical role for interleukin-1beta (IL-1beta) during *Chlamydia muridarum* genital infection and bacterial replication-independent secretion of IL-1beta in mouse macrophages. Infect Immun 77(12):5334–5346. doi:10.1128/IAI.00883-09

Punnonen R, Terho P, Nikkanen V, Meurman O (1979) Chlamydial serology in infertile women by immunofluorescence. Fertil Steril 31(6):656–659

Qu Y, Frazer LC, O'Connell CM, Tarantal AF, Andrews CW Jr, O'Connor SL, Russell AN, Sullivan JE, Poston TB, Vallejo AN, Darville T (2015) Comparable genital tract infection, pathology, and immunity in rhesus macaques inoculated with wild-type or plasmid-deficient *Chlamydia trachomatis* serovar D. Infect Immun 83(10):4056–4067. doi:10.1128/IAI.00841-15

Ramsey KH, Soderberg LS, Rank RG (1988) Resolution of chlamydial genital infection in B-cell-deficient mice and immunity to reinfection. Infect Immun 56(5):1320–1325

Ramsey KH, Sigar IM, Rana SV, Gupta J, Holland SM, Byrne GI (2001) Role for inducible nitric oxide synthase in protection from chronic *Chlamydia trachomatis* urogenital disease in mice and its regulation by oxygen free radicals. Infect Immun 69(12):7374–7379. doi:10.1128/IAI.69.12.7374-7379.2001

Rank RG, Soderberg LS, Barron AL (1985) Chronic chlamydial genital infection in congenitally athymic nude mice. Infect Immun 48(3):847–849

Riley MM, Zurenski MA, Frazer LC, O'Connell CM, Andrews CW Jr, Mintus M, Darville T (2012) The recall response induced by genital challenge with *Chlamydia muridarum* protects the oviduct from pathology but not from reinfection. Infect Immun 80(6):2194–2203. doi:10.1128/IAI.00169-12

Russell AN, Zheng X, O'Connell CM, Taylor BD, Wiesenfeld HC, Hillier SL, Zhong W, Darville T (2015) Analysis of factors driving incident and ascending infection and the role of serum antibody in *Chlamydia trachomatis* genital tract infection. J Infect Dis. doi:10.1093/infdis/jiv438

Satterwhite CL, Torrone E, Meites E, Dunne EF, Mahajan R, Ocfemia MC, Su J, Xu F, Weinstock H (2013) Sexually transmitted infections among US women and men: prevalence and incidence estimates, 2008. Sex Transm Dis 40(3):187–193. doi:10.1097/OLQ.0b013e318286bb53

Schautteet K, De Clercq E, Jonsson Y, Lagae S, Chiers K, Cox E, Vanrompay D (2012) Protection of pigs against genital *Chlamydia trachomatis* challenge by parenteral or mucosal DNA immunization. Vaccine 30(18):2869–2881. doi:10.1016/j.vaccine.2012.02.044

Schoborg RV (2011) Chlamydia persistence—a tool to dissect chlamydia–host interactions. Microbes Infect/Institut Pasteur 13(7):649–662. doi:10.1016/j.micinf.2011.03.004

Schust DJ, Ibana JA, Buckner LR, Ficarra M, Sugimoto J, Amedee AM, Quayle AJ (2012) Potential mechanisms for increased HIV-1 transmission across the endocervical epithelium during *C. trachomatis* infection. Curr HIV Res 10(3):218–227

Scidmore MA, Fischer ER, Hackstadt T (2003) Restricted fusion of *Chlamydia trachomatis* vesicles with endocytic compartments during the initial stages of infection. Infect Immun 71 (2):973–984

Scurlock AM, Frazer LC, Andrews CW Jr, O'Connell CM, Foote IP, Bailey SL, Chandra-Kuntal K, Kolls JK, Darville T (2011) Interleukin-17 contributes to generation of Th1 immunity and neutrophil recruitment during *Chlamydia muridarum* genital tract infection but is not required for macrophage influx or normal resolution of infection. Infect Immun 79(3):1349–1362. doi:10.1128/IAI.00984-10

Shah AA, Schripsema JH, Imtiaz MT, Sigar IM, Kasimos J, Matos PG, Inouye S, Ramsey KH (2005) Histopathologic changes related to fibrotic oviduct occlusion after genital tract infection of mice with *Chlamydia muridarum*. Sex Transm Dis 32(1):49–56

Shin H, Iwasaki A (2012) A vaccine strategy that protects against genital herpes by establishing local memory T cells. Nature 491(7424):463–467. doi:10.1038/nature11522

Sowa S, Sowa J, Collier LH, Blyth WA (1969) Trachoma vaccine field trials in The Gambia. J Hyg 67(4):699–717

Stary G, Olive A, Radovic-Moreno AF, Gondek D, Alvarez D, Basto PA, Perro M, Vrbanac VD, Tager AM, Shi J, Yethon JA, Farokhzad OC, Langer R, Starnbach MN, von Andrian UH (2015) VACCINES. A mucosal vaccine against *Chlamydia trachomatis* generates two waves of protective memory T cells. Science 348(6241):aaa8205. doi:10.1126/science.aaa8205

Stephenson I, Zambon MC, Rudin A, Colegate A, Podda A, Bugarini R, Del Giudice G, Minutello A, Bonnington S, Holmgren J, Mills KH, Nicholson KG (2006) Phase I evaluation of intranasal trivalent inactivated influenza vaccine with nontoxigenic *Escherichia coli* enterotoxin and novel biovector as mucosal adjuvants, using adult volunteers. J Virol 80 (10):4962–4970. doi:10.1128/JVI.80.10.4962-4970.2006

Su H, Raymond L, Rockey DD, Fischer E, Hackstadt T, Caldwell HD (1996) A recombinant *Chlamydia trachomatis* major outer membrane protein binds to heparan sulfate receptors on epithelial cells. Proc Natl Acad Sci USA 93(20):11143–11148

Su H, Feilzer K, Caldwell HD, Morrison RP (1997) *Chlamydia trachomatis* genital tract infection of antibody-deficient gene knockout mice. Infect Immun 65(6):1993–1999

Subbarayal P, Karunakaran K, Winkler AC, Rother M, Gonzalez E, Meyer TF, Rudel T (2015) EphrinA2 receptor (EphA2) is an invasion and intracellular signaling receptor for *Chlamydia trachomatis*. PLoS Pathog 11(4):e1004846. doi:10.1371/journal.ppat.1004846

Van Voorhis WC, Barrett LK, Sweeney YT, Kuo CC, Patton DL (1997) Repeated *Chlamydia trachomatis* infection of Macaca nemestrina fallopian tubes produces a Th1-like cytokine response associated with fibrosis and scarring. Infect Immun 65(6):2175–2182

Wang S, Fan Y, Brunham RC, Yang X (1999) IFN-gamma knockout mice show Th2-associated delayed-type hypersensitivity and the inflammatory cells fail to localize and control chlamydial infection. Eur J Immunol 29(11):3782–3792

Wang J, Zhang Y, Lu C, Lei L, Yu P, Zhong G (2010) A genome-wide profiling of the humoral immune response to *Chlamydia trachomatis* infection reveals vaccine candidate antigens expressed in humans. J Immunol 185(3):1670–1680. doi:10.4049/jimmunol.1001240

Wizel B, Nystrom-Asklin J, Cortes C, Tvinnereim A (2008) Role of CD8(+)T cells in the host response to Chlamydia. Microbes Infect/Institut Pasteur 10(14–15):1420–1430. doi:10.1016/j.micinf.2008.08.006

Xu W, Liu J, Gong W, Chen J, Zhu S, Zhang L (2011) Protective immunity against *Chlamydia trachomatis* genital infection induced by a vaccine based on the major outer membrane multi-epitope human papillomavirus major capsid protein L1. Vaccine 29(15):2672–2678. doi:10.1016/j.vaccine.2010.12.132

Yu H, Jiang X, Shen C, Karunakaran KP, Jiang J, Rosin NL, Brunham RC (2010) *Chlamydia muridarum* T-cell antigens formulated with the adjuvant DDA/TDB induce immunity against infection that correlates with a high frequency of gamma interferon (IFN-gamma)/tumor necrosis factor alpha and IFN-gamma/interleukin-17 double-positive CD4+ T cells. Infect Immun 78(5):2272–2282. doi:10.1128/IAI.01374-09

Yu H, Karunakaran KP, Kelly I, Shen C, Jiang X, Foster LJ, Brunham RC (2011) Immunization with live and dead *Chlamydia muridarum* induces different levels of protective immunity in a murine genital tract model: correlation with MHC class II peptide presentation and multifunctional Th1 cells. J Immunol 186(6):3615–3621. doi:10.4049/jimmunol.1002952

Zhang YX, Stewart S, Joseph T, Taylor HR, Caldwell HD (1987) Protective monoclonal antibodies recognize epitopes located on the major outer membrane protein of *Chlamydia trachomatis*. J Immunol 138(2):575–581

Zhang H, Zhou Z, Chen J, Wu G, Yang Z, Zhou Z, Baseman J, Zhang J, Reddick RL, Zhong G (2014) Lack of long-lasting hydrosalpinx in A/J mice correlates with rapid but transient chlamydial ascension and neutrophil recruitment in the oviduct following intravaginal inoculation with *Chlamydia muridarum*. Infect Immun 82(7):2688–2696. doi:10.1128/IAI.00055-14

Zhong G, Berry J, Brunham RC (1994) Antibody recognition of a neutralization epitope on the major outer membrane protein of *Chlamydia trachomatis*. Infect Immun 62(5):1576–1583

The manufacturer's authorised representative in the EU is Springer Nature Customer Service Centre GmbH, Europaplatz 3, 69115 Heidelberg, Germany. If you have any concerns regarding our products, please contact ProductSafety@springernature.com

Printed and bound by CPI Group (UK) Ltd, Croydon, CR0 4YY

22/09/2026

02220990-0006